LORE OF NUTRITION

CHALLENGING CONVENTIONAL DIETARY BELIEFS

TIM NOAKES
& MARIKA SBOROS

PENGUIN BOOKS

Published by Penguin Books
an imprint of Penguin Random House South Africa (Pty) Ltd
Reg. No. 1953/000441/07
The Estuaries No. 4, Oxbow Crescent, Century Avenue, Century City, 7441
PO Box 1144, Cape Town, 8000, South Africa
www.penguinrandomhouse.co.za

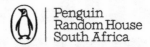

Penguin
Random House
South Africa

First published 2017

1 3 5 7 9 10 8 6 4 2

Publication © Penguin Books 2017
Text © Tim Noakes and Marika Sboros 2017

Cover image of Tim Noakes © Sofia Dadourian

PUBLISHER: Marlene Fryer
MANAGING EDITOR: Ronel Richter-Herbert
EDITOR: Bronwen Maynier
PROOFREADER: Ronel Richter-Herbert
INDEXER: Tessa Botha
COVER AND TEXT DESIGNER: Ryan Africa
TYPESETTER: Monique van den Berg

Set in 10.5 pt on 14 pt Minion

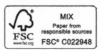

Printed by **novus print**, a Novus Holdings company

MIX
Paper from
responsible sources
FSC
www.fsc.org   FSC® C022948

ISBN 978 1 77609 261 1 (print)
ISBN 978 1 77609 262 8 (ePub)

Contents

I dedicate this book to the sacred few who unselfishly gave of themselves – their wisdom, their humanity, their graciousness and their love – to lead me safely through the trials described herein. They are:

My wife, Marilyn Anne.
Our children, Travis Miles Noakes and Candice Amelia Noakes-Dobson.
My sister, Mandy Ruysch van Dugteren, and the memory of our parents, Reginald Austin ('Bindy') and Mary Wendy Noakes.

The three Archangels, Attorney Adam Pike, Advocate Dr Ravin 'Rocky' (brother) Ramdass and Mike van der Nest SC.

The three Angels, Nina Teicholz, Dr Zoë Harcombe PhD and Dr Caryn Zinn PhD.

– **Professor Tim Noakes**

I dedicate this book to Bruce Cohen, my husband, my greatest fan and critic, and a much better writer than I could ever hope to be; my darling daughter, Demi Bender, uber-organised artist, muso and 'finance whizz'; my beloved son, Joshua Cohen, ever-energetic food-wallah, seeker and wanderer; and my precious grand-children, Jethro and Indiana Bender Tait, who generously shared their Yiayia with the computer for so many months. You all gave me time, space and confidence to revel in the vital, riotous scientific ride that is this book.

– **Marika Sboros**

Acknowledgements

I survived, sanity intact, the unfathomable cruelty of the bigotry, bullying and betrayal described in this book only because a small group of gracious and tenacious heroes – 'the righteous and the holy' – was guiding my train.[*] I can never repay the debt that I owe them. My words cannot adequately convey the unreserved love, joyful thanks and eternal gratitude that I feel for each one of them.

Without the resolute courage, objective counsel and loving support of my thoughtful, strong-willed and super-intelligent wife, Marilyn Anne, I would not have made it through. The forces arrayed against us wholly underestimated the strength of the single person for whom they were no match. For the six years of our personal inquisition, she has stood resolute, refusing to succumb. She was the foundation on which we built our joint defence and on which we ultimately defeated the worst efforts of the 'gamblers', 'wheeler dealers' and 'big shot ramblers'.

Our children, Travis and Candice, were equally resolute and unflinching in their support. They, too, refused to be bullied. Now that it is over, I can begin to repay them for their love and loyalty while I inhabited that other, distracted world.

My sister, Amanda-Louise 'Mandy' Ruysch van Dugteren, has been a pillar of

---

[*] A reference to the traditional American gospel song, 'This train is bound for glory', with new words by Woody Guthrie. © 1958 (renewed) by Woody Guthrie Publications, Inc.

'This train is bound for glory,
Don't carry nothing but the righteous and the holy.
This train is bound for glory, this train.

…

This train don't carry no gamblers,
Liars, thieves, nor big shot ramblers,
This train is bound for glory, this train.

…

This train don't carry no con men,
No wheeler dealers, here and gone men,
This train don't carry no con men, this train.'

strength. She understood exactly what the 'trial' would have meant to our parents, and her unqualified support was a daily reminder that my father and mother would have been in the front row cheering all of us on.

The ultimate irony is that Amanda had adopted the LCHF diet with great success after she discovered *The Low Carbohydrate Diet* by E.L. Fiore, published in 1965, while living in London in the swinging 60s. But she would only share her secret with me after my Damascene moment, explaining that I was the qualified medical 'expert' and that she was not about to tell me I had it all wrong! It would take me 36 years to begin to catch up with her advanced knowledge of practical nutrition.

Attorney Adam Pike directed what I now know as the best legal team in South Africa. Adam's obsessive eye for detail was apparent in the 26 days of flawless presentation that he orchestrated with unbridled passion, focused intelligence, steadfast confidence and irreverent humour. Not for one instant did he falter or misstep.

In terms of their brilliance, benevolence, honesty and desire to see justice prevail whatever the personal cost, senior counsel Mike van der Nest and Advocate Dr Ravin 'Rocky' Ramdass (who by mutual consent is now my 'brother') are in a league of their own. I cannot recall meeting two more remarkable men. Their compassion in recognising a fellow human (and family) in severe distress and their offer to defend me without thought of financial reward are evidence of their astonishing humanity and humility.

The author Jeffrey Archer wrote: 'Some people stand by you in your darkest hour while others walk away; only a select few march towards you and become even closer friends.' I had to survive the dark moments to understand Archer's meaning, for in my darkest hour, Mike and Rocky marched towards me, becoming my superheroes. And my eternal friends.

The three Angels – Dr Zoë Harcombe PhD, Nina Teicholz and Dr Caryn Zinn PhD – who joined our glory train from Wales, the United States and New Zealand respectively, are quite simply three of the bravest and most important minds fighting the disinformation that fronts as modern global 'heart-healthy' dietary advice. In Chapter 13, Marika Sboros accurately captures the massive impact their assured poise, personal integrity and honest testimony had on the conduct and outcome of my trial. Their presence attested to another defining characteristic of the luminaries of the LCHF revolution: their ambition is not personal; it is to advance a cause much greater than themselves.

I met Dr Andreas Obholzer in the first week of my medical training in February 1969; he has been a constant friend and source of inspiration ever since. He and his wife, Dr Karin von Wenzel Obholzer, flew in from Windhoek for each session of the hearing to support Marilyn and me during our hours of need. Again, your best friends are those who march to you to share your darkest moments.

ACKNOWLEDGEMENTS

At his own cost and in his own time, Glen Thomas filmed the trial and big-heartedly allowed The Noakes Foundation to post the material online at https://www.thenoakesfoundation.org/news/videos. Thanks Glen – your kindness and generosity ensured that the trial was recorded for posterity, as it actually happened.

Emeritus Professor J.P. van Niekerk kindly consented to contribute the foreword. As dean of the UCT Faculty of Health Sciences, and despite concerted criticisms that it is not and never will be a science – it is simply too 'Mickey Mouse' – J.P. had the vision (and courage) to champion the introduction of sports science into his faculty in 1981. He appointed me a sports science lecturer that same year. Neither of us would ever have believed that 36 years later we would still be on the same side, continuing the fight against witlessness masquerading as intelligence.

Marika Sboros has correctly acknowledged the brilliant editing skills of Bronwen Maynier, with which I concur absolutely. Marika herself has many kind words to say about me in her acknowledgements. The reality is that without her contribution, this book would have been a lame shadow of what it has become. Like J.P. van Niekerk, Marika represents the skills, the training, the integrity and the social conscience of a bygone era. When she turned those unique skills to reporting the hearing on Twitter (@MarikaSboros) and on Foodmed.net, she ensured that the world would know the truth about what was actually happening. Her work helped keep everyone honest.

Finally, I would like to acknowledge the support of the hundreds of thousands of people all around the world who have adopted the Banting/LCHF diet and who have expressed their thanks especially through social media, such as the 800 000-plus strong Banting Seven Day Meal Plan Facebook page begun by Rita Venter.

In the end we are all fighting this cause for you, for your health and for that of your families.

Your support confirms that it is worth the discomfort.

This train is indeed bound for glory.

TIM NOAKES

Acknowledgements

There's an old saying in the East that when the student is ready, the teacher will appear. Appropriately enough, Professor Tim Noakes appeared on my Skype screen in early 2014. It was clear from the start that he was a natural-born teacher and slayer of nutrition's dogma dragons. He started rocking my worldview and hasn't stopped. Thus began the remarkable journey it is my privilege to travel with him today. He has taught me that most of what I thought was right about nutrition, medicine, disease, health, hearts and healing was wrong. As American journalist and satirist Henry Mencken once said: 'Explanations exist; they have existed for all time; there is always a well-known solution to every human problem – neat, plausible, and wrong.'

I have learnt lots else from Tim: about the power of truth, about integrity, whistleblowing, challenging conventional 'wisdom', facing bullies, and that universities are not always hallowed halls of learning. They can be shark-infested waters, teeming with conflicts of interest and professional jealousies. And in early 2017, when he invited me to co-author this book, I leapt at the chance to document his fight for scientific truth.

Through Tim, I have gained many new friends and guiding lights in nutrition and medical science. Among them are Tim's Angels, Dr Zoë Harcombe, Nina Teicholz and Dr Caryn Zinn, all formidable intellects, women of integrity and courage, beautiful from the inside out. They flew from far-flung lands to testify for him. My guides have also included Tim's legal brothers in arms, the Archangels, as we call them: Michael van der Nest SC, Dr Ravin 'Rocky' Ramdass and Adam Pike. They came well equipped with weaponry to temper the ferocity of the forces trying to silence him for his views on butter, eggs, bacon and broccoli. Watching the brothers at work, I was relieved not to be on the receiving end of their sharpened, shining legal swords. It helped, of course, that Tim has right and robust science on his side.

Watching over us all throughout this never-ending journey has been Tim's wife, Marilyn Anne. Another beautiful spirit from the inside and as brilliantly fierce a Guardian Angel as he could wish to have on the hard road the trial forced him to travel. I am proud to call this remarkable couple my friends.

My thanks also to Penguin Random House's wonderwomen publishing team:

Marlene Fryer, Ronel Richter-Herbert and Bronwen Maynier. Your guidance, input and perceptive corrections are gratefully accepted.

Last but not least, I give thanks to my first guiding lights, my beloved parents: my mother Nora Sboros and my late father Demetrius 'Jimmy' Sboros, and to Dr Ann Childers in the wings.

MARIKA SBOROS

Foreword

Humans seek happiness, health and longevity. Food is an important item on the road to achieving these aims and was at the forefront of the professional conduct inquiry of Professor Tim Noakes. The marathon trial was spread over three years and 25 days of hearings. Most were mystified why it took place at all, but once started, it snowballed into a fascinating drama of its own.

From the lodging of the initial complaint by Association for Dietetics in South Africa (ADSA) president Claire Julsing Strydom to the inquiry itself, hostile attitudes and actions towards Noakes and his views on diets were clearly evident.

The entire process was incredibly demanding emotionally and financially on Noakes and his family. His personal, professional and scientific standing were under threat. He could simply have taken himself off the Health Professions Council of South Africa's medical register (he has not practiced as a doctor for many years) and avoided the anguish, as the HPCSA cannot investigate anyone who is not registered with them. However, Noakes felt that there were important matters of principle to be addressed for the benefit of wider society, and he was prepared to take on the costs, challenges and potential consequences. He was fortunate in obtaining the *pro bono* services of Dr Ravin 'Rocky' Ramdass and Michael van der Nest SC, who were prepared to stand by him whatever it took.

Because of the considerable public interest in the inquiry, the media provided regular reports that focused largely on aspects that were perceived as more dramatic. An exception was Marika Sboros, one of South Africa's most well-known and respected health journalists, who followed and reported on the entire proceedings. She elicited material beyond the trial in a quest for scientific truth and to provide context for her reports. From the start, she saw through the attacks to the man and his scientific mission. With her experienced reporter's eye, she helps readers to do the same in this book.

The inquiry was part of a long-standing battle against the views on diet propagated by Noakes. As a mechanism to demolish his views and to silence him, it backfired spectacularly. The HPCSA, medical and dietetic professionals, and ADSA, who opposed him, have been embarrassed and have lost face and standing. Instead of silencing him, the inquiry provided Noakes with a platform to publicly and convincingly put his case. The publicity during and after the inquiry has been overwhelmingly positive in his favour.

Worldwide major moral and socio-economic battles have raged over the past centuries. Among these, slavery was abolished in the 19th century; the 20th century saw the resolution of women's rights, and the end of prohibition in the United States and apartheid in South Africa; and, more recently, gay rights have largely been addressed in mature democracies. These all took decades to resolve, during which intimidation, violence, prejudice and demonising on all sides were features. The two big worldwide battles being waged at present are the war on drugs and nutrition, both of which are showing significant movement away from previous beliefs.

Change is invariably accompanied by resistance. In 1983, the economist Bruce Yandle coined the term 'Bootleggers and Baptists' relating to the prohibition days in the US – groups with differing moral positions opposed the abolition of prohibition: preachers demanded prohibition to make alcohol illegal, while the criminal bootlegger wanted alcohol to remain illegal to stay in business. This is a model of politics in which the opposite moral positions lead to the same vote. In the Noakes case, professionals opposed to his views wish to protect their beliefs about what is good for their patients, while the beverage, food and pharmaceutical industries don't want to lose business. For ADSA and its members there is the additional consideration of turf wars and of the potential erosion of their profession, unless they are prepared to change their beliefs.

Changing beliefs is incredibly hard, as they are fixed firmly in our limbic system and are not readily amenable to our thinking brain. Confirmation bias protects our beliefs from any opposing and uncomfortable facts. But a fundamental characteristic of science is to constantly challenge beliefs. Noakes bravely confessed the errors of his previous beliefs about carbohydrates when he started studying evidence that was new to him.

While Noakes has celebrity (or demonic) status in South Africa, his views detailed in this book are a reflection of a worldwide re-examination of the basis of the beliefs in 'conventional' nutrition. Findings have included the faulty science of Ancel Keys, who demonised fats; the political opportunism of US President Richard Nixon in supporting the corn industry; the malevolent influence of the beverage and processed (junk) food industries on policy, practice and beliefs; and the rogue role of Big Pharma influencing doctors (think cholesterol and statins, and antibiotics with their effects on the gut organisms).

Such research has shifted the ground, and 'conventional' nutrition increasingly finds itself needing to provide evidence to defend its innocence in contributing to the worldwide obesity and diabetes pandemics instead of Noakes needing to provide the evidence that defends the 'unconventional'.

Medical and other healthcare professionals who oppose Noakes's views would benefit from reviewing the depth of evidence that was so thoroughly provided during the inquiry and is now presented in this book, before dismissing it as inappropriate. Or they need to provide a convincing rebuttal.

After the Noakes inquiry there were rumours that the HPCSA wished to engage on a retrial. My memory of challenged HPCSA cases runs to two: the Steve Biko and Wouter Basson cases, in both of which the council bowed to outside pressures. Should the HPCSA decide to challenge the outcomes of their failed case, this would raise more questions. Would it signify that the HPCSA considered their team to have been incompetent? Should the members, who pay all of the HPCSA costs, not question further, possibly fruitless, expenditure?

Since few cases have been more exhaustively examined, what is there still to be explored? Who would make this decision and on what grounds? If they fail again, should those whose decision it was to proceed not be personally responsible for the costs on both sides? Would this also not seem like a religious persecution of those of another persuasion? Finally, such inquiries are not the appropriate mechanism to resolve such major and complex academic debates.[*]

J.P. DE V. VAN NIEKERK
EMERITUS PROFESSOR (FORMER DEAN) UCT FACULTY OF HEALTH SCIENCES
EMERITUS EDITOR *SAMJ*

---

* The foreword was published in the *Cape Doctor* in September 2017.

Preface

'Few will have the greatness to bend history itself, but each of us can work to change a small portion of events, and in the total of all those acts will be written the history of this generation.'

'Each time a man stands up for an ideal ... he sends forth a tiny ripple of hope, and crossing each other from a million different centers of energy and daring, those ripples build a current which can sweep down the mightiest walls of oppression and resistance.'

'... only those who dare to fail greatly, can ever achieve greatly'.

– Robert F. Kennedy, Ripple of Hope Speech, delivered in Jameson Hall, University of Cape Town, Cape Town, South Africa, 6 June 1966

'... as the skilled and professional people of South Africa and the world, you will be largely removed from contact with the hungry and the deprived, those without ease in the present or hope in the future. It will require a constant effort of will to keep contact, to remind ourselves everyday that we who diet have a never ceasing obligation to those who starve.'

– Robert F. Kennedy, speaking at the University of Stellenbosch, Stellenbosch, South Africa, 7 June 1966

Once upon a time, long, long ago, in another world, I was considered quite a good scientist. Since 2004, the South African National Research Foundation (NRF) has rated me an A1 scientist for both exercise science and nutrition. That is the NRF's highest possible rating, signifying that the foundation judges me to be a world leader in my fields.

I have published more than 500 scientific papers, many in leading international peer-reviewed journals, and have been cited more than 17 000 times in the scientific literature. My scientific H-index stands at over 70 for all my research outputs and at over 40 for those publications dealing exclusively with nutrition. (The H- or Hirsch index is a measure of the impact of the work of a particular scientist.)

I have also won several important scientific awards, including a South African Presidential Order, the Order of Mapungubwe (Silver), and an NRF Lifetime Achievement Award, making me one of few at my alma mater, the University of Cape Town (UCT), to have won this award. For 25 years – an unusually long time – I directed a research unit funded by the South African Medical Research Council (SAMRC). During all that time, the SAMRC regularly rated that unit among the top two or three in its group. I am also a bestselling author of books, including *Lore of Running*, which became known as the 'runners' bible'. Publishers rated it globally as the ninth best ever in its category.

Together with Springbok rugby legend Morné du Plessis, in 1995 I co-founded the Sports Science Institute of South Africa. This would become a beacon of South African excellence for the application of science in the practice of sport.

Perhaps more significantly, during that former life, I challenged accepted medical and scientific dogma six times. Each time, I was proved to be correct, and my view eventually became accepted mainstream teaching.

The most significant of these contributions was to disprove the prevailing dogma that during all forms of exercise, a catastrophic failure of human whole-body physiology, beginning in our exercising muscles, imposes significant limits on human performance. This theory, which British Nobel laureate Professor Archibald Vivian Hill advanced as a novel idea in 1923, had dominated the exercise sciences and had survived uncontested by successive generations of exercise scientists. That was before I became the first to challenge it decisively in 1996.

Remarkably, Hill published very little experimental proof to support his hypothesis. His work deftly confirmed the principle that a new theory requires much less evidence for its original acceptance than its ultimate refutation would demand. In my new and what some have considered pseudo-scientific life after 2010, I would learn that there is no better example of this 'truth' than Ancel Keys's diet-heart hypothesis.

Yet through a series of logical deductions and relatively simple experiments, I led a research team that disproved Hill's hypothesis with relative ease. Instead, we proposed that the human brain determines our athletic performance by anticipating what lies ahead, from the moment any exercise bout begins. According to those predictions, our brain then sets the limits of how hard it will allow us to push ourselves. It does this to ensure that we reach the finish of all exercise sessions with some physical reserve – and still alive!

Our model, grandly titled the Central Governor Model of Exercise Regulation, represents perhaps one of the more important advances in the exercise sciences of the past century.

I then led our team to disprove the Dehydration Myth. That was the industry-driven fallacy that unless we humans drink 'as much as tolerable', we risk our health every time we exercise, especially when in the heat. Our publication in

1991 established beyond doubt that this advice can be deadly.[1] It may even cause the novel, potentially fatal but utterly preventable medical condition known as exercise-associated hyponatraemic encephalopathy (EAHE) in some suscept- ible humans. As I detailed in my book *Waterlogged: The Serious Problem of Overhydration in Endurance Sports*, EAHE has caused the avoidable deaths of scores of athletes and military personnel since 1981.[2] That was when we were the first to recognise and describe the condition.

Importantly, sports medicine authorities ignored our definitive 1991 evidence that simply ensuring that athletes do not over-drink during exercise will pre- vent EAHE. Indeed, an industry seemingly intent on selling as much product to athletes as possible still disregards those definitive findings, ostensibly oblivious of the consequences.

We have made other, rather less spectacular scientific advances. These include disproving an improbable theory first advanced in the early 1970s that running 42-kilometre marathons confers lifelong immunity from coronary heart disease; our finding that catastrophic neck injuries in the sport of rugby are not random chance events but rather occur under predictable circumstances; and that the dehydration that naturally occurs during exercise does not cause the occasional cases of exercise-associated heatstroke in running and other similar sports (as a result, encouraging athletes to drink more during exercise – another false feature of the Dehydration Myth – will not prevent cases of heatstroke).

During that former life, I also convinced Jake White, coach of the 2007 Rugby World Cup–winning Springbok rugby team, to rest key players at crucial peri- ods in the final year before the 2007 competition. This advice was profoundly unconventional and provoked indignant attacks on me in the press and on social media. How could I, who clearly knew so little about the sport, possibly suggest that professional rugby players needed to rest? After all, they are paid – too much, according to some – to play rugby; it is their job.

The error these critics made was a failure to understand the delicate balance between winning major competitions, such as the Rugby World Cup, which hap- pens every four years, and playing just enough competitive rugby in the preceding four years.

My unconventional approach came from the best source: it was based on what I had learnt from studying athletes in other sports. In the end, according to Coach White, I contributed significantly to the Springboks' ultimate victory. He later kindly wrote: 'I had full faith in what Tim said, because I knew he genuinely wanted South Africa to win. I always had the feeling in every meeting we had that he genuinely wanted to find ways in which we could have the edge over the opposition. And he never gave me reason to doubt him. He never said to us, "Don't do it like that, do it like this." He always gave you options and the pros and cons of both options.'[3]

Another previously overwhelmingly unpopular position I adopted, albeit cautiously in public for fear of retaliatory action, was that cyclist Lance Armstrong was the most doped athlete in the history of sport. An editorial I wrote in the *New England Journal of Medicine* began with the question: 'Is it possible for the "natural" athlete who competes without chemical assistance to achieve record-breaking performances in sports requiring strength, power, speed, or endurance?'[4]

My answer in the article was a resounding 'No!' My closing argument featured the story of Werner Reiterer: 'In disclosing his own drug-enhanced performances, former Australian world discus champion Werner Reiterer, who chose to retire rather than risk winning a tainted medal in the 2000 Olympic Games in Sydney, has written, "There was something pathetically wrong with the fact that a packed home arena – an entire country – would urge me on without any concept of the truth behind my ultimate athletic achievement, or of the sham of which they were unwittingly a part."'

I concluded: 'Our burden is that no longer do we share this ignorance. We can no longer pretend that we do not know.'

Seven years later, Lance Armstrong was exposed as, well, yes, the mastermind responsible for 'the most sophisticated, professionalized and successful doping program that sport has ever seen'. That was according to the US Anti-Doping Agency report[5] that finally exposed him.

In my mind, the most incriminating evidence against Armstrong was not what he said; it was what he failed to say. Not once did he complain that other cyclists were doping. If he was truly competing without the aid of drugs, surely he should have emphasised repeatedly that he was winning despite competing at a significant disadvantage? But he never did, confirming his guilt – to me, at any rate.

In time, I realised that any such failure to state the obvious is also a definitive test of the true allegiance of individuals or organisations outwardly committed to making us healthier. Those who refuse to state that the monopoly of companies responsible for the toxic modern food environment are the primary drivers of ill health, confirm that they have no interest in our health. Whether witting or unwitting, these individuals and organisations will usually prove to be nothing other than hired hands for those interests that benefit the most from rising rates of global ill health. I return to this theme in Chapter 17.

But there is another lesson from the Armstrong saga. David Walsh, who had concluded in 1999 that Armstrong was a fraud – 'Lance Armstrong perpetuated what may well be the most outrageous, cold-blooded and elaborate lie in the history of sport' – spent the next 13 years pursuing the truth.[6] Of his experience he wrote: 'How can you reveal the truth if those to whom you are speaking don't want to hear? The UCI [Union Cycliste Internationale] didn't want to know their sport was diseased; the Tour de France preferred to turn a blind eye to the circus the race had become, and too many of the fans couldn't bear to be told the saints were sinners.'[7]

Walsh wrote of the small group of whistleblowers who finally ensured that the truth was exposed: 'What set Emma O'Reilly, Betsy Andreu, Stephen Swart and Greg LeMond apart was their willingness to tell the truth at a time when there was nothing in it for them except vilification and other forms of bullying.'[8] Whistleblowers, my experience would teach me, should expect no favours.

Between 2004 and 2007, I used my medical and scientific skills to assist UCT graduate Lewis Pugh to become the first person in history to swim one kilometre in water of minus 1.8 °C at the geographical North Pole.[9] One outcome was that the United Nations Environment Programme named Pugh 'Patron of the Oceans'. In 2016, after five years of negotiations, he successfully convinced the Russian government to remove their veto and support his campaign to have the Ross Sea in Antarctica declared a Marine Protected Area. That has made the Ross Sea the largest protected area on land or sea. In his negotiations with the Russians, Pugh became known as the 'Speedo diplomat'. In the Antarctic summer of 2016/17, he turned his attention to swims off the Antarctic Peninsula, hoping to add the seas off East Antarctica, the Weddell Sea and the Bellingshausen Sea to the list of Marine Protected Areas by 2020.

As a result of some of these contributions, at least two – *Waterlogged* and the Central Governor Model of Exercise Regulation – considered seminal, UCT bestowed on me its highest degree, Doctor of Science, at age 53.

According to a developing fable, all that ended on 13 December 2010, when, as a new generation of critics claimed, I apparently turned my back on my former life of dedicated, hard-core science. After that day, I began my 'descent into quackery'.

Because of this narrative, beginning in 2011, I converted overnight into just another self-aggrandising celebrity impostor, a snake-oil salesman promising miracle cures to a gullible public. Critics seemed to believe that the nutrition path I was now advocating was based on nothing more than anecdote and my misleading suggestions of a placebo effect without any biological basis.

According to this account, to boost my profile, I had begun to work tirelessly to cherry-pick data and suppress any information that disproved my dogma about the benefits of low-carbohydrate, high-fat (LCHF) diets. I did so, according to their theory, in part by attacking my opponents publicly. My goal, apparently, was to berate, humiliate and silence anyone brave enough to challenge my opinions.

And so, in a few short months, I morphed from a distinguished scientist with a globally acknowledged reputation into a faith-based nutrition activist, ruthlessly advocating an unproven, clearly dangerous 'fad' diet.

The reality, as I explain in this book, is rather different. My scientific conversion came about after what I call my 'Damascene moment'. It happened after I came face to face with compellingly robust evidence that contradicted everything I believed was true about optimum nutrition to treat and prevent serious diseases, such as obesity, diabetes and heart disease.

I started to question whether much of what my professors at medical school had taught me as incontrovertible nutrition truths were, in fact, no more than myths – lies, even. Much like with the other six myths that I had disproved when I was still a perfectly ordinary, hard-core scientist, I challenged two deeply held dogmas: the role of carbohydrate in nutrition and the diet-heart hypothesis that saturated fat causes heart disease.

I was left facing an ethical dilemma of monumental proportions: I had spent the better part of 34 years disseminating nutritional advice both locally and internationally to patients and athletes, not least through the pages of *Lore of Running*, that I now knew to be wrong. Not just wrong, but in all likelihood harmful to many, especially those with insulin resistance (IR) and pre-diabetes.

I had two options: I could either continue preaching these wrong and potentially harmful lies and maintain the scientific nutrition status quo, the so-called conventional 'wisdom', or I could admit my errors, try to correct them and deal with the consequences. For me, there was no choice. I had been raised by parents who viewed honesty, truthfulness and taking responsibility for your actions as ethical absolutes. I knew that to honour their lives, I had no option other than to acknowledge my errors and to live with the consequences.

In my mind, I was just doing what any good scientist does when faced with incontrovertible evidence that contradicts a view, no matter how deeply held: I changed my mind.

I expected that my colleagues in the medical profession – I am also a medical doctor, although I have not practised clinical medicine for more than 17 years – and in academia, including my own university, would be intrigued. They would want to know why I had changed my mind. They would be open to dialogue on matters of science and evidence-based medicine. They would want to learn.

I could not have been more wrong.

The results of my personal choice would prove to be brutal for myself, my wife and the rest of our family, beyond anything I could possibly have imagined.

In the beginning, the earliest criticisms seemed to be nothing more than gentlemanly disagreements between consenting academics. But these were covers for more devious actions, the implications of which would become apparent only much later. Prominent doctors, in particular cardiologists, began criticising me by name in public. That was probably to be expected, since I was going against one of the most enduring dogmas of cardiology, the diet-heart hypothesis and its close cousin, the lipid hypothesis.

Endocrinologists followed suit, as did academics from my own university.

On reflection, my biggest error was to start asking inconvenient questions of my profession – questions that doctors and academics appeared to want to keep hidden from public scrutiny, preferably forever.

I soon realised that I was up against a solid, seemingly impenetrable wall of opposition to what I was proposing. What I found most difficult to understand was not the reluctance of my colleagues to consider anything that went against conventional nutrition 'wisdom', but rather the venom with which critics began attacking me personally and publicly. They seemed intent not just on shooting the messenger, but also on savagely slaying and flaying the messenger publicly until not a shred of my scientific reputation remained intact.

It was as if they were intent, for no rational reason that I could fathom, to maintain the status quo for treatment protocols, in particular for obesity, diabetes and heart disease. Those treatment protocols are based on the pharmaceutical model of disease. They demonstrably do not work, as global epidemics of all those conditions have shown. They have worked only to fill the coffers of the drug-makers.

I was challenging those vested interests. It is probably no surprise then that within a year I had become the focus of a concerted effort to humiliate me publicly by showing first the South African public, and then the rest of the world, that I had lost my mind, had turned my back on science and had become a 'medical impostor', a quack and a danger to the public.

At that stage, I had no idea who or what was behind the campaign to discredit me. It was not long before I began to see a game plan emerging: with my scientific legacy destroyed and appropriately humiliated in the court of public opinion, the critics would effectively silence me. And ensure that no one else would ever again risk doing what I had done.

The coordinated attacks would continue relentlessly for the next six years. Many would originate from medical and dietetic colleagues at UCT – the very same university that I had served with honour and distinction for more than four decades.

The attacks against me began to take on a curiously cultish and religious tinge. Critics said I had morphed into a medical messiah, an evangelist no longer interested in the pursuit of the truth of hard science. I was now a 'zealot' on a 'crusade', using 'extremism' to 'demonise' sugar, 'bend' patients to my will and force my views on them.

They said I was practising 'bad' or 'pseudo' science by oversimplifying complex issues such as obesity and by promoting a 'fad' diet. For someone who developed the 'complex' model of exercise regulation, they said that I should 'be horrified with such reductionistic, simplified thinking'.

They began to predict that my end was nigh. As a result of all my considerable failings, and because of 'significant doubt and criticism from the scientific community' about my views on nutrition, my scientific legacy was under serious challenge and was unlikely to survive.

A former PhD student got in on the act, even advising me how I could still escape the trap into which my manifest professional and personal character weaknesses and failings had somehow impelled me. He said I needed to curb the passions and enthusiasms that were driving me 'to extreme viewpoints on complex phenomena'. I should become 'more nuanced, less dogmatic' and more conciliatory towards doctors practising their particular form of medicine – even though it was one I realised was killing people.

A leitmotif in all these attacks was that I had 'lost my way'; that orthodox doctors and dietitians were on the 'right path' of 'balanced, healthy, high-carbohydrate, low-fat diets'. They needed urgently to do something drastic to bring me 'back into the fold' and save the public from my madness.

Critics said I should 'stop resorting to weak anecdotes that constitute poor science' because they undermined my position. Instead, they counselled me to 'apply the rigour of scientific thinking that shook so many fallacies in fatigue and dehydration to your OWN arguments. Your good messages will be stronger for it.'

Not surprisingly, cardiologists who are intellectually and commercially wedded to the diet-heart and lipid hypotheses were prominent critics. They included UCT cardiology professor Patrick Commerford. He led a group of Cape Town professors and cardiologists who wrote an open letter to the media in 2012, calling me a cholesterol denialist and a 'danger to the public'. Johannesburg cardiologist Dr Anthony Dalby expressed similar sentiments, predicting that I would end up killing people with my diet, which is, in his opinion, 'criminal'.

Endocrinologists took particular exception to the message I was beginning to promote. It was one I thought would excite all doctors: that type-2 diabetes mellitus is not necessarily a chronic degenerative condition. Not all diabetics would need to take drugs for the rest of their lives and risk blindness, kidney failure, heart disease and limb loss. Simple dietary change could control the condition and, in some cases, eliminate the need for medication altogether.

You would have thought I was telling patients to commit slow suicide, so virulent was the response to the evidence I was trying to share.

Another critic even suggested that were I to wake up to the error of my ways, South Africa could become 'the first nation to reject hyped up, fad/cultish thinking and become the world leader in healthy eating, with balance'. Ironically, I guess in a nutshell that is pretty much what this book is all about.

Attacks were not always from deep inside the medical or dietetic professions.

Professor George Claassen is the brother of former Springbok rugby captain Wynand Claassen, and the son of the 1961 winner of the Comrades Marathon, George Nicolaas Claassen. In his academic career, Claassen was professor and head of journalism at the University of Stellenbosch.

In his book *Quacks, Whims and Disease*,[10] originally written in Afrikaans,

Professor Claassen devoted two of the first nine text pages to what he presumably meant as a dispassionate analysis of why I had become a quack. The problem with my opinion on the low-carb, high-fat diet, he said, is that it is 'widely reported ... without performing any clinical tests or double-blind experiments'. He then argued that my scientific publication on the self-reported data of 127 subjects[11] was a classic example of 'confirmation bias'. By way of explanation, he said that because the subjects lost weight and improved their blood sugar concentrations after adopting the diet, it was 'confirmation bias' to conclude that the weight loss and improved blood sugar concentrations were a result of the dietary change.

The logic of his argument continues to elude me, as it probably escapes others in the scientific nutrition community globally. However, that is how Professor Claassen explained it in his book.

One thing sets Professor Claassen apart from many other critics: he clearly knows the value of covering his back. He concluded his summary of why he had afforded me quack status with the following: 'The final word has yet to be spoken about the Noakes dispute. Sometime in the future clinical research may show him to be correct, but by following the incorrect scientific route he has set himself up for accusations of quackery that have damaged his reputation.'

Over the following six years, a host of prominent South African doctors and medical and scientific organisations would echo many of these sentiments and add their own creative words of negative criticism. The attacks are all detailed in Chapter 7. Perhaps the most personally devastating, however, was the letter to the *Cape Times* from UCT and my colleagues in its Faculty of Health Sciences in 2014. The concluding paragraph stated: 'UCT's Faculty of Health Sciences, a leading research institution in Africa, has a reputation for research excellence to uphold. Above all, our research must be socially responsible. We have therefore taken the unusual step of distancing ourselves from the proponents of this diet.'

A month later, the HPCSA would use that letter to charge me with unprofessional conduct. My public humiliation was, it seemed, complete.

The end result was that in a few short years I had been reduced in the public mind and in the mind of my profession from a world-leading scientist in exercise science and nutrition to a quack embarking on a voyage of personal destruction. Others might argue that I had become the most publicly humiliated doctor in South African medical history.

In this book I try to understand how, and more importantly, why this happened. How was it possible for me to spend 40 years becoming a world-leading scientist, only to descend into quackery within a few short months? And all, as I will explain, because I chose simply to change my mind when I realised that the evidence, as I understood it, had changed.

At first I did not realise it, but gradually a perplexing idea crept into my mind, an idea that, with time, would take on sinister implications: while all I had done was change my opinion in response to my altered understanding of the evidence, my colleagues in the medical and scientific professions had, in response, begun to act as if they were party to a communal vow of silence. It was as if they had been forewarned of dire consequences should they ever express even an inkling of support for my opinions. Would they face immediate academic excommunication should they suggest that, just perhaps, my new dietary ideas be treated with a degree of deference, befitting my status as a highly rated scientist, and not with unreserved contempt?

And so the thought popped uninvited into my mind that my critics were acting as if they were loyal to a medical and scientific omertà.

Omertà is the Italian word for 'manhood', but it more popularly refers to the code of silence taken by members of the Mafia. In its extreme version, it is the vow that Mafiosi take in refusing – to the death – to talk about criminal activity and give evidence that would be helpful to the authorities investigating organised crime. I had begun to feel as if I was starring in a B-grade Hollywood gangster movie set in the medico-scientific world.

Of course, I am not the first to compare modern medicine and its pharmaceutical-science model to organised crime. Danish physician Dr Peter Gøtzsche did it first in a ground-breaking book, *Deadly Medicines and Organised Crime: How Big Pharma has Corrupted Healthcare*.[12] It is a compelling, disturbing read; perhaps the most disquieting book about my profession that I have ever read.

So I begin this book by detailing the case that my colleagues and assorted hangers-on have made against me. It began in the media and ended in a sensational 26-day 'trial' brought against me by the HPCSA on a charge of disgraceful professional conduct. I have become the first medical scientist in modern medical history to be prosecuted for his views on nutrition.

Not for nothing has the public dubbed the case against me 'the Nutrition Trial of the 21st Century'. They have compared me to Galileo.

The case against me shows in stark relief what happens when a familiar scientist dares to threaten convention. This is especially the case if that convention is built on the exploitation of science for commercial gain.

A large part of my contribution to this book describes why I believe what I do. It explains why I believe so strongly in the science that I was prepared to subject myself to the stresses of this campaign, despite the intense emotional discomfort it caused me, my wife and our children – not to mention the exorbitant financial costs that we incurred. By simply deregistering as a medical doctor, I could have made the trial go away. The HPCSA would no longer have had jurisdiction over me. The dietitian who first complained about me for a single tweet would have had no recourse.

In retrospect, embarking on this journey was not something my family and

I did lightly. We certainly did not choose it. But once our enemies threw down the gauntlet in the most public way that they did, my wife and I were not going to go quietly into the night. Our opposition, the prosecution, has learnt that to their considerable cost. If ever there was an illustration of the lesson in unintended consequences, then the case against me is the classic example.

My message to you, dear reader, is that all people are entitled to their own opinions. But not to their own set of facts. So do not believe what you want to believe. Believe what the facts tell you is the truth.

For in the context of junk diets, embedded scientists, corrupt – or simply ignorant – doctors and dietitians, human health and omertàs, what you believe about your personal nutrition will determine not just how you live, but also how you die.

TIM NOAKES
CAPE TOWN
SEPTEMBER 2017

Preface

'Those who will not reason, are bigots, those who cannot, are fools, and those who dare not, are slaves.'
— **Lord Byron, English poet**

In 2014, I began researching and writing about Professor Tim Noakes and his nutrition 'Damascene moment', as he calls it. At the time, I was a vegetarian and had been for more than 25 years. Actually, I wasn't a 'real' vegetarian for all those years. With a perfectly straight face, I would tell anyone who asked that I was a 'biltong-eating vegetarian'. If you don't know what biltong is, you're not South African. It's our dried-meat version of American beef jerky, only nicer – at least to me.

I wore my 'no meat' badge with pride for my health's sake. I also studiously avoided dairy products, including cheese and yoghurt, which I loved. I refused to eat low-fat yoghurt, though. My Greek background makes it an oxymoron. I actually loathed the taste of many low-fat foods. However, thanks to expert advice and my own research, I was firmly fat-phobic.

I stuck to low-fat, high-carbohydrate foods because doctors and dietitians I trusted told me I should. In fact, they said everyone should eat that way. They said that it would significantly reduce the risk of life-threatening lifestyle diseases, such as obesity, diabetes, heart disease and even cancer. With the wisdom of hindsight, I now marvel at how ignorant and blindly trusting I was, especially considering my natural scepticism – and cynicism – as a health journalist.

I believed in the diet-heart hypothesis that saturated fat causes heart disease as if it were gospel. Cardiologists I trusted said it was written in stone. I believed them. Why wouldn't I? They were clever, omniscient creatures – god-like, really. They had lots of fancy letters after their names. I was fully in the thrall of eminence-based medicine. I never thought to question their conventional nutrition 'wisdom'. I therefore avoided 'fad' diets. I knew about Atkins. I believed it to be a 'dangerous fad' because cardiologists told me it was. And anyway, it seemed counterintuitive that you could eat fat to get thin. It seemed reasonable that fat in the diet would equal fat in the arteries.

I wrote about many different diets and tried most of them – for well-being, not weight loss. I was never overweight, although I was also never happy with my weight. It always seemed to yo-yo. I wasn't a slave to the scale. Instead, my clothes were my slave master. When they grew too tight, as they often did, I immediately ate less. I would simply starve myself into submission. I believed wholeheartedly in the calories-in, calories-out model of obesity. I arrogantly believed that obese people were mostly just slothful gluttons. They ate too much and moved too little – at least that's what the experts said.

I tried a vegan diet once, but found it too much like hard work. In my hippie incarnation, I tried the macrobiotic diet, eating lots of grains. I liked the idea of plant-based diets, but never felt good on them. I also tried an Ayurvedic diet. Ayurveda is the ancient Indian traditional healing system that promotes eating according to 'doshas'. I loved the delicious Ayurvedic desserts, especially rice pudding. I also once ate only raw food for five months – fresh fruit, vegetables, nuts and seeds. But I was always hungry.

Once or twice a year, I went on punishing water-only fasts. I believed the promise of a 'detox' to my system that would leave me 'good and clean and fresh' – much like the soap-powder commercial. I would feel grim for a day or two on water only. Then I would become energised, literally out of nowhere. The longest I ever lasted was eight days. I emerged looking cadaverous, but feeling fine. However, as soon as I reverted to my 'normal' low-fat, high-carb way of eating, my energy levels dropped and any weight I had lost piled back on.

None of the diets made me feel good physically or even mentally. If anyone had told me that the *real* fad was the low-fat, high-carb diet I was eating, I would have instantly suffered a severe bout of confirmation bias. Confirmation bias is when we discount or ignore any evidence that flatly contradicts a deeply held belief. US physician and LCHF specialist Michael Eades tells me that confirmation bias suffuses us all – including him. It's how we manage the bias that counts, he says.

I didn't even know that I had confirmation bias until I started researching LCHF, or 'Banting' as it's known in South Africa. As far as I was concerned, I was doing all the 'right' things according to conventional nutrition 'wisdom'. Feeling below par was normal for me. Over the years, I put my frequent mood swings down to pregnancy, motherhood and menopause, then just age. After all, the 'experts' say that ageing and declining health are constant companions. Those are the same experts who tell patients with type-2 diabetes that their condition is chronic, degenerative and irreversible. (This book proves that it isn't.) I never made the connection between what I was eating and how low I often felt in body and mind.

Of course, I knew about Noakes. He is, after all, one of the most well-known and well-respected South Africans in the global medical scientific community. Recently retired UCT deputy vice-chancellor Danie Visser has called him a 'force in the world'. Former South African Comrades Marathon king Bruce Fordyce has described him as 'a national treasure, one of the most important South Africans of all time'. When I first heard about his spectacular about-turn on nutrition in 2010, I was in and out of the country and unable to focus on the story. I thus only began to research Noakes and his new ideas on dietary carbs and fats in early 2014, and then mainly because of what people were saying about him in the media.

His peers in the medical profession (Noakes is also a medical doctor) were making statements that seemed to me to be defamatory. Even academics at UCT and other universities appeared to be defaming him with impunity. They were demonising him using cultish, religious terminology. They called him a zealot, a heretic, messianic, a 'celebrity' scientist, a quack peddling dangerous snake oil to unsuspecting followers. They painted a picture of him as dangerous and devilish, the closest thing to a nutrition antichrist that modern medicine has ever seen. They said that he had lost the scientific plot and was practising pseudo-science.

Noakes had clearly made enemies in the highest echelons of medical and academic establishments. He was probably lucky he wasn't living in medieval times. His peers would have burnt him at the stake as a heretic for challenging orthodoxy.

I became aware of cardiologists, in particular, banding together to discredit him. In September 2012, UCT cardiology professor Patrick Commerford and colleagues had co-authored an open letter in which they accused Noakes of 'Cholesterol Denialism'.[1] They described his views on diet as 'dangerous and potentially very harmful to good patient care'. The previous month, Johannes-burg cardiologist Dr Anthony Dalby had been quoted in a media report calling Noakes's dietary advice 'criminal'.[2]

Noakes has infuriated drug companies and raised many a cardiologist's blood pressure with his antipathy to the cholesterol-lowering drugs known as statins. Statins are the most prescribed drug on the planet. Drug companies that make them have made billions in profits. Yet research shows that the risks of statins far outweigh the benefits.

The frequency and virulence of attacks by cardiologists left a lingering impression on me. It's why I later speculated in Foodmed.net that cardiologists may lie at the heart (pun intended) of the HPCSA's case against him.

Cardiologists were not the only ones suggesting that Noakes would end up killing people with his dietary views, and on a scale close to genocide. I found that claim extraordinarily shocking and hyperbolic. After all, I had known Noakes for decades, not personally, but as an interview subject in my journalistic career. I had interviewed him many times, ironically, as it turned out, on the use of high-carb, low-fat diets for athletic performance. I had always found him to be a scientist of formidable intellect, as well as a caring medical doctor. He is charismatic, but I'd never considered that a crime. And anyway, Noakes always appeared to me to be sincere and have integrity of purpose.

Yet here were all these doctors, dietitians and assorted academics naming and shaming him in public, and the media enthusiastically baying for his blood. I wondered if the distinguished, world-renowned scientist could possibly have gone 'rogue'.

I contacted Noakes to ask for a Skype interview. He agreed, and the next day we spoke for hours. I tried hard to keep the scepticism out of my voice as I peppered him with questions. I'm Greek. I gesticulate a lot. My Mediterranean background makes me passionate about issues close to my heart. It also makes me a very bad poker player. It lets my confirmation bias run riot at times. I was trying to understand if Noakes had any solid science to support what he was now proposing.

He was his usual polite, patient self. He explained that there was nothing new to what he was saying, that the evidence had been there for years, and that those in positions of power and influence over public nutrition advice had either ignored or suppressed this evidence. He directed me to scientific people, papers and places I didn't even know existed.

I ended the conversation feeling unsettled. Noakes sounded eminently rational, reasonable and robustly scientific. I started reading all the references he gave me. I read the work of US physician-professors Stephen Phinney and Eric Westman, and Professor Jeff Volek. I read Eades; US science journalist Gary Taubes, author of *Good Calories, Bad Calories* and *Why We Get Fat* (and most recently *The Case Against Sugar*); and one of British obesity researcher Dr Zoë Harcombe's many books, *The Obesity Epidemic*. I also read *The Big Fat Surprise* by US investigative journalist Nina Teicholz. That book thoroughly rocked my scientific worldview, as it has done for countless others.

The *Wall Street Journal* said of Teicholz's book: 'From the very beginning, we had the statistical means to understand why things did not add up; we had a boatload of Cassandras, a chorus of warnings; but they were ignored, castigated, suppressed. We had our big fat villain, and we still do.' Former editor of the *British Medical Journal* Dr Richard Smith wrote about *The Big Fat Surprise* in a feature for the journal in 2014, titled 'Are some diets "mass murder"?' LCHF critics have suggested that prescribing a diet restricted in carbohydrates to the public is 'the equivalent of mass murder'. Smith gained a very different impression after ploughing through five books on diet and some of the key studies to write his feature. The same accusation of 'mass murder' can be directed at 'many players in the great diet game', Smith said. In short, he said, experts have based bold policies on fragile science and the long-term results 'may be terrible'.[3]

For her book, Teicholz researched the influential US dietary guidelines, which were introduced in 1977 and which most English-speaking countries, including

South Africa, subsequently adopted. She discovered that there was no evidence to support the guidelines' low-fat, high-carb recommendations when they were first introduced, and that any evidence to the contrary was ignored or suppressed for decades.

My research into LCHF left me uneasy. As a journalist, I'm a messenger. I began to wonder whether I had been giving the wrong messages to my readers for decades. Had I unwittingly promoted advice that harmed people suffering from obesity, diabetes and heart disease? Among those was my father, Demetrius Sboros, who suffered from heart disease for many years before his death in 2002. Had I given him advice and information that shortened his life?

I put those worries aside and wrote up my interview with Noakes. The backlash was instant. On Twitter, total strangers called me irresponsible, unscientific, unethical and biased. Astonishingly, some were medical doctors, mostly former students of Noakes. They said that I was Noakes's 'cheerleader', and even accused me of having a 'crush' on him. Some said that Noakes must have been paying me handsomely to say nice things about him. (For the record, he has never paid me anything, nor would he think to offer to pay me or I to accept.) Others said I was a 'closet Banter', as if that was the worst possible insult.

At first I was irritated. After all, I had quoted Noakes accurately. I had reflected what critics said about him, to ensure that I gave both sides. And anyway, I readily confess to bias, but only in favour of good science. I've always said that if anyone can show me robust evidence that Noakes is wrong about LCHF, I will publish it. Knowing him as I do, so will he.

Most of all, though, I was shocked at the venom behind the attacks on Noakes. He had simply done what any good scientist does when faced with compelling evidence that contradicts a belief: he had changed his mind. I've never seen much sense in having a mind if you can't change it.

The attacks against him grew more gratuitously vicious and libellous. Then, in July 2014, researchers at UCT and the University of Stellenbosch published a study in *PLoS One* that became known as the Naudé review.[4]

In August 2014, four of Noakes's UCT colleagues published a letter in the *Cape Times*. Dubbed the UCT professors' letter, it accused him of 'making outrageous unproven claims about disease prevention' and of 'not conforming to the tenets of good and responsible science'.

After repeatedly being accused on social media of being a 'closet Banter', I eventually decided I might as well at least try the diet everyone said I was on. I figured that, like all the other diets I had tried, I wouldn't feel any different on this one. But then at least I could write honestly to say that LCHF hadn't worked for me. And it might get some of the trolls off my back.

It was in late 2014 that I began experimenting with eating LCHF foods. I have obsessive-compulsive tendencies, so when I start something, I tend to go 'all in'.

I observed all the basic Banting rules to the letter. I cut all bread, pasta, pizza, rice, potatoes, chocolates, sweets and other processed carbs from my diet.

It took about a week before I started noticing changes. The first was mood, in particular the afternoon 'slump' that I experienced daily at around two or three p.m. I would always feel suddenly ravenous at that time of the day, like I had to eat something, anything, preferably high carb, if I wanted to live. But on LCHF, the afternoon slump vanished, never to return.

My sugar and other carb cravings reduced rapidly too. It took at least three days before I stopped longing for my next sugar 'fix'. I hadn't ever thought of myself as genuinely addicted to sugar. I knew I had an unquenchable sweet tooth, but I never thought of myself as a real, live sugar addict. Of course, I always knew that bread and other carbohydrate foods turned to glucose in my bloodstream, just as sugar did. But I didn't see that as a threat.

I felt other positive changes on LCHF. My energy levels were up. I felt as if I was concentrating better and for longer periods. Most of all, I wasn't feeling hungry, depressed or deprived with this new way of eating. The only variable that had changed in my lifestyle was the food I was eating. Of course, I know that it is anecdotal evidence, but it made me sit up and take notice.

Today, while my sugar and carb addiction is well under control, it hovers ever on the periphery of my consciousness. After all, I nurtured it over a lifetime. I sometimes break the rules and fall off the 'Banting wagon'. However, the benefits have become sufficient positive reinforcement to get me back on track every time.

It also helps that Noakes and all the other LCHF experts I have since interviewed are open in their views on optimum nutrition. They don't say that LCHF is the only way or a one-size-fits-all approach. They do say that anyone who is obese, diabetic, has heart disease or has otherwise become ill on a high-carb, low-fat diet should try LCHF before drugs or invasive bariatric surgery. That sounds reasonable and rational to me. They also say that LCHF is a lifestyle, not a diet.

As I continued my research, it became apparent why so many doctors, dietitians, and food and drug industries want to silence Noakes. He threatens their businesses, reputations, careers, funding and sponsors. And cardiologists and endocrinologists are not the only ones at risk of class-action lawsuits if, or more likely when, LCHF diets become mainstream, especially to treat health problems such as obesity, diabetes and heart disease. All doctors and dietitians may be at risk if it is shown that they knew about LCHF but deliberately chose not to offer it as an option to their patients.

When the HPCSA eventually charged Noakes in late 2014 with allegedly giving unconventional advice to a breastfeeding mother on Twitter, I began to prepare to report on the hearing. The deeper I dug, the more unpleasant the experience became. In 2015, for example, I was having what I thought was a relatively civil phone call with Johannesburg cardiologist Dr Anthony Dalby. I asked for comment on research suggesting that the diet-heart hypothesis was unproven. 'If you believe that, then I leave it to you,' he said, and hung up on me. Other doctors, academics and dietitians followed suit, avoiding my emails, or slamming the phone down if I ever managed to get past their gatekeepers.

Teicholz told me of similar experiences while doing research for *The Big Fat Surprise*. In response to a question on fat, an interviewee suddenly said, 'I can't talk about that,' and hung up. Teicholz was shaken. 'It felt as if I had been investigating organised crime,' she said. The analogy was apt for her then. It became apt for me too.

The wall of silence I came up against while reporting on the HPCSA hearing should not have surprised me. I had a good working relationship with Claire Julsing Strydom, the dietitian who laid the initial complaint against Noakes – that is, until I started writing about her role in the whole affair. Strydom was president of the Association for Dietetics in South Africa when she lodged the complaint. Once I began asking uncomfortable questions, she stopped talking to me. ADSA executives and academics have followed suit, clearly acting on legal advice.

Like many, I enjoy a good conspiracy theory. However, at the first abortive attempt at a hearing session in June 2015, I wasn't convinced of an organised campaign to discredit Noakes. By the trial's end, I was.

Strydom and ADSA deny a vendetta against Noakes. Yet the signs were always there. Another ADSA executive member, Catherine 'Katie' Pereira, lodged a complaint with the HPCSA against Noakes in 2014 that was even more frivolous than Strydom's. During an interview for a newspaper, Noakes had said that he didn't know of any dietitian who told poor people not to drink Coca-Cola and eat potato crisps. (Most orthodox dietitians I know tell people that it's fine to eat and drink these products as long as they do so 'in moderation'.) The journalist made that comment a focus of the published interview. Pereira was offended on behalf of the entire dietetic profession. The HPCSA initially – and sensibly, to my mind – declined to prosecute. Strydom then intervened and pleaded with the HPCSA to charge Noakes. That case is still pending.

Nevertheless, to me, Strydom and ADSA have always looked more like patsies – proxies for Big Food and other vested interests opposed to Noakes. And this book turned into not so much a 'whodunnit' than a 'why they dunnit?'.

When I first started writing about Noakes and LCHF, I also wasn't convinced that he was on the right scientific track, persuasive though his arguments were. I needed time to absorb all that I was learning. That would come later, after I attended the 'world-first' international low-carb summit in Cape Town in 2015. The summit was an important pit stop on this remarkable journey with Noakes and many other LCHF experts as my guides. I have learnt much from them about good and bad nutrition science. I have also learnt how best to deal with gratuitous attacks on my character and credibility as a journalist. I have only had the tiniest taste of what his opponents have subjected him to for years.

I have put into practice the many lessons I have learnt as a student of traditional Chinese and Japanese martial arts under internationally renowned instructor Edward Jardine. One of Jardine's favourite sayings is: 'Everything in moderation, including moderation.' Oscar Wilde said it first, but Jardine says it with deeper wisdom. He teaches that the most important opponent you have to overcome in life is yourself. My training in martial arts has shown me the wisdom in strategic silence: that it is one of the hardest arguments to refute.

And in *The Art of War*, Sun Tzu writes: 'If you wait by the river long enough, the bodies of your enemies will float by.' This book proves it, and more.

MARIKA SBOROS
LONDON
SEPTEMBER 2017

Introduction

'In a time of universal deceit, telling the truth is a revolutionary act.'
– **Unknown**

This is the story of a remarkable scientific journey. Just as remarkable is the genesis of that journey: a single, innocuous tweet.

In February 2014, a Twitter user asked a distinguished and world-renowned scientist a simple question: 'Is LCHF eating ok for breastfeeding mums? Worried about all the dairy + cauliflower = wind for babies??'

Always willing to engage with an inquiring mind, Professor Tim Noakes tweeted back: 'Baby doesn't eat the dairy and cauliflower. Just very healthy high fat breast milk. Key is to ween [*sic*] baby onto LCHF.'

With those few words, Noakes set off a chain of events that would eventually see him charged with unprofessional conduct, caught up in a case that would drag on for more than three years and cost many millions of rands. More difficult, if not impossible, to quantify is the devastating emotional toll that the whole ordeal has taken on him and his family, as critics attacked his character and scientific reputation at every turn.

At the time, it was open season on Tim Noakes. Doctors, dietitians and assorted academics from South Africa's top universities had been hard at work for years trying to discredit him. They did not like his scientific views on low-carbohydrate, high-fat foods, which he had been promoting since 2011. His opinions contrasted sharply with conventional, orthodox dietary 'wisdom', and the tweet provided the perfect pretext to amp up their attacks and hopefully silence him once and for all.

Within 24 hours of his tweet, a dietitian had reported him to the Health Professions Council of South Africa for giving what she considered 'incorrect', 'dangerous' and 'potentially life-threatening' advice. To Noakes's surprise, the HPCSA took her complaint seriously.

Noakes is one of the few scientists in the world with an A1 rating from the South African National Research Foundation (NRF) for both sports science and nutrition. In his home country, he has no equal in terms of expertise in and research into LCHF. Few can match his large academic footprint – quantified by an H-index of over 70. The H- or Hirsch index is a measure of the impact of a scientist's work. Noakes's impact is significant. He has published more than 500 scientific papers, many of them in peer-reviewed journals, and over 40 of which deal exclusively with nutrition. He has been cited more than 17 000 times in the scientific literature.

Yet, remarkably, the HPCSA chose to back the opinion of a dietitian in private practice over an internationally renowned nutrition research scientist. They charged him with 'unprofessional conduct' for providing 'unconventional advice on breastfeeding babies on social networks' and hauled him through the humiliating process of a disciplinary hearing.

The public quickly dubbed it 'the Nutrition Trial of the 21st Century'. I've called it Kafkaesque. The HPCSA insisted that it was a hearing, not a trial, but the statutory body's own conduct belied the claim.

At the time of Noakes's tweet, I wanted to give up journalism. After more than 30 years of researching and writing about medicine and nutrition science, I was frustrated and bored. People were growing fatter and sicker, and the medical and dietetic specialists I wrote about weren't making much difference to patients' lives. Neither was my reporting.

Then I started investigating and writing about the HPCSA's case against Noakes. The more questions I asked, the more walls of silence came up around me, and from the most unexpected sources. There's an old saying that silence isn't empty, it is full of answers. I found that the silence was loudest from those with the most to hide. I could not have foreseen the labyrinthine extent of vested interests ranged against Noakes, or the role played by shadowy proxy organisations for multinational sugar and soft-drink companies in suppressing and discrediting nutrition evidence.

It took a US investigative journalist to join many of the dots I had identified. Russ Greene's research led to the International Life Sciences Institute (ILSI), a Coca-Cola front organisation. In an explosive exposé in January 2017, Greene showed how the ILSI has worked to support the nutrition status quo in South Africa, as well as the health professionals and food and drug industries that benefit from it. It has opened a branch in South Africa and has funded nutrition congresses throughout the country. It has also paid for dietitians and academics opposed to Noakes and LCHF to address conferences abroad.*

Of course, it might be coincidence that so many doctors, dietitians and academics with links to the ILSI became involved, directly and indirectly, in the HPCSA's prosecution of Noakes. Then again, maybe not.

Many people suggested that I write a book about Noakes's trial, for a trial it

---

* Russ Greene, 'Big Food vs. Tim Noakes: The Final Crusade', *The Russells*, 5 January 2017, available at https://therussells.crossfit.com/2017/01/05/big-food-vs-tim-noakes-the-final-crusade/

was. I was the only journalist to cover all six sessions over 25 days. I sat through all the evidence from the HPCSA's six witnesses. I listened as Noakes and his three witnesses testified. Noakes himself spoke for almost 40 hours, showing nearly 1200 slides and citing 350-odd publications and other materials. I also saw first-hand the toll the trial was taking on him, even as he was strong in scientific and academic spirit.

And when – and out of the proverbial blue – Noakes invited me to co-author a book he was writing on the trial, I accepted in a heartbeat. I knew it would be a remarkable journey, even if it was not one of his choosing. Thus, I became one of this book's two narrators. Noakes provides the background to the HPCSA hearing and discusses the all-important science behind the LCHF/Banting diet. He speaks passionately about why he champions this lifestyle despite the constant persecution and efforts to silence him. I cover the hearing and the hype from my perspective as a journalist and an outsider.

The HPCSA's conduct throughout the hearing and since its conclusion has been revelatory. To a large extent, it confirms the premise of this book: that those in positions of power and influence in medicine and academia were using the case to pursue a vendetta against Noakes. The trial highlighted the inherent perils facing those brave enough to go against orthodoxy. It is in Noakes's DNA as a scientist to seek truth and challenge dogma. He has done it many times before and has been proved right every time. I have no doubt that this time will be no different. On this latest journey, he has demonstrated the unflinching courage, integrity and dignity that are his hallmarks as one of the most eminent scientists of his time.

The trial has also become an object lesson in unintended consequences on social media. It is not only social media marketing gurus who must come to grips with the pleasures and pitfalls of networking in the disruptive digital era. Social media is a double-edged sword: an invaluable tool for building reputations, careers, businesses and livelihoods, but with the potential to be equally destructive.

With his invitation to be a co-narrator on this journey, Noakes reignited my passion as a journalist. For that, I am grateful. I am also grateful for the privilege of travelling this road with him and meeting the many other brave scientists, writers and activists who are his companions and supporters. They don't all speak with one voice. All are forging a powerful new path in nutrition science, one that puts patients before profits. As a journalist, I choose to tread this irresistible path. As a scientist, Noakes is destined to be on it.

PART I

THE LOW-CARB REVOLUTION

1

The Low-carb Summit

'He that takes medicine and neglects diet,
wastes the time of his physician.'
— Ancient Chinese proverb

When I flew from Johannesburg to Cape Town on 19 February 2015, I had a feeling I wasn't on just another assignment. I was in for a real scientific treat. I was off to the Cape Town International Convention Centre to cover a health summit that the organisers had billed as unique. They said it could change the world for the better, nutritionally speaking. They had brought together under one roof, from all corners of the globe and for the first time on an international stage, 15 experts in the science and controversy behind the low-carbohydrate, high-fat lifestyle being used to treat and prevent the life-threatening chronic diseases plaguing South Africa and the rest of the planet.

Professor Tim Noakes was to be the conference host. The organiser and visionary behind it was beautiful South African former model Karen Thomson. Thomson is a recovered alcoholic, and a former cocaine and sugar addict. She is also the bestselling author of *Sugar Free! 8 Weeks to Freedom from Sugar and Carb Addictions*, in which she documents her personal experience of the ravages of addiction to alcohol and various types of 'white stuff', and recounts her recovery. Her grandfather was the late heart-transplant pioneer, Professor Christiaan Barnard. It was Barnard and his team's actions that first inspired Tim Noakes to become a medical doctor.

Thomson first heard Noakes speak about sugar and addiction in the same breath in a TV documentary in 2014. It was as if he had shone a light on the darkness of her addictions. Before then, she had no idea that there was such a thing as sugar addiction. Many doctors and dietitians wedded to conventional nutrition 'wisdom' insist that there isn't. Thomson realised that she had replaced her addiction to alcohol and cocaine with sugar and other carbohydrate foods – these were her new drugs of choice. She was determined to quit her sugar habit for good.

Thomson contacted Noakes about opening a sugar addiction centre, and the two bonded instantly. Thus, she began her LCHF journey with Noakes as her guide and mentor. He inspired her to write the book and develop the Healthy Eating & Lifestyle Program in 2012. HELP was the first of its kind in the world, a 21-day, in-patient programme that treats sugar and carbohydrates as an addiction using an LCHF nutrition approach.

The real driver behind the Cape Town LCHF summit was Thomson's distress and growing fury at the venomous personal and professional attacks on Noakes in the media. The feeding frenzy had grown more intense in the wake of the announcement that the Health Professions Council of South Africa intended hauling him in for a disciplinary hearing. The HPCSA had charged Noakes with unprofessional conduct for his February 2014 tweet to a breastfeeding mother, in which he advised weaning babies onto LCHF foods.

The public attacks on Noakes brought back painful memories for Thomson. 'I knew what it was like to grow up in a famous family and have total strangers take swipes at us in the media,' she told me. 'When I was 10, a newspaper published an interview in which the reporter said awful things about my grandfather. It upset me deeply. I never forgot it. It's not right that people can just say these things about someone and the media publish them to sell more newspapers and get more visitors to their websites.'

Thomson wanted to do something constructive to counter the attacks on Noakes. What better weapon, she thought, than good science. Her vision started out small. She would hold a one-day seminar and invite a few experts from abroad to speak up for Noakes by presenting the scientific evidence for the LCHF lifestyle.

To this end, she invited the two men widely acknowledged as the 'fathers' of the LCHF movement in the US: Professor Stephen Phinney and Dr Eric Westman. She also invited Canadian physician Dr Jay Wortman and American LCHF blogger Jimmy Moore. All immediately accepted.

From there, Thomson's vision took on a life of its own. She and Noakes started inviting other LCHF experts from around the globe. Low Carb Down Under had invited Noakes to speak in Melbourne, Australia, in 2014. His reception there was positive and in stark contrast to the criticism back home. Australian doctors, among them Low Carb Down Under co-founder Dr Rod Tayler, expressed a desire to attend Thomson's seminar.

The stellar list of speakers that Noakes and Thomson eventually assembled included internationally renowned medical doctors, scientists and researchers. Among the medical doctors were a cardiologist, a nephrologist, a psychiatrist, a bariatric surgeon and an orthopaedic surgeon. All said they would come, many at their own expense, to show support for Noakes and to spread the word to the world about the growing evidence for the safety and efficacy of LCHF diets.

The only invited expert who couldn't attend was Nina Teicholz, the US author of *The Big Fat Surprise: Why Butter, Meat and Cheese Belong in a Healthy Diet*. Her invitation arrived just a few hours after she had committed to another event. She told Noakes and Thomson that she would be with them in spirit.

At a dinner in Cape Town before the conference, Noakes met the former owner and CEO of the Fleet Feet franchise in the US, Tom Raynor. Raynor leaned over and asked: 'If there was one additional person you would like to have at your summit, who would that be?' Without hesitation, Noakes replied: 'That's easy. Gary Taubes.' Taubes is an American science writer and the author of bestsellers such as *Good Calories, Bad Calories, Why We Get Fat and What To Do About It* and *The Case Against Sugar*. Raynor responded: 'You have your wish. I will fund his attendance at your meeting.'

Response to the conference was positive and exceeded even Thomson's expectations. The growing list of speakers and delegates wanting to attend required a venue change. She chose the Cape Town International Convention Centre, which is not exactly cheap. Noakes broached the issue, which he and Thomson had blithely ignored until then, of how they would finance the conference. He had visions of them both ending up seriously out of pocket, if not impoverished.

Thomson is a glass-half-full kind of person. She had no such reservations. She gave Noakes what he called a 'Barnardesque response'. 'Prof, you are always telling everyone to believe in the outcome,' she told him. 'So, you should just follow your own advice. Believe in the outcome. It will happen.'

And happen it did. Thomson and Noakes managed a coup of sorts. They secured significant financial support from a wholly unexpected source: the country's top international investment, savings, insurance and banking group, Old Mutual.

Old Mutual was an inspired choice of partner for the venture. It ensured that the summit avoided compromising ties with Big Food and Big Pharma, and any other companies or people with a vested interest on either side of the divisive nutrition debate.

Old Mutual chief medical officer Dr Peter Bond was keenly aware of the risk the company was taking in supporting the conference and, by association, Noakes. From the outset, the conference was a direct challenge to orthodoxy and the powerful vested interests behind conventional nutrition 'wisdom'. Bond therefore chose his words very carefully in his opening address to the conference. Old Mutual was 'not endorsing a particular diet or way of eating', he said. The company was simply acknowledging that health crises around the world, including in South Africa, showed that 'new approaches are necessary'. There was a need to 'elevate preventative medicine to the level it deserved', and to not only do it, but, more importantly, also have the desire to do it. 'We have clearly failed to date,' Bond said.

He presciently added: 'We believe that when you get the right critical mass behind the topic, you can make big changes and difference. Part of the reason this conference is taking place is the contribution towards a critical mass behind preventative measures which will alter the course of serious non-communicable diseases [NCDs] that affect people in this country.'

Old Mutual executive general manager Marwan Abrahams was more direct: 'We are extremely proud to be associated with this conference and to have the calibre of thought leaders that we have in this room today.'

The conference eventually became known as the Old Mutual Health Convention, although many referred to it informally as the Cape Town low-carb summit. With so many speakers, Thomson extended the conference programme to four days: three for health professionals, and the fourth and final day for the lay public.

All doctors, dietitians and related healthcare practitioners have to register with the HPCSA in order to practise in South Africa. The HPCSA requires its members to update their professional knowledge and skills each year, and to this end has implemented a Continuing Professional Development (CPD) programme. Healthcare practitioners are required to accumulate 30 CPD points annually. With the calibre of speakers and the content of their presentations, Thomson easily secured 19 CPD points from the South African Medical Association (SAMA) for conference attendees.

It wasn't long before around 600 people had registered. More than 400 of them were health professionals – local and some foreign medical doctors, dentists, dietitians, nutritionists, psychologists and complementary medicine practitioners.

But the conference nearly didn't happen.

Nine days before the scheduled 19 February opening, SAMA withdrew the CPD points after a group of ADSA dietitians objected. They cited the by-now oft-repeated canard that there is no evidence base for the safety or efficacy of LCHF diets. The paradox, of course, was that evidence was exactly what the summit would provide for the first time in South Africa. Without CPD points, many of the 400 health professionals would no longer be willing or able to attend the event. Thomson and Noakes faced the prospect of the summit's imminent collapse, with all the financial implications.

The dietitians, however, did not anticipate Thomson's fighting spirit. Through her lawyer, she instructed SAMA that its withdrawal of the CPD points was 'irrational, unlawful and falls to be set aside as an unjust administrative action'. She pointed out that a SAMA official had informed her in writing that she could market the conference as one for which CPD credits would be available. She would therefore apply for an immediate urgent injunction from the High Court for reinstatement of the CPD points.

SAMA was not exactly an unbiased or disinterested party on this occasion. On the contrary, it was riddled with conflicts of interest and bias against Noakes and LCHF.* UCT psychiatry professor Dr Denise White (since deceased) had been a member of the HPCSA Preliminary Committee of Inquiry that had made the decision to charge Noakes over his tweet. White had a long association with SAMA and, in fact, would be elected as its president in October 2015.

SAMA wisely backed down in the face of Thomson's threat of an urgent interdict, reinstating the points and granting two more. In trying to sabotage the conference, the dietitians had helped Thomson gain extra CPD points. It was the first of many lessons in unintended consequences for die-hard opponents of Noakes and LCHF.

In the build-up to the summit, Thomson issued an open invitation to all Noakes's critics to attend for free and debate the science with him and other experts. She even offered to cover the travel costs of those who felt they could not afford it. Among those she invited were the authors of the UCT cardiologists' and academics' letters published in 2012 and 2014 respectively (see Chapters 3 and 5). Thomson also invited Strydom.

Unsurprisingly, none accepted the invitation to debate the science at the summit, coming up with a variety of excuses. The blanket avoidance of public debate took on a coordinated air.

The conference themes were many and varied. Chief among them were alternative theories on the causes of obesity, diabetes, heart disease and many other NCDs (also called lifestyle diseases) that are now epidemic across the globe. In particular, the conference looked at the role of insulin resistance. Speakers showed how these diseases, which they say would be better described as nutritional diseases, are just the tip of the iceberg and that underneath them all lies IR. They also demonstrated the role that a high-carbohydrate diet plays in laying the groundwork for IR to develop in susceptible individuals.

With little preamble, speakers embarked on the ritual slaughter of sacred nutrition cows. Chief among them was the diet-heart hypothesis that saturated fat causes heart disease. Another was the calories-in, calories-out (CICO) model of obesity, which holds that people are fat because they eat too much and move too little.

The diet-heart hypothesis and CICO are the pillars on which the influential official Dietary Guidelines for Americans rest. The guidelines were another major focus of the conference. In particular, speakers looked at the available science, or rather lack thereof, when the US introduced the guidelines in 1977.

Gary Taubes was one of the first to dissect CICO at the conference and reveal its terminal flaws. In his presentation, titled 'Why we get fat: Adiposity 101 and

---

* In 2016, SAMA invited Noakes to speak at its annual conference. A few weeks later, an embarrassed SAMA executive called Noakes to say he was no longer invited. Then president Denise White claimed not to know why her organisation had uninvited him.

the alternative hypothesis of obesity', he argued that the global epidemics of obesity and diabetes were not caused by people eating too much and moving too little, or 'human weaknesses such as ignorance or indulgence'. Calling CICO the 'original sin' of obesity research and the 'biblical equivalent of greed and sloth', Taubes said that research now shows that the key driver of obesity is hormonal imbalance. In particular, science has identified dietary carbohydrates that drive insulin, which in turn drives fat.

Swedish physician Dr Andreas Eenfeldt, who is known as Sweden's Diet Doctor, was equally critical of CICO. Eenfeldt is the visionary behind Sweden's biggest and fastest-growing health blog. He is also the author of *Low Carb, High Fat Food Revolution: Advice and Recipes to Improve Your Health and Reduce Your Weight*. After eight years of successfully treating obese and diabetic patients with LCHF diets, Eenfeldt quit his medical practice in 2015 to run his website in the hopes that by reaching more people, he could change the status quo. In order to stay free from advertisements, product sales and industry sponsorship, his blog is fully funded by the public via an optional membership.

Eenfeldt told the conference that CICO is like saying a 'Homer Simpson virus' has spontaneously spread across the world. It doesn't make sense to say that people have suddenly become lazy gluttons, he said. According to him, CICO is little more than marketing. It's what the junk-food industry wants us to believe.

'They spend billions of dollars trying to convince you of that because it absolves them and their products of any guilt in causing the obesity epidemic,' Eenfeldt said. For proof, you just have to look at what food and drink companies get up to. For example, in the US, Coca-Cola, Pepsi and Kellogg's have all sponsored the country's largest association of nutrition professionals, the Academy of Nutrition and Dietetics (AND). In Canada, Coca-Cola sponsored Ontario's 2012 Healthy Kids Strategy, the goal of which was to reduce childhood obesity by 20 per cent over five years.

In 2016, the US *Observer-Reporter* revealed how Coca-Cola bought off top scientists and funded millions of dollars' worth of research to downplay the link between sugary beverages and obesity. Instead, the company used its massive financial muscle to demonise fat.[1] Coca-Cola has also continued to promote the idea that, provided people exercise enough, they can eat (and drink) whatever they like – including sugar-sweetened beverages.[2]

Eric Westman got straight to the point at the start of the second day with a presentation titled 'LCHF treatment of obesity and metabolic syndrome'. As an academic and associate professor of medicine at Duke University in Durham, North Carolina, Westman is at the coalface of the fight against obesity and related diseases. His research interest is disease prevention. Because smoking and obesity are the major causes of morbidity and mortality in modern society, his research involves clinical trials of new therapies for smoking cessation and obesity. He also runs a weight-loss clinic at Duke. In his extensive research, Westman has described the clinical use of LCHF for the treatment and prevention of both obesity and metabolic syndrome.

Westman said that people are always demanding to see the science for LCHF eating, yet the evidence is all there. 'It is not hard to get this information,' he said. 'It's out there.' He presented significant evidence from clinical trials demonstrating the efficacy of LCHF diets compared to Mediterranean-style, low-fat and low-GI diets. One of the best studies, at the time, to support LCHF diets was the Israeli-led, multi-year DIRECT study, published in the *New England Journal of Medicine* in 2008, which showed improvements in carotid thickness – a measure of atherosclerosis – on an LCHF diet.[3] Westman also referred to a comparison of four diets – Atkins (low carb), Zone, Weight Watchers and Ornish – published in the *Journal of the American Medical Association (JAMA)* in 2005. It showed that Atkins achieved the most weight loss at six and 12 months.[4]

Westman's second presentation on the final day of the conference was titled 'Practical implementation of a low-carb diet'. While less scientific and more entertaining, it was just as compelling and informative as his previous talk. Donning a white coat and addressing the members of the audience as if they were his obese patients, he took them step by step through the basics of LCHF for weight loss and maintenance thereafter. His message was as simple as it was key to nutrition and health: for long-term health and weight control, a conscious reduction in carbohydrate intake is essential. He also made the case for 'real food' – asking the audience: 'Have you ever seen a bread or pasta tree?' – but made it clear that he is no fan of fruit because of its high sugar (fructose)' content. Fruit, Westman said, is 'nature's candy'.

Next up was Canadian nephrologist (kidney specialist) Dr Jason Fung, who focused on another powerful conference theme: why so many doctors and dietitians still tell patients that diabetes is a chronic, degenerative, irreversible and ultimately incurable disease. Fung used to believe that, too. He said the driver for change was his own professional frustration after 10 years of religiously adhering to orthodox treatment protocols for his diabetic patients. When he looked back, Fung told the audience, he realised that he had not helped his patients much – he had just made them fatter, sicker and more reliant on drugs.

Fortunately for his patients, Fung doesn't suffer from cognitive dissonance. Cognitive dissonance occurs when a person who is confronted with compelling evidence that contradicts a deeply held belief chooses to ignore the evidence in favour of belief. Fung started researching alternatives. He came across evidence on the role of insulin and IR in diabetes that flatly contradicted his beliefs. He changed his mind to accommodate the evidence, and began advising his diabetic patients to ditch the conventional low-fat, high-carbohydrate dietary advice, and try LCHF. Fung said that he was amazed by the results. In most cases, his patients showed a significant reduction in symptoms. Better still, some patients were able to do without medication altogether.

Fung began his presentation by asking how resistance develops in a biochemical system. After all, the body is naturally designed to function properly, so why does it sometimes become unable to fend off resistance? He told the audience that just as taking antibiotics is the precursor to developing antibiotic resistance, so insulin is the precursor to IR.

Fung said that there are two 'big lies' in the treatment of type-2 diabetes mellitus (T2DM). The first is that type-2 diabetes is a chronic, progressive disease that can't be cured. The second is that lowering blood sugar is the primary goal. The truth, Fung said, is that diabetes is a 'curable' dietary disease. That's because it is a disease of high insulin resistance, which can be treated, and eventually reversed, by lowering that resistance. Conventional treatment with ever-increasing doses of insulin simply worsens the patient's state of IR, he said.

Fung took the audience down the intriguing new path of the insulin theory of obesity, which he has documented in his book *The Obesity Code: Unlocking the Secrets of Weight Loss.* In his presentation, Fung painted a chilling picture of a vicious cycle in which insulin drives IR, which in turn drives obesity. He explained that obesity is not the cause of diabetes. Rather, it is excessive insulin levels over time that causes both obesity and T2DM. And the cause of all that insulin? Not just carbohydrates, Fung said. Bad dietary advice to the general public, and especially to diabetics, which prescribes 'grazing' on carbohydrates, was also to blame. (British obesity researcher and speaker Dr Zoë Harcombe had caused much mirth in her presentation when she said, 'Don't graze, unless you are a cow or want to be the size of one.')

Fung's message was one of the most important to come out of the conference. He made a clarion call for doctors and dietitians to recognise that diabetes is curable, or at the very least reversible. He also said that diabetics should avoid not just carbohydrates, but also insulin. In an ideal world, even type-1 diabetics should have so little carbohydrate that the need to take insulin is at least drastically reduced, perhaps in a few cases even eliminated.

Insulin resistance quickly became a leitmotif at the conference. Speaker after speaker explained why doctors, dietitians and patients should all take IR seriously. They emphasised that high-carbohydrate diets increase the likelihood of IR developing. Noakes, for example, argued that ignoring IR undermines the practise of chronic medicine. If all the conditions attached to IR are linked to nutrition, as he believes they are, then patients don't need drugs. Obesity, diabetes, heart disease and many other life-threatening conditions are not caused by a lack of pharmaceutical drugs, he said. 'They are caused by too many carbohydrates in the diet. We fuel the fire with carbohydrates and try to put it out with pharmacologic drugs that don't work.'

Other speakers focused on the urgent need for a revision of the official dietary guidelines that favour LFHC foods. Harcombe presented the results of her research for her PhD, a meta-analysis of the evidence for dietary guidelines in the US and the UK.[5] The timing couldn't have been better. *Open Heart* had published her first paper on the topic a week before the summit. Harcombe's conclusion: there was no evidence from randomised controlled trials (RCTs) – the supposed 'gold standard' of scientific research – to support the official dietary guidelines when the US and the UK introduced them in 1977 and 1983 respectively.[6]

The official guidelines affected the health of more than 270 million people at the time, said Harcombe. That number is likely to have risen to billions in the interim, she concluded.

American physician Dr Michael Eades was another speaker who focused on the weaknesses of the conventional guidelines. Eades has practised bariatric, nutritional and metabolic medicine since 1986. In his presentation, he gave evidence from his book *Protein Power* and other research showing how studies biased against saturated fat worked their way into government recommendations.

British consultant cardiologist Dr Aseem Malhotra also took broad aim at the guidelines[7] and the diet-heart hypothesis.[8] Malhotra is science director of Action on Sugar, a group in the UK comprising respected scientists and doctors who campaign to reduce the public's sugar consumption and raise awareness of the ubiquitous presence of sugar in many processed foods.

Malhotra spoke eloquently of the basic conditions necessary for efficient healthcare to exist. These demand that both doctors and patients are informed, he said. He referred to the 'seven sins' that contribute to a lack of knowledge on both sides. These sins include biased funding of research (i.e. research funded because it is likely to be profitable, not because it will be beneficial to patients), financial conflicts of interest, a culture of 'defensive medicine', and a corresponding attitude that 'more treatment is better'.

Malhotra also spoke about the benefits of a Mediterranean diet – but only if it is high in good fats and low in carbohydrates.

A conference sub-theme around the diet-heart hypothesis was the overuse and abuse of cholesterol-lowering drugs known as statins. Noakes is also not a fan of statins. He has called them the 'single, most ineffective drug ever invented'.[*]

Another vocal statin critic was American family physician Dr Jeffry Gerber, who is known as Denver's Diet Doctor. He gave a lively presentation titled 'Cholesterol OMG!'. He used the catchy title, he said, to make people realise that there are some issues related to the non-standard LCHF diet and concerns about cholesterol, cardiovascular risk and health. Traditionally, dating back even to the

---

[*] Noakes is not alone in believing that his views on statins lay at the heart of the attacks on him by cardiologists, and were why so many doctors so enthusiastically aided the HPCSA in prosecuting him.

days of Dr Robert Atkins, doctors tried to scare people off LCHF diets and onto statins by saying that their levels of low-density lipoprotein (LDL) – the so-called bad cholesterol – would go up. The idea was that Atkins and similar diets would clog the arteries and cause fatal heart attacks and strokes.

Gerber predicted that statins have passed their sell-by date. Despite being the most prescribed drug on the planet, they will probably be 'gone in 10 years', he said.

Another major focus of the conference was the benefits of fat adaptation: being able to use fat rather than glucose from carbohydrate metabolism as an energy source. An expert on this topic is Stephen Phinney, an American physician-scientist and emeritus professor of medicine at the University of California, Davis. One of Phinney's presentations covered the benefits for sports performance – and overall health – of nutritional ketosis. Much of his presentation was taken from his book *The Art and Science of Low Carbohydrate Performance*, co-authored with Professor Jeff Volek. Phinney coined the term 'nutritional ketosis' 30 years ago. He did so, he said, because of confusion and fear around ketones, ketosis induced by dietary carbohydrate restriction (nutritional ketosis), and ketosis caused by an absence of insulin (a condition known as ketoacidosis, which can be fatal).

He explained that many doctors and dietitians are fearful of ketosis and ketones, and that they instil this unnecessary fear and anxiety in their patients. It's all down to ignorance, Phinney said. Doctors and dietitians are still class-ically taught that ketones are 'toxic by-products of fat metabolism'. That can be true, but only in the case of extremely high levels of ketones coupled with a complete absence of insulin. In that case, it is ketoacidosis, which occurs in type-1 diabetics and more rarely in end-stage type-2 diabetics. For the rest, Phinney showed why ketosis is an essential, normal and benign bodily state.

Intriguing insight into the addictive properties of sugar and other carbohy-drate foods came from adult and paediatric bariatric surgeon Dr Robert Cywes. Cywes was born in South Africa but now lives and works in the United States. He pointed to a disturbing health pattern. Sixty years ago, experts were wringing their hands about the rise in lung cancer, heart disease and emphysema. They completely ignored and argued against the evidence that tobacco was the cul-prit. Today, they sit wringing their hands about obesity, diabetes, cholesterol and hypertension while ignoring what Cywes called the 'culprit' drugs. 'The most prevalent chronic NCDs killing us as a species are a consequence of drugs not well tolerated by human systems,' he said. These drugs are alcohol, tobacco and the obesogenic drug – carbohydrates.

One of many strengths of the low-carb summit was that speakers often spoke personally and from the heart. Canadian physician Jay Wortman is a public-health specialist and clinical assistant professor at the University of British Columbia's Faculty of Medicine. His research was featured in the hit Canadian

Broadcasting Corporation news documentary, *My Big Fat Diet*. Wortman told the summit how he reversed his own T2DM in 2002 by going on an LCHF diet while waiting for advice from his orthodox peers on what medication to take. He said that he has been free of any evidence of the condition ever since. He also addressed concerns about the safety of LCHF regimens for children and pregnant women, saying that his extensive research into traditional diets shows that there are no safety issues.

Australian nutrition therapist Christine Cronau told how she lost weight and eliminated serious health issues on an LCHF diet. She dispelled many myths that still exist about the LCHF lifestyle.

United States Air Force veteran and psychiatrist Dr Ann Childers told of how she developed metabolic syndrome and subsequently reversed all her symptoms by going on a ketogenic diet (an extreme form of LCHF). Childers explained that metabolic syndrome is an umbrella syndrome that encompasses a cluster of problems, including heart disease, lipid (blood fat) problems, hypertension, T2DM, dementia, cancer, polycystic ovary syndrome and non-alcoholic fatty liver disease (NAFLD). As an adult and child psychiatrist, Childers has a special interest in nutrition and mental health. She has researched the effects of nutrient-poor, high-carbohydrate diets, as well as high-grain diets, through the ages. These foods don't just contribute to weight gain, Childers told the conference, they are also not good for body or brain.

And despite what many dietitians still believe and teach, Childers said, fats, including saturated fats, are the brain's best foods, not carbohydrates. She also criticised food companies for changing health patterns with their processed foods. 'The bottom line is their obligation to their stockholders,' she said. 'They do what they need to do to make a profit. They embed themselves in nutrition organisations.'

Eades and Childers also looked at LCHF from an evolutionary perspective. Eades recalled how he had first been alerted to the dangers of the 'conventional' LFHC diet when he came across research showing that the Ancient Egyptians, the first population to attempt this diet between 2500 BC and AD 395, were anything but healthy. 'The fondness of Egyptians for bread was so well known that they were nicknamed "artophagoi" or eaters of bread,' he said. 'Their diet consisted primarily of bread, cereals, fresh fruit, vegetables, some fish and poultry, almost no red meat, olive oil instead of lard, and goat's milk for drinking and to make into cheese.' Eades called these foods a 'veritable [modern] nutritionist's nirvana'.

If these foods were so healthy, then 'the Ancient Egyptians should have lived forever or at least should have lived long, healthy lives and died of old age in their beds', he said. But did they? On the contrary. Eades found 'an Egyptian populace rife with disabling dental problems, fat bellies and crippling heart disease … Sounds a lot like the afflictions of millions of people in America today, doesn't it?'

The Egyptians did not eat much fat or refined carbohydrate. They ate almost nothing but wholegrains, fresh fruit and vegetables, and fish and fowl. Yet they suffered from the same diseases that afflict modern man. 'The same modern man,' Eades said, 'who doctors and dietitians advise to eat lots of wholegrains, fresh fruits and vegetables, to prevent or reverse these diseases.'

Australian orthopaedic surgeon Dr Gary Fettke gave one of the most exciting and controversial presentations to the conference, on cancer and nutrition. Fettke is a senior lecturer at the University of Tasmania and a cancer survivor. He is another who has paid a heavy price for daring to go against nutrition orthodoxy. In 2016, the Australian Health Practitioner Regulation Agency (AHPRA) banned Fettke for life from talking to his patients about sugar. That was after a dietitian complained about the dietary advice he was giving to his patients. Fettke has sensibly chosen to ignore the ban. He continues to advise patients with obesity and T2DM to reduce their intake of sugar and other carbohydrates. By doing this, he tells them, they can significantly reduce their risk of limb loss.

In his presentation, titled 'So you think you need sugar? Your cancer needs it even more!', Fettke looked at the science behind the metabolic model of cancer therapy, which is based on the work of Nobel Prize–winning German biochemist Dr Otto Warburg in the 1930s.[9] Fettke presented research suggesting that dietary intervention, in particular a ketogenic diet, is the cancer treatment of the future.

One of the strengths of the summit was that it included a lay speaker. Jimmy Moore runs the hugely successful Livin' La Vida Low-Carb blog. In his presentation, he described his momentous decision in January 2004 to lose the weight that was literally killing him. At age 32 and weighing 410 pounds (185 kilograms), he began eating LCHF. Within a year, he had lost 180 pounds, shrunk his waist by 20 inches (50 centimetres), and dropped his shirt size from 5XL to XL. Moore started his blog and related podcast in response to a flood of requests from family and friends for help and information. It hasn't all been plain weight-loss sailing for Moore. He is open about his battles to stay at a healthy weight and the new approaches he has tried.

Feedback from the conference was generally positive. Many doctors and dietitians who attended said that the compelling science that the speakers presented was a game-changer. The barbs that did come were from the few LCHF critics in attendance. One was Jacques Rousseau, a lecturer at the UCT Faculty of Commerce. I make a detour here to talk about Rousseau because of his family background and his active opposition to LCHF and Noakes. His father, Professor Jacques Rossouw, is a UCT graduate who works for the National Institutes of Health (NIH) in the US. He is also one of Noakes's most implacable foes.

Rousseau has an honours degree in philosophy and a master's in English. He has co-authored a book with clinical psychologist Caleb Lack, titled *Critical Thinking, Science and Pseudoscience: Why We Can't Trust Our Brains*, and he writes a personal blog called Synapses. Rousseau lectures on critical thinking and ethics.

I first became aware of Rousseau in 2014. By then he had written 15 blog posts attacking Noakes. That number has since nearly doubled. I can probably count myself lucky that Rousseau devoted only one nasty post to me, and only after I started writing about Noakes. In my opinion, he demonstrates an unhealthy obsession with Noakes and LCHF science. Recently, though, Rousseau has begun back-pedalling, as have many other LCHF opponents in the face of the evidence. He now plaintively claims that he always said that Noakes could be right. He also claims never to have accused Noakes of bad science. Yet in a blog post from 2013, titled 'Lessons in bad science: Tim Noakes and the *SAMJ*', he did just that, accusing Noakes outright of practising bad science.[10] Three days later, in a post titled 'More lessons in bad science (and reasoning) from Noakes', Rousseau again accused Noakes of willingly ignoring the 'basic principles of good science'.[11]

Rousseau's critics on social media have at times questioned why he does not declare his significant conflict of interest (that his father is Professor Jacques Rossouw) when attacking Noakes. Rossouw's antagonism towards Noakes is well known and is covered elsewhere in this book (see Chapter 4). Critics have also challenged Rousseau (junior) on why he spells his name differently from his father. I once asked him about it via email. I found his explanation naive at best. He said that he changed his name legally 25 years ago because he did not want anyone to link him to the country's then ruling National Party, the architects of the apartheid regime that had made South Africa the pariah of the world. I wondered if Rousseau genuinely believed that people automatically assumed that anyone with an Afrikaans name supported apartheid.

Then there is Rousseau's wife, Dr Signe Rousseau, an academic in the same faculty as him at UCT. She has a doctorate in film and media. In 2015, she wrote an article in the journal *Food, Culture & Society* titled 'The celebrity quick-fix: When good food meets bad science'.[12] No prizes for guessing who she thinks is practising bad science. In the article, Signe parrots much of what her husband says about Noakes. Like him, she invokes a straw-man argument against Noakes, claiming that the sole evidence Noakes uses to advocate the LCHF diet is anecdotal. Thus: 'As the revelation about his personal health may suggest his initial evidence was based on a sample of one – himself.' She doesn't think to mention her conflict of interest: that she is the daughter-in-law of Professor Jacques Rossouw.

Both Rousseau and his wife appear oblivious of the fact that Noakes adopted the LCHF diet only after extensive research of both the scientific and popular literature. And Rousseau appeared not to understand much of the scientific evidence presented at the Cape Town conference. Afterwards, he made much about the fact that some speakers preferred to talk of a 'healthy-fat', rather than a 'high-fat' diet, as if he thinks Noakes is promoting a high intake of unhealthy fats.[13]

Critics of the summit predicted from the outset that it would be an LCHF 'echo chamber'. It was anything but. The speakers agreed on some major points of LCHF theory, but disagreed on others. They differed in how low in terms of carbohydrates LCHF diets have to go for maximum benefit. All agreed, however, that LCHF is not a fad diet. The real fad, they said, is the low-fat, high-carb diet prescribed by the official guidelines for decades. None of the speakers said that LCHF is a one-size-fits-all way of eating.

Some differences turned out to be little more than semantics. Harcombe, for example, said that she does not call the nutrition advice she promotes 'LCHF'. However, she also said that when people eat 'real food' – unprocessed, unadulterated food that is as close to its natural state as possible – they tend to eat LCHF.

The only criticism of the conference that stood up to any scrutiny was a lack of question time for the audience. That was mostly a function of speakers having so much science to present and contextualise. The speakers made up for it, however, by making themselves available during breaks and over lunchtime to answer questions.

The conference produced a consensus statement, which all speakers signed – except for Taubes, as he had engagements that meant he could not stay until the end. The statement read:

> The mainstream dietary advice that we are currently giving to the world has simply not worked. Instead, it is the opinion of the speakers at this summit that this incorrect nutritional advice is the immediate cause of the global obesity and diabetes epidemics.
>
> This advice has failed because it completely ignores the history of why and how human nutrition has developed over the past three million years. More importantly, it refuses to acknowledge the presence of insulin resistance (carbohydrate intolerance) as the single most prevalent biological state in modern humans.
>
> Persons with insulin resistance are at an increased risk of developing a wide range of chronic medical conditions if they ingest a high carbohydrate diet for any length of time (decades).

Noakes closed the summit on 22 February with a powerful presentation. Titled 'The way forward', it was a compelling mix of the personal, professional and scientific. In it, Noakes showed who he thinks is really practising junk science and endangering people's health.

'The key problem,' he said, 'is that both sides believe the facts sit with them. Either they are right or I am right. We can't both be right.'

The right thing to do, Noakes said, is to look at all the evidence and especially the quality of the evidence. That's good science, according to the rules laid down by the late Sir Austin Bradford Hill, the man revered as the 'father of medical statistics'. Scientists who choose to ignore the RCTs and other evidence that dispute their theories are not practising good science.

Since Bradford Hill's death in 1991, many researchers have ignored his criteria and 'flipped into a model of junk science', said Noakes. These scientists 'are more interested in getting funding and more work, not making people healthier'. They have dropped the bar to the lowest level of performance achieved in a cross-sectional (associational) study. This means that just about anything can be proved to cause something. It demonstrates a move from hard science to junk science.

'We have generated a whole discipline of nutritional science [ignoring Bradford Hill's criteria],' said Noakes, 'and we wonder why we have got it all so very wrong.' He then quoted British physicist Stephen Hawking, who is clear on what to do if the facts don't fit the theory: 'Abandon the theory.'

Noakes also quoted from Hawking's book *In Black Holes and Baby Universes and Other Essays*: 'In practice, people are very reluctant to give up a theory in which they have invested a lot of time and effort. They usually start by questioning the accuracy of the observations. If that fails, they try to modify the theory in an ad hoc manner. Eventually the theory becomes a creaking and ugly edifice. Then someone suggests a new theory, in which all the awkward observations are explained in an elegant and natural manner.'[14]

Noakes said that the Cape Town conference had exposed the creaking, ugly edifice of conventional wisdom on nutrition, and had explained an alternative in an elegant and natural manner.

For Noakes, the summit was ultimately the realisation of a dream. 'It allowed us to make the message global and to show people the facts about nutrition, fats and carbohydrates in the diet,' he said afterwards. Taubes said that the summit gave 'validity' to those attending – a platform to 'entertain the idea that something they may have believed all along was wrong and that there is a better way of doing it'.

'We have two choices,' Noakes said in his closing remarks. 'Either we can continue to ignore the evidence presented at this summit, and go on blaming the obese and diabetic for their sloth and gluttony [that is supposedly the sole cause of their obesity and diabetes]. Or, if we are ever to reverse this epidemic that has become the greatest modern threat to human health, we need to admit that we have been wrong for the past 40 years, and must now change.'

Experts, Noakes said, can continue to apply a failed model to a growing global health crisis in the 'utterly irrational hope that what has not worked in the past will suddenly, miraculously, produce a different result'. That, as Einstein noted, is the true marker of insanity – doing the same thing over and over again and expecting different results.

Alternatively, said Noakes: 'If we have the individual and collective courage, we can acknowledge our insanity, admit our errors and start the healing process by adopting the solutions presented by the speakers at this summit.

'Our greatest hope is that this summit will serve as the global tipping point for the final acceptance that what we have prescribed and practised as healthy nutrition for the past 40 years is not only *not* based on any good science, but tragically has been profoundly damaging to human health on a global scale.'

Noakes ended his presentation with a quote from Professor Christiaan Barnard: 'I have saved the lives of 150 people through heart transplantations. If I had focused on preventative medicine earlier, I would have saved 150 million people.'

Noakes said that it was his hope that Barnard, the man who gave South Africa its greatest medical moment in history, would have his wish posthumously: 'That is to bring health and healing to billions of humans through the provision of dietary advice that is appropriate because it is scientifically based. It understands the biological consequences of our human evolution. It recognises the widespread presence of insulin resistance in most populations across the globe.'

At that, the assembled delegates and speakers from around the world gave Tim Noakes a lengthy standing ovation. Harcombe later noted: 'There was hardly a dry eye left in the house.' It augured well as Act I in the coming drama, the Kafkaesque 'Theatre of the Absurd', as I later called the HPCSA hearing against Noakes.

2

The Most Important Experiment of My Life

'When my information changes, I change my mind.
What do you do, sir?'
– John Maynard Keynes, British economist

When I matriculated from a Cape Town high school in December 1966, all of my classmates, and the girls with whom we associated, were lean – with one exception: a larger boy who would today be labelled obese. So uncommon was his appearance that we assumed he had a rare disease, perhaps cancer.

We were, of course, the generation that would become known as the Baby Boomers – the children of the so-called Greatest Generation, the generation that had fought the war against Nazism and had returned to build the most prosperous period in human history.

Because our parents had lived through the deprivations of a world war, they were necessarily frugal. There was no excess and there was no waste. Our parents fed us the foods on which their parents had raised them – in my case, good, wholesome, real farm foods.

In our adolescence, we Baby Boomers spawned the hippie movement. We grew up on the music of Elvis, the Beatles, the Rolling Stones and the Byrds, and the folk poetry of now Nobel laureate Bob Dylan, and Simon & Garfunkel. We were surrounded by leanness. It was not because we exercised to excess. On the contrary, there were no commercial gyms, and our generation had yet to discover the joys of marathon running. That would happen only after 1976.

Today, when I speak to matriculating high-school students in South Africa, I see quite a different picture. Leanness is uncommon except, paradoxically, sometimes in the pupils at wealthier schools. In the schools serving the poorer communities, the outlook is depressing. Adolescent obesity is rampant.

Global trends in the same period match my personal experience of the complete transformation in the appearance of the youth of today, compared to the norm 50 years ago.

When I completed my undergraduate medical training at UCT in 1974, fewer of our patients were obese, and T2DM was an uncommon condition. I recall treating only one case of diabetic ketoacidosis in the six months of my medical internship, and I observed very few limb amputations as a result of diabetic peripheral artery disease (PAD).

Today, the situation is entirely different. Indeed, my home town of Cape Town is at the centre of an escalating South African T2DM epidemic. What could possibly have happened in the intervening four decades?

The answer, it turns out, is not difficult to uncover. It is predicted in at least seven published works by credible medical scientists over the past century: Englishmen Major General Sir Robert McCarrison MD DSc (*Nutrition and Health*), Dr Thomas L. Cleave (*The Saccharine Disease*) and Professor John Yudkin (*Pure, White and Deadly*); Scotsman Dr Walter Yellowlees (*A Doctor in the Wilderness*); Canadian Dr Weston Price (*Nutrition and Physical Degeneration*); American Dr Benjamin Sandler (*How to Prevent Heart Attacks*); and South African Dr George D. Campbell (*Diabetes, Coronary Thrombosis and the Saccharine Disease*). Of these books, only those by Price, Yellowlees and Yudkin are still readily available.

As far as I can tell, none of these books are prescribed reading for either medical or dietetics students, yet the totality of the proof that they present is compelling. It is so convincing that anyone with a mind even slightly open to the authors' inconvenient conclusions would have to ask why they were never presented with this evidence, and why they have been so thoroughly misinformed. I review the work of these pioneers in Chapter 16, and look at why it does not make sense to accuse ancient foods of suddenly causing the epidemics of modern diseases currently sweeping the globe.

Perhaps Yellowlees's book provides the best personal narrative of how dramatically the diseases to which modern humans are now prone have changed in the past 50 years.

Yellowlees graduated in medicine from Edinburgh University in 1941. He served with the Royal Army Medical Corps during the latter years of the Second World War, winning the Military Cross for outstanding bravery 'for tending the wounded under heavy fire ... and for being the last to leave the battlefield'. For 33 years after the war he worked as a medical practitioner in a traditional, rural Scottish farming community, retiring in 1981.

In 1993, he wrote his autobiography to record the precipitous deterioration in the health of the community he had served. He wanted to explain what he considered to be the real causes of this decline, and to express his frustration that no one in his profession seemed particularly concerned to expose them. 'If a GP lives up to the traditions of his calling,' Yellowlees wrote, 'he must forever seek to understand why this particular patient is suffering from this particular complaint.'[1]

The modern approach is quite different. Doctors now have another option:

they can continue to take, as Yellowlees put it, the 'much wider view which encompasses not only the patient's disease, but his way of life, food, relationships and environment. The latter attitude, in the Hippocratic tradition, assumes that health is the normal inheritance of mankind and seeks to know what has gone wrong to disturb that inheritance.' Or they can view the patient's illness as 'an unfortunate happening, a haphazard quirk of fate'.[2]

In choosing the first option, Yellowlees discovered a perplexing paradox. He struggled to understand why, during the 20th century, 'thanks to better sanitation, clean water, preventive inoculation and improved housing, the incidence of infective diseases caused by bacteria or viruses has greatly diminished', yet, in his own medical lifetime, he had personally observed a dramatic increase in the incidence of degenerative diseases, the so-called diseases of lifestyle, which he concluded could not be conveniently rationalised by 'better methods of diagnosis or the ageing of the population'.[3]

His conclusion was that this alarming deterioration was the result of a change in diet, as sugar, refined flour and processed foods had replaced the traditional foods on which his people had lived for centuries:

> Food and drink, highly processed and degraded by a multitude of additives, consumed by an ever expanding urban-based population inevitably brings a heavy load of degenerative disease. In Scotland, especially, refined sugar and constipating white flour are still consumed in huge quantities. Obesity and diabetes are rife; the overall incidence of cancer increases.[4]

Yellowlees was not one to desert the battlefield before the last shot had been fired. Like many of us, he wanted to understand why something so obvious to him was apparently beyond the understanding of almost all others.

There were, he wrote, three reasons for the 'wilderness of confusion' about the true causes of the rising ill health he encountered in rural Scotland and which mirrored my experiences in Cape Town, South Africa. The first, he suggested, was 'the frailty of human nature on the part of scientists, engaged in nutrition research, who get hold of an idea and refuse to accept any evidence, however compelling, which casts doubt on its veracity'. The second was 'the dominant role of commercial interests in determining the dietary habits of consumers, as well as in shaping developments in agriculture and in medical practice'.[5]

'Food manufacturers,' Yellowlees observed, 'equipped with their immensely powerful weapons of mass advertising, join the fray; they do so either openly to the consumer or through a more subtle approach to doctors and dieticians by financing research, publications or conferences.'[6]

The HPCSA trial against me bears brutal testimony to the extent to which this has happened in South Africa.

As to the third reason, Yellowlees suggested that the medical profession had capitulated in the face of these commercial forces. Doctors, he argued, 'are meant to be scientists and science is supposed to reveal the truths of the material world'. Instead, they have forsaken Christian values and become too scared to be deemed either 'judgmental' or 'moralizing'. The result:

> The third and daunting part of my wilderness is the spiritual darkness which, in the second half of this century, has cast a deepening shadow over all our affairs. By darkness I mean the loss of loyalty, honesty, integrity and decency without which human transactions revert to the violence and inhumanity of the beast. These sad trends follow the retreat of Christianity and the rise of humanist false prophets who preach the supremacy not of God, but of human reason; they seek to rule the world, not by God-given wisdom, but by the power of money.[7]

Finally, he asked: 'Are doctors to remain silent when they believe the truth is being perverted?'[8]

Perhaps the major error that I made after December 2010 was to imagine, like Yellowlees before me, that my first professional responsibility was to expose those medical or scientific 'truths' I believed to be false. It never occurred to me that my colleagues and peers would react to the outcomes of my personal search for truth as if they had sworn an oath of silence, a scientific omertà aimed at suppressing the evidence I had accumulated for a new nutrition paradigm.

When I experienced what I call my Damascene moment, I had no inkling of the descent into a spiritual wilderness it would precipitate, or of the heartlessness and lack of humanity I would experience at the hands of many of my senior professional colleagues. But, as one of my favourite rugby coaches always used to say, in the toughest of times when all appears lost, 'it is what it is'.

It helped that I had learnt a lot from sport – especially that you play every moment as if your life depends on it until the final whistle; only then may you stop. That is the way I have learnt to live my life. It is what led Winston Churchill to implore of the British people, including my parents, in the darkest hours of the Second World War: 'Never give in. Never, never, never, never – in nothing, great or small, large or petty – never give in, except to convictions of honour and good sense. Never yield to force. Never yield to the apparently overwhelming might of the enemy.'

In the face of scientific evidence, it was simply not an option to yield to dogmas on treatment methods that clearly were not working to improve people's health.

So this is my story.

I have spent my scientific life conducting experiments on others. I began perhaps my most important experiment, on myself, when I was already 61 years old.

On the evening of Sunday 12 December 2010, I put the final touches to a body of scientific work on which I had toiled for almost 30 years. It was the 27th and final revision of a manuscript that would appear as the book titled *Waterlogged: The Serious Problem of Overhydration in Endurance Sports*. My last act of the day was to email the final version of the manuscript to my American publisher.

That research had brought me into direct conflict with PepsiCo, one of the iconic companies in the US, because I had challenged a body of scientific thinking used to promote the sale of their segment-leading sports drink, Gatorade. As a result of my unpopular opinion, many of my sports-science colleagues, especially those funded by PepsiCo, had publicly questioned my intelligence.

My response was to write a massive tome in which I laid out the whole truth, as it appeared to me, in minutest detail. Happy that my completed manuscript properly presented my iconoclastic position, I switched off my computer and retired to bed.

The sense of release was extraordinary. I was certain that the facts presented in the book would prove that I was not the one who was crazy. More importantly, the mountain of evidence I had collected would, I was sure, reduce the risk of more endurance athletes dying from the potentially fatal but entirely preventable condition called exercise-associated hyponatraemic encephalopathy that I and my colleagues had been the first in the world to describe. Our research had established that these deaths are the result of a belief in a false model of how the human body works, a model that had been skilfully marketed as a global truth, not, in my opinion, to promote athletes' health, but to increase sports-drink sales.

In the middle of the night, my brain woke me with a new instruction: 'Get up tomorrow morning at 6 a.m. and run,' it said. 'And make sure that you run on most days for the rest of your life.'

I have learnt to trust my subconscious brain's infrequent instructions. The last time my brain spoke to me so directly was in March 1968, when it instructed me to apply for admission to the medical faculty at UCT. Besides marrying my wife, Marilyn Anne, that was the most important decision of my life.

So shortly before 6 a.m. on Monday 13 December 2010, I dutifully rose from my bed, dressed in my running gear and dragged myself half-asleep around the shortest (five kilometres) and flattest running route in my neighbourhood. I had never stopped running, but over the years I had begun to run progressively less. By the time I completed *Waterlogged*, I was running only about 20 kilometres each week, very slowly. That, compared to the 120–220 kilometres per week I had often run in preparation for my favourite ultra-distance race, the 88-kilometre Comrades Marathon. Running had simply become too much of an unpleasant effort. I continued only because I believed it was good for my health.

On that flat, five-kilometre run, only with the greatest difficulty was I able to average seven minutes a kilometre, even when running at an average heart rate of 135 beats per minute. Worse, it felt as if the two tiny rises along the route took more out of me than the monster hills of the Comrades Marathon ever did. By the final kilometre, I had slowed to eight minutes, little better than a fast walk. Clearly, something had to be done if I was going to run on most days for the rest of my life. I might be over 60, but I was not as old as those few tiny hillocks made me feel that Monday.

I resolved that to run better, I would have to begin by losing some of the extra weight I had accumulated, especially over the previous 10 to 15 years. But in my youth, I had only ever lost a significant amount of weight when training extra hard for many, many months. Even then, despite any weight loss so hard achieved, I would regain it all within a few weeks of returning to my more normal training. Indeed, my 41 years of running, including over 70 marathons and ultra-marathons, had taught me that, while running produces a wide array of physical and emotional benefits, sustained weight loss is definitely not one of them.

I already knew from personal experience that the conventionally prescribed weight-loss diets are ineffective because they work only when people are sufficiently active to burn all the extra (redundant) calories needed to satisfy exaggerated hunger. But the moment their activity level returns to a more sustainable level, hunger returns, and they tend to ingest more calories than required and rapidly regain all the lost weight. No one had ever bothered to tell me that perhaps the excessively high carbohydrate content of my diet was driving my hunger. And so, always hungry, I was perpetually eating more calories than my body really needed, except for those few months of my life when I was able to burn off the excess carbohydrate calories by training for two or more hours a day.

I also knew that even when I was able to lose some weight using this conventional, exercise-more, eat-less approach, the process was unbearably slow and frustrating, requiring mammoth amounts of discipline and will power. That is to be expected of a treatment prescribed to punish the slothful and gluttonous obese.

As a result of my own experience, and like most of my medical colleagues who were unable to regulate their body weights, I had never felt sufficiently confident to express any opinions on the causes, treatment and prevention of obesity. Nor could I make any sense of the voluminous obesity literature. Instead I chose to ignore the topic, leaving it to the experts. The proof is that there is no reference to any methods of weight loss in any of the first four editions of *Lore of Running*, which I wrote between 1981 and 2002.

And so, as I struggled through that final kilometre on the morning of 13 December 2010, pondering my dire state, I really had no idea how to address my growing obesity and declining health. I was now much older, less physically able and indeed unwilling to train for up to two hours a day as I would have 40 years earlier. I was beginning to think that only divine intervention could save me.

Providence was close at hand, for at that very moment the sole solution to my predicament was finding its way to me via the internet.

It came in the form of an email advertising a new book, *The New Atkins for a New You* by doctors Eric Westman, Stephen Phinney and Jeff Volek. The book promised 'The Ultimate Diet for Shedding Weight and Feeling Great', and claimed that it would allow me to lose six kilograms in six weeks 'without hunger'. Since I was scheduled to speak to a group of elite Swedish ultra-marathon runners in Stockholm in a few weeks, the idea was attractive. What if I could lose six kilograms by the time I appeared before that lean, athletic audience?

My initial curiosity was short-lived, soon to be replaced with dismay. I was appalled that these three supposedly serious scientists could allow their names to be associated with Dr Robert Atkins, the madman who, in the 1970s, had encouraged us all to eat more saturated fat and less carbohydrate, wilfully misleading the world with his dangerous dietary non-science. I knew this to be true because it is what I had been taught since 1976, when I began my scientific education in Professor Lionel Opie's heart research unit at UCT. Thanks to the wisdom of a range of authority figures, including the US government, those of us who were properly educated 'knew' that this advice could only kill us.

I knew that, beginning in 1972, Atkins had caused a global stir with his book *Dr Atkins' Diet Revolution*, in which he proposed that the healthiest diet was one that included as much fat, including saturated fat, as one's appetite dictated. His book sold more than 10 million copies, but it garnered Atkins few medical friends. Instead, he was demonised and his diet labelled a fad. Every heart association on earth and all the world's most eminent cardiologists hastened to inform us that the Atkins high-fat diet was the direct cause of heart disease.

Undeterred by collegial disdain and his growing notoriety, Atkins developed a money-losing medical practice specialising in weight loss on New York's Upper East Side. I would later learn that his clinic, highly successful at curing obesity and T2DM, was sustained by the proceeds from his book sales. Criticised for not using that money to study the effects of his revolutionary diet, in the early 2000s Atkins began funding the research of Westman, Phinney and Volek. That research would ultimately lead to their book and the email in my inbox announcing its publication.

Putting aside my dismay, I realised that regardless of what I might think or know about Dr Atkins, I also knew that all three authors are exceptionally good at what they do. Take, for example, Stephen Phinney, an outstanding and innovative scientist who in 1983 published the world's first scientific study of the effects of long-term adaptation to a high-fat diet on human exercise performance.[9]

Inspired by that research, our exercise-research group at UCT had been among the first to perform similar studies.[10] My former PhD student, Professor John Hawley, also contributed a series of significant studies in the early 2000s.[11]

But there was another, even more important reason why I had great faith in Phinney and his colleagues. Shortly after the publication of Phinney's original paper in 1983, I had received a call from Paula Newby-Fraser, an expatriate Zimbabwean then plying her profession as an Ironman triathlete in the US. She had just heard of Phinney's study and wanted to know what I thought of it.

'It makes logical sense,' I told her. 'Why don't you try it?'

I meant that she should add more fat to her diet, not that she should abandon carbohydrates. Three decades later, after Newby-Fraser had dominated the world of Ironman triathlons, winning a total of 28 Ironman races, including the World Championship in Kona, Hawaii, an unmatched eight times, and after she had been selected as the Triathlete of the 21st Century, she told me that the recommendation to eat a carbohydrate-restricted, high-fat diet was the single most important piece of advice she had ever received in her athletic career.

The irony, of course, is that while Paula Newby-Fraser was becoming one of the world's greatest endurance athletes, following, on my advice, a high-fat diet, in *Lore of Running* I was advising all athletes to eat high-carbohydrate diets. Can I explain this? The answer is no.

So, on the balance of the available evidence, I decided to give the authors of *The New Atkins for a New You* the benefit of my scepticism. Perhaps Westman, Phinney and Volek had sold out to commercial interests, as is common. But what if they were also correct? What if they had discovered a truth hidden behind others' dogmas and conflicts of interest? Phinney especially had advanced knowledge, having studied a high-fat diet in athletes. What could I possibly lose by investigating their claims more fully?

I got up from my desk and drove the three kilometres to the nearest bookshop to search for their book. Fortuitously, there was a single copy. I was home within 20 minutes, and began reading despite a healthy scepticism. I still doubted that anyone could seriously propose weight loss 'without hunger'. After all, we all 'know' that there is one absolute when it comes to dieting: to lose weight, you must submit to perpetual hunger. Regardless of the scientific credentials of the three authors, I was fairly certain that their outrageous assertion would prove to be bogus, and that the whole thing would be just another fad diet.

After reading a few pages, I was suddenly less certain. I sensed that Westman, Phinney and Volek were advancing a crucial health message, one based on a body of hard science of which I was completely ignorant.

An hour later, I had read enough to suggest that here was something worth considering. I wondered how I had missed all the work from which Dr Eric H. Kossoff MD, director of the Ketogenic Diet Center in the Division of Pediatric

Neurology at Johns Hopkins Hospital, Baltimore, Maryland, had concluded: 'In more than 150 articles, these three international experts on the use of low-carbohydrate diets to combat obesity, high cholesterol, and type 2 diabetes have led the way in repeatedly proving how a low-carbohydrate approach is superior to a low-fat one.'[12]

By lunchtime, I had read enough to make my Damascene decision: I would ignore my scepticism, ingrained by 40 years of medical 'education', and put the advice of Westman, Phinney and Volek to the test.

As they suggested, I embraced the idea that eating fat is a healthy choice. I immediately stopped eating the carbohydrate-laden 'foods'* that I had consumed in increasing amounts after I began running seriously in 1972, leading to my full adoption of the low-fat, supposedly heart-healthy, 'prudent' diet after 1977. That LFHC diet was the same one that I had described in Lore of Running as the essential dietary basis for all great athletic achievements.

All that was now in the past. A new future beckoned.

There would be no more bread, potatoes, bananas, rice, porridge or boxed breakfast cereals, including muesli. No more fruit juices or soft drinks. No more cakes, sweets, chocolates, ice cream or, indeed, any desserts. I would slowly remove all sugar and other sweeteners from my tea and coffee. I would focus on seven foodstuffs: meat, fish, eggs, dairy produce, nuts, leafy vegetables and a restricted range of low-carbohydrate fruits, mainly berries.

And so began probably the most important experiment of my life.

For that first lunch, I snacked on biltong (a form of dried meat, similar to beef jerky in the US, which is a delicacy in South Africa), cheese and high-fat

---

* I put the word 'foods' in inverted commas because, in time, I would discover that most of the foods I had removed from my diet are not real foods. Rather, they are highly processed 'food-like substances', which are all specifically designed to be high in addictiveness – sometimes confused with palatability – and low in nutritional value. The boxed cereals that the world's most sophisticated advertising campaign had led me to believe were so highly nutritious are, I learnt, just a toxic combination of rapidly digestible carbohydrate laden with sugar. Compared to eggs, sardines and liver – three of the most nutritious foods known to humans – these foods are nutritionally barren. The only thing that sustains them is an advertising campaign that spends more money on the promotion of breakfast cereals than on any other single food group. I now appreciate that a typical bowl of breakfast cereal provides an oversupply of glucose and sugar, neither of which is necessary for human existence. Real foods are those like eggs, meat, nuts, fish, dairy, vegetables and fruits that are unprocessed and which exist in a natural state in our environment. They are foods that 'have been alive until quite recently'. Only later would I begin to comprehend that, whatever the contrasting advertising claims, foods are processed for two principal reasons, with one shared goal: to sell more of a very cheap product at maximum profit. The industry achieves this by making foods so palatable that they become 'irresistible' – a term food marketers choose in preference to the real description, 'addictive'. The food industry also makes products long-lasting so that they can survive on shop shelves for months, if not years. It took me at least a year to understand why these highly refined, food-like substances are at the core of the epidemics of obesity, diabetes and ill health that have engulfed the world in the last 30 years.

nuts, especially macadamias. These would become my staple snack foods. I soon added tinned fish, especially pilchards and sardines, chicken and dairy products in the form of butter, milk, cream, cheese and full-cream yoghurt. I ate little fruit and vegetables to begin with, and had yet to discover the value of eggs and organ meats such as liver, kidneys, hearts and brains. I was unable immediately to remove all the sugar from my diet – it would take another 14 months before I could finally drink tea and coffee without added sugar. It was another five years before I stopped adding milk to my tea.

Despite my advanced age, within weeks I saw an improvement in my health, well-being and running ability that I can still only describe as astonishing. The first obvious change was that my enthusiasm for running returned. Within a week, I could not wait to exercise each day, slow and wobbly as those first runs continued to be. I could feel the changes in my body and they were telling me that something remarkable was happening.

Within the first seven days, my weight had dropped from 101 kilograms to 99 kilograms. Remarkably, as Westman and his colleagues had promised, I had absolutely no hunger – whenever I felt like eating, I would snack on biltong, cheese or nuts. A few mouthfuls and I would be ready to continue without the need to think about food again for another few hours.

Within two days, I had lost any cravings for the 'foods' that I now choose to avoid. Instead, the nutritious foods that had become the focus of my eating satisfied my hunger in a way that I could not remember since my youth. I now realise that I had simply rediscovered the foods of my childhood.

Three weeks later, at the start of 2011, I was down to 96 kilograms – a loss of five kilograms in three weeks. By the time I arrived in Sweden five weeks later, my weight had fallen to 90 kilograms for a total loss of 11 kilograms in the eight weeks I had been on the eating plan. I had dramatically exceeded Westman and his colleagues' improbable promise of six kilograms in six weeks. They were clearly not selling snake-oil nutrition science. Thereafter, my rate of weight loss slowed substantially. I reached an initial plateau weight of 86 kilograms at the start of June 2011, a weight loss of 15 kilograms after just 24 weeks on the eating plan.

Fourteen months later, after I had increased the fat content of my diet and begun to use the diabetic drug Glucophage (to better control my errant blood glucose concentration) and to include intermittent fasting, my weight dropped further, to between 80 and 81 kilograms. It has remained here ever since, and all without hunger.

Even more exciting, my running began to improve, at first almost imperceptibly, but then quite dramatically. On my trip to Stockholm, in one 12-hour period I ran a total of 27 kilometres, including an 18-kilometre run in minus 15 degree Celsius weather. Eight weeks earlier, this would have been unimaginable.

Within 12 weeks, I had reduced the time for my usual five-kilometre course by six minutes, and my longer 12-kilometre mountainous run by 40 minutes. In April 2011, I ran the Two Oceans 21-kilometre half-marathon 40 minutes faster than the previous year. I failed by just seven minutes to break two hours, and ran two of the final four kilometres at five minutes per kilometre, as fast as I could run in training. Yet, just 14 weeks earlier, I had been unable to sustain a pace of eight minutes per kilometre after only four kilometres of gentle running. Even the winner of the Two Oceans could not have felt as proud as I did at the end.

During this time, I noticed other changes. My chronic dyspepsia (indigestion), which had become increasingly severe over the past decade, magically disappeared within the first month on the new eating plan. I subsequently learnt that Dr John Yudkin's group had performed a controlled clinical trial in 1972 showing that a low-carbohydrate diet can cure dyspepsia.[13] Interestingly, dyspepsia is one of the most common modern human medical complaints. Treatment for it generates billions of dollars annually in the sale of drugs that do not cure the condition, but merely limit the symptoms to some extent. Now it would seem that the only treatment needed to cure this common problem could be to switch to a low-carbohydrate diet.[14] I certainly would have appreciated receiving this information as part of my medical training.

Next, the regular headaches that I suffered at least once a week and for which I took powerful painkillers disappeared completely. In the almost seven years since adopting the eating plan, I have had to take medication only twice to treat a headache. This is understandable if an allergy to wheat gliadin is a common cause of recurrent headaches, as cardiologist Dr William Davis proposed in his bestselling book *Wheat Belly*. Or if a majority of common headaches are caused by gluten sensitivity, as neurologist Dr David Perlmutter suggested in another *New York Times* bestseller, *Grain Brain*.

My condition of allergic rhinitis and bronchitis, which I had always considered to be due to a pollen allergy, also disappeared, as did my occasional attacks of post-exercise wheezing (asthma). For 30 years, I could expect a severe attack at least every three to six months of the year. These attacks were each sufficiently debilitating to require treatment with inhaled corticosteroids. In the past seven years, I have had only two mild attacks of rhinitis/bronchitis. Since the only change I have made to my diet in that time was to remove grains and cereals, I must also assume this condition was due to an allergic response to grains or cereals, or both.

Next, my eyesight improved to the point where I no longer required reading glasses, which I had used since age 15. (This could suggest that my problem with carbohydrates was already present when I was a teenager.)

My wife became overjoyed when, as I lost fat especially around my neck, I stopped snoring, proving, at least to me, that snoring is caused by carbohydrate-induced fat deposition in the upper throat. Perhaps snoring is just another obvious indication that one is overweight and in need of a dietary change.

In time, I discovered that many of these conditions form part of non-coeliac gluten sensitivity (NCGS), a malady that has only been properly recognised in the past five years. The condition is caused by an allergic response to gliadin in wheat and may occur in at least 30 per cent of humans without their knowledge.[15] The evidence that cereals and grains containing gluten and gliadin may be the direct cause of a wide range of medical conditions conflicts with the current dietary guidelines, which promote cereals and grains as the basis for a healthy diet.

Over the past seven years of my most important experiment, I have learnt more about nutrition than I did in the previous 41 years of my medical and scientific training.

Perhaps the most sobering lesson was that this new way of eating is not new at all. It has been around for quite some time – for about three and a half million years, in fact. It therefore makes no sense at all to call LCHF a fad diet. It is the original eating plan, the way nature designed us humans to eat.

Over time, I came across Gary Taubes's monumental works, *Good Calories, Bad Calories* and *Why We Get Fat*, as well as a *New York Times* article that he had written back in 2002, titled 'What if it's all been a big fat lie?'[16] I realised that, like Atkins, Westman, Phinney and Volek, Taubes is one of the most important figures in revealing a dietary history that has been forgotten, perhaps hidden.

Thus it is in *Good Calories, Bad Calories* that Taubes rediscovers the story of how Dr William Harvey cured the obesity of 19th-century London undertaker to the royal family William Banting, by prescribing a low-carbohydrate diet. Banting subsequently described the nature of his cure in probably the world's first diet book, *Letter on Corpulence, Addressed to the Public*, which he self-published in 1863. In the 1880s, German cardiologist Wilhelm Ebstein wrote two books, *Treatment of Corpulence* and *The Regimen to be Adopted in Cases of Gout*, both of which promoted the use of low-carbohydrate diets to the medical profession in Europe. Within another decade, this knowledge had crossed the Atlantic and was the diet that Sir William Osler prescribed for the treatment of obesity in his iconic medical text *The Principles and Practice of Medicine*.

I was left with one overriding question: If this information has been in the medical literature since at least 1882, and if it has helped me improve my health so dramatically, why is it not being taught at medical schools across the globe?

I would find answers to this and other questions only when I began relating my experiment and experience to others.

I knew at the time that everything I was saying was controversial and that many would disagree with me. It is natural and normal in science – or should be. Science is all about the search for truth, after all, and truth is never static. Loud warning bells ring in my head whenever nutrition scientists say that the science 'is settled'. It is not in the nature of science ever to be settled. Nor is science ever about 'consensus'.

I was well aware that I was directly challenging conventional nutrition 'wisdom', particularly South Africa's influential LFHC dietary guidelines and the powerful vested interests in the food and drug industries that have benefited massively from them. South Africa's guidelines are based on those that the US introduced way back in 1977, the very same guidelines that American science journalist Nina Teicholz and British obesity researcher Dr Zoë Harcombe showed to be unsupported by robust science when they were adopted, and which remain so to this day.[17]

I also suspected that some doctors and dietitians would dismiss my experiment and experience as anecdote. However, all good scientists know that all of science begins with anecdote. And my experience simply adds to a subsequent groundswell of anecdotal evidence coming in from people around the globe.

The establishment backlash, when it came, was swift, targeted and ugly, and of a startlingly venomous personal nature. Most alarming of all, however, was the impenetrable wall of silence that rose around the science. My critics were either ill prepared or, for reasons known only to them, not prepared to debate the science in public. Soon, though, from behind that wall began to emerge the roots of what looked like an organised campaign to discredit the evidence for LCHF by demonising and defaming me.

The next chapter chronicles the beginning of the pushback to protect the status quo.

3

The Backlash Begins

'In science it's not a sin to change your mind when the evidence
demands it. For some people, the tribe is more important than the truth;
for the best scientists, the truth is more important than the tribe.'
– Joel Achenbach, American science writer[1]

My epiphany in December 2010 came a few months after I had completed the first edition of my memoir, *Challenging Beliefs*. The physical and spiritual transformations that resulted from my dietary change occurred too late for that story to be included in the first edition of the book. In any case, I was still uncertain whether the new way I was eating would become a lifelong commitment or hold any value for others.

It took me many months to pluck up the courage to take my story to a wider audience. The first chance was a regular column I was then writing for Discovery Health, the company that was generously funding my research and the work of the Sports Science Institute of South Africa (SSISA). In the winter 2011 edition of their health magazine, *Discovery*, I broke my silence, describing for the first time my initial uncertain steps into the world of the low-carbohydrate diet. The title 'Against the Grains' identified the focus – it was a report of how and why I had removed grains and other carbohydrates from my diet.

In the introductory paragraph, I demonstrated that I already knew that what I was writing would be unpopular: 'I am not one to shy away from controversy. But I suspect that this column will attract more unfavourable comment than perhaps anything else I have recently written. Yet the message could be life-changing for some.' The article included the following observations:

- Global obesity rates have risen dramatically since the adoption of the US dietary guidelines, which promote 6–11 daily servings of bread, cereals, rice and pasta.
- Humans have eaten meat for millions of years, but grains for only the last 20 000 years or so.
- Humans developed our large brains by eating 'high-energy' foods like meat and fish. 'Perhaps,' I quaintly proposed, 'humans are closet carnivores.'

- Low-carbohydrate diets produce weight-loss results 'at least as good as those achieved with the traditional low-fat, high-carbohydrate diets'.
- High-protein diets produce satiation, whereas carbohydrates drive hunger. 'This absence of hunger is more likely to encourage compliance and sustained weight loss (in those eating low-carbohydrate diets). In contrast, there may be an addiction especially to rapidly assimilated carbohydrates like sugar and refined carbohydrates, that drives the overconsumption of all foodstuffs, fat included, and hence leads to weight gain.'
- As a result, 'it is the unrestricted intake of especially refined and hence addictive carbohydrates that fuels an overconsumption of calories, not a high fat intake as is usually believed'.

Finally, and in my usual provocative style, I asked why these facts were not apparent to everyone. My conclusion: 'There is a saying that to find the root cause, follow the money trail. If a low-carbohydrate intake is more healthy than we expect, then why is that fact hidden? The answer is that some very large industries, including the soft-drink, sugar and confectionery industries (all of which produce high-carbohydrate products with minimal nutritional value) do not want us to know this.'

That final statement would perhaps prove to be truest, since it would lead to the events described in this book.

One immediate consequence of that first article was that *Discovery* cancelled my regular column, which I had written for many years.

By the end of 2011, the message that I had abruptly reversed my dietary advice was beginning to spread across South Africa. My publisher, sensing an opportunity, approached me to add new material to *Challenging Beliefs*. Bolstered by a growing certainty that I now had a novel dietary message of value for a much larger group of South Africans, I added 35 pages. These are the key themes that I introduced:

- The low-carbohydrate diet cannot be labelled a fad diet, because William Banting described its first successful adoption in the 1860s, more than a century before the real fad diet, advocated by the 1977 Dietary Guidelines for Americans, went mainstream.
- Industries determine what we believe about nutrition. They engineer these beliefs to increase food and beverage sales, not to protect or improve our health. In fact, most of what we have been taught is detrimental to our health.
- Humans can be classified as either carbohydrate tolerant or carbohydrate intolerant (today I prefer the terms insulin sensitive and insulin resistant).
- Dietary carbohydrates, not fat, cause obesity and lead to diabetes in those who are insulin resistant.
- There is no evidence that a high-fat diet is harmful to health.
- Sugar, not fat, is the single most toxic ingredient of the modern diet. It is also

the most ubiquitous foodstuff on the planet. (Today I would add that sugar is not a foodstuff; it is a drug.)

- Cholesterol is not the unique cause of heart disease and may not even be an important factor (especially in women).
- You cannot outrun a bad diet.
- Athletes are not thin because they exercise. Rather thinness begets exercise, whereas obesity causes sloth.
- It is possible to exercise and train vigorously while eating a low-carbohydrate diet. (I added the proviso that it was still unknown whether or not athletes could sustain high-intensity exercise if they did not increase their carbohydrate intake both before and during exercise.)
- I concluded with nine health recommendations for those living with IR.

When I added these ideas in early 2012, I was certain that they were sufficiently correct for me to risk exposing them to a wider audience. I also assumed that because we live in a mature academic democracy in South Africa, these ideas would inspire a grown-up debate in the scientific community, especially among colleagues at my academic home, the Faculty of Health Sciences at UCT.

As a result of that adult debate, I presumed that my colleagues would warmly embrace whatever was of value in these ideas. Equally, after appropriate joint discussions, we would summarily dismiss any ideas that science subsequently disproved. The outcome would be a better understanding of IR, obesity and T2DM (plus a wide range of other conditions), and the development of better, safer ways to more effectively treat many more patients. How exciting if, finally, we could advocate a simple method to prevent and treat the chronic medical conditions that are destroying healthcare in South Africa as elsewhere. And in a way that would not bankrupt patients or medical-aid schemes. What could possibly be more rewarding?

I was in for some rude surprises, the first of which was a series of public criticisms from colleagues at the UCT Faculty of Health Sciences, a faculty that I had first entered in February 1969 and which, in my opinion, I have served honourably ever since.

The first clear public evidence that my challenge to orthodoxy was sparking intense concern among some senior UCT academics materialised on 13 September 2012, when I was awarded the National Research Foundation's Lifetime Achievement Award. This is the highest South African scientific award. The citation to the award stated the following:

This serves to acknowledge Professor TD Noakes who is recognized internationally for his extraordinary contribution to the development of science, what he stands for as a South African, and for the manner in which his work has touched and shaped the lives and views of many South Africans.

Within minutes of receiving the award, at about 9:30 p.m., my cellphone rang. It was a local news reporter who wished to include my comments in a story he was writing about a letter to be published the following morning in his newspaper.

Written by a group of Cape Town cardiologists, headed by then UCT cardiology professor Patrick Commerford and including Professor David Marais and doctors Mpiko Ntsekhe, Dirk Blom, Elwyn Lloyd and Adrian Horak, the letter warned that the prescription in *Challenging Beliefs* of a 'high-fat, high-protein' diet for 'all persons' is 'contrary to the recommendations of all major cardiovascular societies worldwide, is of unproven benefit and may be dangerous for patients with coronary heart disease [CHD] or persons at risk of coronary heart disease'.[2] In addition, the cardiologists were unhappy that I was 'questioning' the value of cholesterol-lowering agents (i.e. statins), because this was 'at best unwise and may be harmful to many patients on appropriate treatment'.

What struck me most about the cardiologists' open letter to the media was its timing. As a result, the front-page story in the following morning's issue of the *Cape Times* was not about my being awarded South Africa's most prestigious science award. Rather it was all about my supposedly unprofessional behaviour in expressing opinions that conflicted with those of the anointed UCT cardiologists. Was the timing of this letter mere coincidence, or had it been planned?

The gist of their complaint appeared to be that the simple act of questioning their cohesive professorial dogma was contrary to the Hippocratic Oath because it might harm patients. Yet one thing my Damascene moment had shown me was that it is our collective failure to question the causes of the global obesity/T2DM epidemic that is truly harming our patients and our nation.

I continue whimsically to believe that the function of universities is to advance knowledge, not to insulate professorial opinions from external scrutiny and thus institutionalise what I call the power of the anointed. I believe the very reason why universities exist is because we do not (yet) know everything. If we did, we would have no reason to invest so much in such costly institutions.

My opinion as an educator is that we are unlikely to foster future generations of inquisitive doctors and cardiologists wishing to improve standards of medical care through innovation and change if we follow these cardiologists' reactionary educational approach. I can think of no favourable outcomes of attempts to suppress the opinions of those with whom we disagree – other than to protect the interests of those who have benefited from the surge in chronic diseases, including heart disease, over the past hundred years.

In the following months and years, the warning that the LCHF/Banting diet 'might' damage health would become the distinctive, recurring theme rallying the attacks directed at me by my professional colleagues. Of course, anything 'might' cause anything. The role of science is to discover what causes what. That is why we have universities, and why universities employ professors: to advance our diligent search for truth by considering any and all opposing opinions.

I interpret these professional attacks as a measure of the extent to which the pharmaceutical industry has captured our profession. Those whose careers have become partially or wholly dependent on a close relationship with the marketing arms of pharmaceutical companies simply will not tolerate anyone who dares question either the need for or the efficacy of any therapeutic intervention involving pharmaceutical products or related medical interventions.

In *Deadly Medicines and Organised Crime*, Danish physician and former Big Pharma insider Peter Gøtzsche writes: 'The pharmaceutical industry does not sell drugs. It sells lies about drugs.'[3] And in exchange for money and prestige, it manipulates its surrogates – embedded medical scientists and physicians – to disseminate those untruths.

Had I become an unwitting target of some of that money?

The UCT cardiologists further used their letter to espouse their expected industry-required advertorial claiming that statin drugs are 'cheap' and 'make you live longer'. They suggested I should only voice my opinions in 'the academic forum and the medical literature where they could be critically evaluated and challenged' by my peers. In other words, there is no place for books written by academics for the general public, unless they regurgitate that which the anointed professors have approved. 'To present these controversial opinions as fact to a lay public, in his un-refereed book, is dangerous and potentially very harmful to good patient care,' they pronounced.

It is not clear to me how opinions can be inherently dangerous, except perhaps to those whose careers require that certain opinions are never heard.

The essential failure of these cardiologists, however, has been their assumption that the general public is wholly uneducated, with no capacity to think for itself. I believe that eventually, through the power of the internet and social media – the wisdom of the crowd – the public will demand to know why the faith and tax money it invested was so misplaced in these academics.

Perhaps it is the natural consequence of living in the ivory tower of academia, surrounded for too long by sycophantic surrogates whose career prospects are so dependent on pleasing their professors, the anointed. Ultimately the anointed become the victims of their own hubris and self-importance, believing they can program, like robots, an ignorant public on what to do and how to think. It is as George Orwell wrote in *1984*: 'The whole climate of thought will be different. In fact, there will be no thought, as we understand it now. Orthodoxy means not thinking – not needing to think. Orthodoxy is unconsciousness.'[4]

After four decades of regular intellectual interactions with the general public, my abiding impression is of the remarkable intelligence of the majority, most of whom have never enjoyed even an informal training in medicine or science. I have also learnt that this aptitude is not a function of social position or economic status.

That two journalists without any formal training in medicine – Gary Taubes and Nina Teicholz – could write the three most important general medical books of the past few decades, far more important than anything any cartel of academic cardiologists has yet contributed to the public discourse, is further evidence that traditionally educated professors do not hold a monopoly on medical wisdom.

The authors of the cardiologists' letter to the media continued: 'We understand some patients are placing their health at risk by discontinuing statin therapy and their prudent diets on the basis of this "expert opinion". Having survived "Aids Denialism" we do not need to be exposed to "Cholesterol Denialism".'

Then, in a final statement of hubris, they said: 'Scientists and clinicians have an ethical obligation to ensure that the information they impart to their patients and the public at large is correct, in line with best available evidence, and will not cause harm.'

Conventionally trained cardiologists never consider that their dietary advice is the direct cause of the greatest medical threat humans have ever faced: the global obesity and T2DM epidemics that began after 1977 with the introduction of the 'heart-healthy', 'prudent' diet. Cardiologists continue to promote this diet unquestioningly on a daily basis to anyone whose blood cholesterol concentration exceeds 5.01 millimoles per litre (mmol/L). I wonder if any ever inform their patients that to prevent one major coronary event or stroke, these supposedly life-saving 'miracle' drugs must be prescribed to 140 low-risk patients for five years.[5] For a single heart attack or stroke to be prevented in the group at lowest risk (but whose blood cholesterol levels are nevertheless above 5.01 mmol/L), 167 patients will require treatment for five years.[6] After a heart attack, statins will need to be prescribed to 82 heart patients to prevent a single fatal heart attack, to 39 to prevent a single non-fatal heart attack, and to 125 to prevent a single stroke.[7] More importantly, in those at low risk, statin therapy has no effect on the really crucial outcome measure: all-cause mortality, which is the measure of deaths from all causes (including, for example, cancer, T2DM and infection).[8]

When the 'average postponement of death in statin trials' (i.e. the extension in lifespan) is calculated, the results are equally unimpressive. In one literature review, Malene Kristensen, Palle Christensen and Jesper Hallas found that the 'median postponement of death for primary and secondary prevention trials were 3.2 and 4.1 days, respectively'. (Primary prevention refers to trials in people without evidence of heart disease at the start of the trial, while secondary prevention trials are in people with established heart disease.) The authors concluded: 'Statin treatment results in a surprisingly small average gain in overall survival within the trials' running time. For patients whose life expectancy is limited or who have adverse effects of treatment, withholding statin therapy should be considered.'[9]

It is of little value to take a drug that might marginally reduce one's risk of suffering a heart attack or stroke if it increases the risk of dying from something else, without any extension in life expectancy. Because statin therapy is not without risk of long-term adverse consequences, including an increased risk to T2DM[10] and perhaps Parkinson's disease,[11] some 'mavericks' suggest that healthy people should not take statins simply because they have an 'elevated' blood cholesterol concentration.[12] Professor John Ioannidis is concerned that, given the prospect of one billion people using statins in the future, with cumulative global sales of statins approaching $1 trillion by 2020, 'crucial evidence is still missing'.[13]

In fact, the evidence is not missing. But like the proven benefits of the LCHF diet in the management of IR and T2DM, the definitive proof that statins do not work is simply not seen. There are now at least 44 cholesterol-lowering trials, including the testing of eight different classes of drugs, all of which establish that lowering cholesterol through diet or drugs 'does not significantly prolong life or consistently prevent CHD'.[14] Thus Robert DuBroff proposes that 'we must accept the empirical record even though it contradicts our long-held beliefs. Other researchers believe this reluctance can be explained by the tendency to "see what you want to see," and ignore what you do not.'[15] Clearly the UCT cardiologists do not want to see that which is so dreadfully inconvenient.

But on what evidence do conventionally trained cardiologists base their certainty in what they do?

Cardiology is responsible for initiating and performing more unnecessary, non-evidence-based and costly medical interventions than perhaps any other medical discipline. For example, the most lucrative therapy, coronary artery bypass surgery, is unnecessary for the vast majority of patients with stable coronary artery disease, including those with more advanced disease.[16] It is also a procedure that carries significant risk of mental impairment. It has been shown that these patients can do extremely well on medical management without coronary artery bypass surgery.[17] Similarly, in a meta-analysis of randomised trials comparing percutaneous coronary intervention (i.e. coronary artery 'stenting' and angioplasty – the unrestrained use of which ensure that cardiology is an especially lucrative medical speciality) with conservative medical treatment, the authors found that: 'In patients with chronic stable coronary artery disease, in the absence of recent myocardial infarction [heart attack], percutaneous coronary intervention does not offer any benefit in terms of death, myocardial infarction, or the need for subsequent revascularization compared with conservative medical treatment.' As a result, 'we believe that many percutaneous interventions that currently are performed in patients with non-acute coronary artery disease are not justified'.[18]

There are essentially two reasons for this conclusion. Firstly, even patients with severe coronary artery disease are not at death's door as we are led to believe. Research has found that these patients have an annual mortality of less than 1.5 per cent. In other words, when receiving standard medical care, 98 out of 100 patients will still be alive at the end of the first year of treatment.[19] Secondly, complications caused by coronary artery disease, including heart attack and sudden death, arise when the coronary arterial plaque ruptures, causing the sudden obstruction of blood flow to the heart.[20] However, the vast majority of these ruptures, perhaps as many as 85 per cent,[21] occur in coronary arteries that are not considered candidates for bypass surgery, 'stenting' or angioplasty because the plaques that ruptured were considered too small to warrant any of these interventions.[22]

In their comment on the case for medical treatment in chronic stable coronary artery disease, Thomas Graboys and Dr Bernard Lown conclude by asking:

> So why the more than 1 million annual invasive coronary procedures? Regrettably, left unmentioned is the factor that trumps scientific evidence – namely, the economic advantage that costly interventions afford to hospitals, to interventionist cardiologists, to cardiac surgeons, and to others. Medicine as a calling would be far better served if criteria for coronary artery interventions were determined by issues that truly matter to patients, such as survival and long-term well-being.[23]

Why are so many patients unaware of these facts? According to Dr Lown, a pioneering cardiologist, members of our profession indulge in 'fear mongering'.[24] Telling a patient he is 'a walking time bomb', 'this narrowed coronary artery is a widow maker' or 'you are living on borrowed time' places the cardiologist in control, establishing a parent–child relationship between doctor and patient. And the child is usually too scared to ask any questions.

Lown eventually decided to stop referring his heart patients for coronary angiography because he understood that, in the 1970s, the sole possible outcome would be coronary artery bypass surgery (today it is angioplasty or 'stenting'). The reaction from his peers was interesting. 'For the first time in my medical career I received phone calls from outraged physicians accusing me of abandoning science or of setting cardiology back to the Dark Ages,' he said. Not much has changed, it seems.

Perhaps cardiologists should take heed of the old dictum that 'those who live in glass houses should not throw stones'. If you make your money prescribing drugs or performing invasive procedures that have little or no proven benefit and which may cause harm, you need to be very wary of accusing others of doing harm. When it comes to the dietary advice that I promote, you should be especially cautious, as there is no published scientific evidence that it causes harm.[25]

My response to the cardiologists' letter was published in the *Cape Times* on 17 September 2012. Titled 'Time to admit that heart disease theory has failed', it read:

Professor Patrick Commerford et al's letter to the *Cape Times* ('Noakes has gone too far', September 14) refers. As I wrote in *Challenging Beliefs*, a 2010 meta-analysis of studies involving 347 747 subjects published in the *American Journal of Clinical Nutrition* found 'no significant evidence for concluding that dietary saturated fat is associated with an increased risk of coronary heart disease or cardiovascular disease [CVD]'. A 2011 report from the Cochrane Collaboration, an organisation that is independent of the pharmaceutical industry, found that 'there was no clear evidence for dietary fat changes on total mortality or cardiovascular mortality'. Thus the scientific evidence is clear: A low-fat diet has no proven role in the prevention of (coronary) heart disease. It is time that cardiologists began to teach this fact in our medical schools.

So if a high-fat diet does not cause heart disease then what does? In carbohydrate-intolerant subjects like myself, a low-fat/high-carbohydrate diet produces all of the following abnormalities, some of which are causally linked to arterial damage and heart disease:

1. *Elevated blood glucose, insulin and glycated haemoglobin (HbA1c) concentrations.* The best predictors of heart attack risk are blood HbA1c and random glucose concentrations. Elevated values in diabetics increase heart attack risk 7-fold. In contrast, an elevated cholesterol concentration increases heart attack risk about 1.3-fold, a value low enough in statistical terms to be potentially spurious.

2. *Low blood HDL [high-density lipoprotein]-cholesterol and high triglyceride and uric acid concentrations.*

3. *Increased numbers of small, dense LDL-cholesterol particles.* In contrast, a high-fat diet increases the number of large, fluffy LDL-cholesterol particles that are not related to heart attack risk.

4. *Elevated blood lipoprotein(a) concentrations.*

5. *Obesity* and, in my opinion but as yet unproven, *elevated blood pressure.*

6. *Elevated ultra-sensitive C-reactive protein concentrations* indicative of a whole-body inflammatory state.

7. *Elevated blood homocysteine concentrations* (due to dietary deficiencies in folic acid, vitamin B6 and B12 found in eggs and meat).

If the cause of heart disease was truly known (as is the cause of HIV/AIDS), then the condition should have disappeared with the universal promotion of the so-called 'heart-healthy prudent diet' and the annual prescription of tens of billions of dollars' worth of cholesterol-lowering drugs globally. Yet one of the leading causes of death in the USA is now chronic heart failure caused by coronary heart disease. To service its burgeoning heart disease problem, the US now requires twice the number of cardiologists currently in practice (17 000). If current dietary and therapeutic advice was effective, cardiology and cholesterol-lowering drugs should be going the way of the dinosaur. Instead both are major growth industries. No wonder both fear 'cholesterol denialists'.

In 1900, when most Americans cooked in lard and ate a diet full of butter and dairy produce, pork and saturated fat in meat (but low in sugar and processed foods), heart disease was so rare that their most famous cardiologist, Dr Paul Dudley White, encountered his first case only in the 1920s (although the disease has since been described in grain-eating Egyptian mummies). Today in a nation that has replaced animal fats and dairy in its diet with 'healthy' carbohydrates, heart disease, like obesity and diabetes, is rampant.

With regard to statin therapy, I advise anyone who does not have established heart disease or genetic hypercholesterolaemia, and who is either already taking or considering using cholesterol-lowering drugs, to read *The Great Cholesterol Con* (2006) by Anthony Colpo. This book should also be required reading for all my colleagues, medical students especially, who are currently prescribing these drugs or who plan to do so in the future.

The theory that blood cholesterol and a high-fat diet are the exclusive causes of heart disease will, in my opinion, prove to be, like the miasma theory, one of the greatest errors in the history of medicine.

It is time to admit that the theory has failed. We need to adopt an open mind if we are ever to discover the real cause(s) of the current global epidemic of obesity, diabetes and coronary heart disease, all of which are likely caused by the same factors.

Four days later, on 21 September 2012, what appeared to be a follow-up attack found its way into the *Mail & Guardian* under the headline 'Is Tim Noakes the Malema of medicine?'[26]

Earlier that month, Dr Martinique Stilwell had interviewed me for the article she was writing for the weekly newspaper. Probably best known for her memoir about growing up at sea, *Thinking up a Hurricane*, Stilwell is a medical graduate of the University of the Witwatersrand and currently works as an anaesthetist. She has no more formal training in nutrition than any other South African doctor.

Stilwell began her article by genuflecting to the complaints of the UCT cardiologists. The gist of her argument was that while I had successfully exposed the non-science behind the sports-drink scam and had developed the Central Governor Model of Exercise Regulation, the sole evidence I had for promoting the LCHF eating plan were my personal experiences, specifically my marked weight loss and the improvement in my running. 'Noakes said he experiments on himself and judges the results by how he feels,' Stilwell wrote. 'He encourages lay people to do the same, which doctors say is irresponsible.'

A more impartial journalist would have reported that my dietary conversion occurred only after I had read the remarkable book by doctors Westman, Phinney and Volek. *The New Atkins for a New You* was full of science about the LCHF diet, much of it derived from a series of world-class, peer-reviewed scientific papers published by the authors over the past 20 years. My personal experience after my December 2010 Damascene moment had simply confirmed the hard science contained in their book. Those experiences also contradicted much of what I had been taught by the anointed professors that Stilwell seemed so keen to champion.

Returning to the cardiologists' complaints, Stilwell said that since I began to question the benefits of statins, there had been 'murmurs among cardiologists that Noakes is the Malema of medicine, a man with a hoarde [*sic*] of followers and considerable media sway, who is capable of producing charismatic, easy to hear and probably irresponsible solutions to very complex problems'.

The fact is that there is nothing complex about the diet-heart and lipid hypotheses promoted by these cardiologists and accepted by Stilwell. They simply boil down to: eating saturated fat raises blood cholesterol concentrations, which clog coronary arteries and lead to death from heart disease. Nothing particularly complex here, except the difficult question that cardiologists choose to ignore: the role of sudden plaque rupture as the decisive event causing heart attack and sudden death in those with even a tiny amount of 'clogging' in their coronary arteries.[27]

Stilwell interviewed a signatory of the Commerford letter, Dr Dirk Blom, who is described as 'an academic at UCT's lipid clinic'. Blom confirmed my contention that most people who suffer heart attacks have normal blood cholesterol concentrations. How do we explain this inconvenient finding if an elevated blood cholesterol concentration is the single most important factor causing heart attack, as Blom and his colleagues endlessly repeat? How can cholesterol cause heart attacks when present in the bloodstream in 'normal' amounts that are too low to justify treatment with cholesterol-lowering statin drugs? The inability to grasp this paradox is known as cognitive dissonance.

In fact, UCT lipid expert Professor David Marais, another signatory of the Commerford letter, was the co-author of a large study of blood cholesterol concentrations and other risk factors in South African men and women living in Soweto. The so-called Heart of Soweto study found that the majority of black South Africans who have had heart attacks have low blood cholesterol concentrations with an average value of only 4.1 mmol/L (see Figure 3.1).[28] Others have reported essentially identical findings in North Americans hospitalised with acute or prior heart attacks.[29]

Figure 3.1

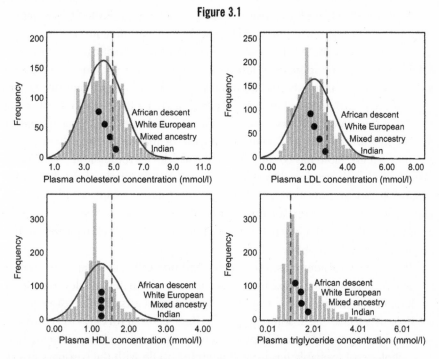

Frequency distributions of total plasma cholesterol, plasma LDL, plasma HDL and plasma triglyceride concentrations (mmol/L) in Sowetan residents of (a) African, (b) White European, (c) mixed and (d) Indian descent treated for heart attack in the Heart of Soweto study. Note that only in the Indian group is the average total plasma cholesterol concentration greater than the value of 5 mmol/L that is considered 'dangerous', requiring the prescription of statin therapy. But in all groups, plasma HDL cholesterol concentrations are low and triglyceride concentrations are elevated, indicating the presence of insulin resistance

These values are too low to qualify for treatment with cholesterol-lowering statin drugs that supposedly reduce heart-attack risk. But if these patients' blood cholesterol levels are too low to justify treatment to prevent heart attacks, what caused their heart attacks? The obvious conclusion is that the cholesterol theory is false. I will discuss this further in Chapter 17.

Using industry-speak designed to obfuscate, Blom attempted to explain: 'If cholesterol is not markedly elevated it is not a sole predictor of heart disease, but it is part of the risk calculation.' Which means what, exactly? In the first place, these patients do not have blood cholesterol levels that are 'not markedly elevated'; they have values that are too low to warrant treatment according to the internationally accepted guidelines developed by Blom and others.

Surely Stilwell should have interrogated his evasion more critically if she were truly intent on providing her readers with intelligently moderated information? She should also have asked Blom to declare any conflicts of interest that might influence his apparent religious devotion to the promotion of this form of drug treatment. My own simple investigation found that since he first became interested in cholesterol and heart disease in 2002, Blom has published 33 articles on the topic, including nine reports on large-scale trials of different statins to which he personally contributed. The results of most of these specific trials were published in world-leading medical journals, indicating that the studies were very well funded. It is fair to say that Blom's research career is dependent on the largesse of the pharmaceutical industry. There is a saying that you do not bite the hand that feeds you. Of course, the UCT Faculty of Health Sciences also benefits financially from Blom's tight relationship with the makers of statin drugs.

Interestingly, Blom has co-authored seven articles on the cholesterol-lowering drug evolocumab, produced by Amgen. A one-month supply of the drug costs around $1 200, and the FOURIER study found that 74 people would need to take evolocumab for two years for just one to show benefit in terms of avoiding a cardiovascular event. Clearly this is not a drug that has much relevance to the greater South African public.

Blom's special academic interest is the condition called familial hypercholesterolaemia (FH), a genetic 'disease', the key feature of which is an elevated blood cholesterol concentration on a familial (hereditary) basis. It is the disease that cardiologists use as the absolute proof that 'bad' cholesterol clogs the coronary arteries, leading to CHD. In Chapters 7 and 17, I present evidence showing that 'bad' cholesterol probably has little, if anything, to do with the coronary artery clogging found in some, but certainly not all, people with FH. The scientific evidence strongly suggests that people with FH develop arterial 'clogging' for exactly the same reasons as everyone else (without FH) – as a result of those with IR eating diets high in carbohydrates, sugar and processed foods. If true, this suggests that cardiologists like Blom should perhaps prescribe low-carbohydrate diets rather than statins for their patients with FH. Not that I suspect the pharmaceutical industry would be too enthusiastic to fund any studies testing this possibility.

In the Stilwell article, Blom continued by saying that statins 'unequivocally' save lives and that those who do not benefit are simply low-risk individuals who should not have been on the drugs in the first place. I have learnt that scientists only use words like 'unequivocal' when the evidence is the opposite – that is, when it is entirely equivocal. As already mentioned, statin drugs produce miniscule benefits with the risk of significant side effects in perhaps as many as 20 per cent of subjects. The drug on which Blom has focused most of his attention is hardly a lifesaver and is not likely to be without worrying side effects.

The benefits for women seem to be even less, perhaps non-existent. Cardiologist Dr Barbara Roberts writes in her book *The Truth about Statins*: 'In women under the age of sixty-five who don't have established vascular disease, we have *zero* evidence that statin treatment lowers their risk for having a cardiac event ... And women experience more side effects from statins than men do.'[30] As a female doctor interested in health promotion, Stilwell should have interrogated her male colleague on this topic. Instead, she allowed him to mislead her into believing that what applies to men must equally apply to women. With regard to statin therapy, this is certainly not the case.

Stilwell went on to quote a cardiologist who wished to remain anonymous: 'I feel sorry for Tim. He likes to take on a challenge, but when it comes to statins I think he's painted himself into a corner.'

I have no doubt that sometime in the not-too-distant future those of us who have warned that the diet-heart and lipid hypotheses are the greatest scams in the history of modern medicine, and that statins are among the most ineffective drugs ever produced by the pharmaceutical industry, will be vindicated.

Stilwell concluded her article with a clarion call to safe orthodoxy:

Noakes has swung from high carbs to no carbs [*this is not true*]. The most widely accepted research suggests something in between. Avoid transfats, sugar and refined carbohydrates, eat a calorie-restricted, balanced diet with whole grains, protein and healthy fats, exercise in moderation and, if you are thirsty, drink water.

I seriously question the merits of Stilwell's dietary advice, taken, as it is, from the classic 1977 US dietary guidelines.

How, for example, does one exist forever on a calorie-restricted diet? By definition, a calorie-restricted diet will cause progressive weight loss leading to relentless hunger and, ultimately, death. The exception is if one is eating LCHF, which in 1970 Professor John Yudkin described as being 'in reality a low-calorie diet'.[31] In Chapter 4, I discuss Ancel Keys's Minnesota Starvation Experiment and what it reveals about the psychological and behavioural effects of trying to live on a low-calorie, low-fat diet of the kind that Stilwell proposes.

The dietary recommendations that Stilwell promotes fail to take into account the role of the brain controller (the appestat) in the regulation of hunger. Carbo-hydrates stimulate hunger, whereas fat and protein satiate it. After 40 years of practice, I think we can finally recognise the traditional dietary guidelines for what they are: a complete failure. As the saying goes, 'however beautiful the strategy, you should occasionally look at the results'.

My suspicion is that Stilwell's article formed part of a game plan directed by, among others, her acquaintance Jacques Rousseau. As described in Chapter 1, Rousseau was using his blog to show me up as a scientist who had 'lost his way'.

Between the release of the updated edition of *Challenging Beliefs* in March 2012 and the first pot shots in the press, on 21 July 2012 I was invited by Professor Diane McIntyre from the School of Public Health and Family Medicine in the UCT Faculty of Health Sciences to speak to faculty members about cholesterol and heart disease. McIntyre has an international profile and has since been appointed executive director of the International Health Economics Association. She had personally adopted the LCHF diet for a time and wanted to give me the opportunity to speak on the scientific reasons why I was no longer advocating a low-fat diet.

I presented a standard, hour-long talk explaining why the epidemiological (associational) evidence linking elevated blood cholesterol concentrations to increased risk of heart disease was, at best, weak; that associational studies linking dietary saturated-fat intake to higher rates of heart disease provided equally weak evidence; and that any associational link was, in any case, disproved by a number of prospective RCTs, all of which showed that low-fat diets do not reduce the risk for developing heart disease. And finally, as fully discussed in Chapter 17, that there was no evidence from autopsy studies that pre-morbid blood cholesterol concentrations predict the extent of coronary artery disease present at death. This material would form the basis for the 25 000-word chapter I would write for *The Real Meal Revolution* a year later, in July 2013.

After the talk, the questions were fairly banal and predictable.

An example: How can you say that blood cholesterol concentrations do not predict heart-attack risk when 'we' (the anointed) know that cholesterol causes heart disease?

As I presented in my talk and as discussed in Chapter 17, markers of IR/T2DM are much better predictors of future heart-attack risk. In any case, T2DM and its associated medical complications, and not heart attacks, are the illnesses that we must prevent if we wish to improve human health and save global medical services from bankruptcy and collapse. However, because the low-fat diet is the most likely cause of the obesity/T2DM epidemic, it is difficult, if not impossible, for those who have advocated this fallacy for the past 40 years to suddenly find the courage to acknowledge and apologise for their gross error.

Another example: How can you prescribe a high-fat diet knowing that it will cause blood cholesterol levels to rise and must therefore increase heart-attack rates?

There is actually no evidence that cholesterol causes heart disease. Instead, as I argue in Chapter 17, the introduction of population-based screening for blood cholesterol concentrations is what leads to arterial disease, because it teaches doctors and dietitians to prescribe high-carbohydrate diets (and statins) to people with normal (i.e. below 7.5 mmol/L) blood total cholesterol concentrations but who are insulin resistant. Prescribing high-carbohydrate diets for those with IR can produce only one result: an epidemic increase in T2DM, with its associated scourge – disseminated obstructive arterial disease of all the key blood vessels in the body.

Another question came from an industry-funded hypertension expert: How can you say that statin drugs are so ineffective when 'we know' that lowering blood cholesterol concentrations with statin drugs reduces heart-attack risk by at least 30 per cent?

My counter-questioning made me realise that the expert had not been taught the difference between the relative (30 per cent) and absolute (~1 per cent) benefits supposedly provided by these drugs. He also did not understand, because he had not been taught to think that way, that both values are meaningless unless one understands an individual's baseline risk for developing the disease of interest. He also did not appear to understand that the only drug effect of real value is whether a specific drug makes people live longer by reducing all-cause mortality (i.e. reduces the risk of dying prematurely from all diseases considered together, not just as a result of suffering a heart attack).

There is no value in taking a drug that reduces the risk of suffering a heart attack if it simply causes people to die at a younger age from something else, such as cancer. A drug that causes death from cancer in all who take it will certainly prevent all deaths from heart attack. But that might not be the best reason to justify prescribing that drug. Unfortunately, this is often the reasoning cardiologists use to prescribe statins – that these drugs marginally reduce one's risk of suffering a heart attack. The key question is whether or not these drugs also reduce all-cause mortality, and it is now abundantly clear that most do not.[32]

Importantly, a 100 per cent increase in baseline risk for developing a particular disease is irrelevant if the risk is trivial. Certainly, buying two Lotto tickets increases the chance of winning the jackpot by 100 per cent. But the probability of winning even with two tickets is still only one in tens of millions. Similarly, if anyone has a one in 1 000 chance of suffering a heart attack in the next five years, using a drug that (allegedly) reduces that risk by 100 per cent (to one in 500) still means that 499 of 500 people will receive no benefit from the use of that drug. Yet all 500 will be exposed to the detrimental effects of that drug, whatever those might be.

Typically, the pharmaceutical industry lavishes money on its industry-friendly key opinion leaders, of which the hypertension expert was one, to promote the 'benefits' of their drugs by using relative benefits (the larger number). When talking about the risks of these drugs, however, they either ignore the topic or use absolute risk (the much smaller number). And no one ever talks about baseline risk, because for all diseases – even lung cancer in smokers – for any single individual, the risk is usually quite low.

For example, people considered at highest risk for a future heart attack experience only nine events per 10 years per 100 subjects, and those at lowest risk just two per 10 years.[33] Which means that after 10 years, 91 of the 100 people considered to be at highest risk for a cardiac event will not have experienced any such event. And 98 of those 100 considered to be the healthiest will also not have experienced any cardiac problems.

Perhaps predictably, predictive models used by cardiologists to estimate future risk overestimate risk by as much as 150 per cent in men, but less in women (up to 67 per cent).[34] Naturally, the effect of such overestimation will be twofold: more healthy patients will be terrified that they are about to drop dead in the next few days because their blood cholesterol concentrations have suddenly risen above 5.01 mmol/L; and the over-prescription of a lifetime of statin drugs to healthy people, the majority of whom will not ever suffer cardiac events.

I came away from the lecture satisfied that I had made my points and that no one in the audience had punched any holes in my arguments. The reception was not overtly hostile and was certainly not a portent of things to come, when four months later I would lock horns with Professor Jacques Rossouw in the hubristically termed 'Centenary Debate' organised by the same faculty, in front of an audience oozing animosity.

4

The Centenary Debate

'If you must criticize scholars whose work challenges yours,
do so on the evidence, not by poisoning the land on which we all live.'
– Alice Dreger, *Galileo's Middle Finger*[1]

In November 2012, I hosted Swedish physician Dr Andreas Eenfeldt and health coach Monique Forslund in Cape Town to launch the English version of Forslund's book *Low-carb Living For Families*. We used the occasion to have both speak at an evening seminar at the UCT Faculty of Health Sciences. The audience was riveted. Eenfeldt has been a key figure in the global LCHF movement since he began to promote the LCHF lifestyle in his medical practice in Karlstad, Sweden. He currently hosts the world's most widely accessed, well-researched and well-referenced LCHF website, Diet Doctor.

Over dinner one evening, I happened to mention that UCT had invited me to debate Professor Jacques Rossouw in its Faculty of Health Sciences Centenary Debate in a few days' time, on 6 December 2012. Eenfeldt immediately asked: 'Do you know that the most important finding from his paper on the Women's Health Initiative is a single sentence hidden deep in the text and not repeated in the abstract?'

I did not know. Eenfeldt pulled out his computer and showed me the evidence. There, on the seventh page of a 12-page article in a 2006 issue of *JAMA* was the key line: 'The HR [hazard ratio] for the 3.4% of women with CVD at baseline was 1.26 (95% CI [confidence interval], 1.03-1.54).'[2]

This means that the women in the trial who had suffered a previous heart attack and who were randomly selected to eat the 'heart-healthy' low-fat diet for the duration of the trial were at a 26 per cent increased (relative) risk of experiencing further heart problems during the eight years of the trial compared with those on the supposedly unhealthy, artery-clogging, higher-fat diet. Although this was the sole significant finding of the diet component of a $700-million study, no one paid any attention. Instead, the authors simply buried it, out of sight, out of mind.

Next, Eenfeldt drew my attention to Figure 3 on the ninth page. 'See here,' he said, 'there's a phrase missing. It's the line identifying the increased risk for women with previous heart disease.' Thus, if you missed the key sentence buried in the article and only looked at this table, you would never know about the study's only significant finding.

Another paper, published in 2011, five years after the original publication, reported that within as little as a year, the condition of those women who started the trial with T2DM and who were randomised to the low-fat diet had worsened. The authors were sufficiently transparent to acknowledge this, for they wrote that 'women with diabetes at baseline did experience adverse glycemic effects of the low-fat diet, which indicated that caution should be exercised in recommending a reduction in overall dietary fat in women with diabetes unless accompanied by additional recommendations to guide carbohydrate intake'.[3]

However, they should have said that their data showed that patients with T2DM should not be treated with a low-fat diet. These adverse effects were reported after only the first year of an eight-year trial. To my knowledge, the final eight-year outcome data for women with T2DM has never been published. If diabetic outcomes worsened after only one year on a low-fat diet, how much worse might those outcomes have been seven years later?

If the Women's Health Initiative trial had been properly designed to detect this adverse outcome, I wondered whether the researchers should have taken women with T2DM off the low-fat diet after the first year of the study. Those women would have presumed that their health would not be allowed to deteriorate as a result of participation in an ethical trial. Of course, terminating that part of the trial would have had major consequences for those who promote the low-fat diet dogma.

Convinced that exposing this new information about the concealed aspects of the Women's Health Initiative study, which Rossouw had directed, would swing the Centenary Debate decisively in my favour, I set about finalising my presentation. I was certain that my UCT colleagues would want to hear the truth.

Clearly, I was still unaware of the power of the omertà.

I have known Rossouw since the 1980s. In those years, I was a peripheral member of a research team under his direction that completed a population intervention trial in three towns in the Western Cape, the so-called Coronary Risk Factor Intervention Study (CORIS). The goal was to determine whether an intensive, hands-on, 'heart-healthy' intervention programme in one town, Robertson, would produce better long-term health outcomes than a less intensive intervention in a second town, Riversdal.

In Riversdal, the sole source of 'heart-healthy' information was what the project organisers sent through the mail. Robertson, the intensive, hands-on town, received the same 'heart-healthy' information focusing on a low-fat diet and physical activity, but also specific interventions to improve blood pressure control, and reduce stress and blood cholesterol concentrations, especially in those at highest risk. A third town, Swellendam, served as the control. Swellendam received only the general health information available to all South Africans at that time through radio, television and the printed press.

Four years later, the researchers returned to measure the effects of the intervention in the different towns. Surprisingly, they found the outcomes were essentially the same in the two intervention towns. In other words, the more intensive programme targeting high-risk individuals in Robertson had not produced any additional benefits than those measured in Riversdal.[4]

Eight years later, a second follow-up found that although the risk-factor profiles had continued to improve in all three towns, the extent of improvements in the low-intervention (Riversdal) and control (Swellendam) towns were greater than in Robertson, the town receiving the most intensive intervention. The authors' final conclusion was that the low-intensity intervention was the most successful.[5]

So, according to the scientifically revered null hypothesis,[*] this study actually proved that a 'heart-healthy', hands-on intervention was no better than simply giving general health advice through the mail, or letting participants educate themselves on the basis of what they hear or read in the media. But how could this possibly be true if the intervention in Robertson was based on the best available, evidence-based medical practices?

An inconvenient conclusion would have been that the 'best' evidence-based medical practices available in 1980 caused harm. However, this was not how Rossouw and his colleagues – including, by association, me – presented the study outcomes. Instead, they concluded that such intervention trials can no longer measure the 'truth', positing a new post-hoc theory:[†] that already by the early 1980s, all the dietary and other information necessary to improve a community's health was freely available in the popular media. Thus, providing yet *more* information, even accompanying an intensive, hands-on approach to those at greatest risk, could not produce a better outcome.

However, objective science does not allow such post-hoc interpretations. That possibility should have been included in the original hypothesis. The original hypothesis was whether or not the intensive intervention programme would improve health outcomes more than doing little or nothing in Riversdal and Swellendam. It did not. According to the null hypothesis, the only scientifically legitimate conclusion was that the intensive intervention – including the

---

[*] No scientist is God, therefore no scientist can ever be certain that s/he has designed the utterly perfect experiment to discover a novel, irrefutable truth. Scientists must assume that the single variable they are studying in their experiments, whatever it may be, will not make any difference to the experimental outcome. We call this the null hypothesis.

[†] Modifying a theory to explain why an expected experimental outcome did not happen is known as post-hoc (after the fact) revision.

promotion of the 'heart-healthy' low-fat diet – failed to make any difference, and might even have caused harm. To admit this conclusion would be to break the omertà. Rather than tell the truth, the researchers chose to invoke the code of silentce.

Importantly, a key focus of the intervention was the promotion of a 'heart-healthy' low-fat diet to lower blood cholesterol concentrations. In these farming communities, which would, at least in the past, have eaten a higher-fat (although not necessarily a lower-carbohydrate) diet, this might have meant quite a large change from their more traditional farmers' diet.

What if the 'heart-healthy' diet had been adopted more widely in Robertson than in the other two towns? And what if this diet produced an adverse outcome that outweighed other health benefits produced by the other interventions promoted exclusively in that town? Interestingly, the diet had little effect on weight in any of the towns, as weight increased over the 12 years in men, but fell marginally in women.[6] Without a change in body mass towards more healthy values, it would be unlikely that long-term health would change significantly in a community at risk from a whole range of IR conditions.

Perhaps the key conclusion from this study was that the 'heart-healthy' low-fat diet had failed to improve the health of the people living in Robertson. Had that lesson been learnt, it might have influenced the planning of the most expensive diet trial ever undertaken, the $700-million Women's Health Initiative Randomized Controlled Dietary Modification Trial (WHIRCDMT) in the US, funded by the National Institutes of Health. It was a study with which Rossouw would soon become intimately involved.

In 1989, shortly after completing the initial phase of the CORIS, Rossouw immigrated to the US and in time became an American citizen. In 1991, he was placed in charge of the WHIRCDMT, an eight-year RCT involving more than 48 000 post-menopausal women. It included elements of the CORIS writ very, very large.

Rossouw's involvement in the study would initially do no harm to his international reputation. In 2006, *Time* magazine named him one of its 100 most influential persons in the world. A special event to acknowledge this achievement was held at UCT in May 2006. His son, Jacques Rousseau, represented him. Rousseau said of his father: 'What drives him is doing his bit to decrease ignorance and confusion, and he'll continue to hold that committed attitude for as long as he's got something useful to say – regardless of whether it's appreciated or not.'

I suspect that the NIH funded the WHIRCDMT specifically to prove that the low-fat diet was the perfect eating plan for all humans. It was an attempt by the US government, through its medical research agency, the NIH, to prove once and for all that the 1977 United States Department of Agriculture (USDA) Dietary Guidelines for Americans, which promote the consumption of cereals and grains, seed (vegetable) oils and, in practice but not by design, high-fructose corn syrup (HFCS), were fully justified.

Enjoying such an unprecedented level of institutional support, senior research-ers involved in the WHIRCDMT, including Rossouw, might reasonably have begun to dream that perhaps even a Nobel Prize was within their grasp.

This then was the man that the UCT Faculty of Health Sciences had lined up as my opponent in the Centenary Debate. They may have assumed that it would not be a close contest; the WHIRCDMT Goliath would not fall to this David, a mere 'sports scientist/general practitioner'.

The topic for the debate was 'Cholesterol is not an important risk factor for heart disease and current dietary recommendations do more harm than good'. I had no input in the choice of topic. My interest is the role of high-carbohydrate diets in causing a constellation of chronic diseases in people with IR, and the reversal of those conditions with carbohydrate restriction.

I opened the debate in a packed lecture theatre. I had recently returned from a lecture trip to the Eastern Cape, where two university audiences had visually and verbally expressed their enjoyment of my lectures. On my home turf, in front of my own faculty, I expected a similar response, even though I knew it was not going to be an easy encounter.

The first surprise came in the week before the debate, when UCT's chosen moderator, Professor Jimmy Volmink, dean of the Faculty of Medicine and Health Sciences at the University of Stellenbosch, asked for a copy of my slides and notes. He needed them, he told me, to prepare his closing remarks. Volmink is also director of the South African Cochrane Centre at the South African Medical Research Council (SAMRC).

At the time, I was unaware that his institute had already been commissioned, ostensibly by the Heart and Stroke Foundation of South Africa (HSFSA), to prepare a meta-analysis of studies of low-carbohydrate diets, of which Volmink turned out to be the senior co-author. The clear goal of that meta-analysis, as I discuss in Chapter 6, was to prove that LCHF diets are of no medical value and are likely very dangerous.

Therefore, already in December 2012, Volmink was not an independent party to this debate. Published in 2014, the study would become known as the Naudé review, named after its first author, Dr Celeste Naudé.[7] The study would play a pivotal role in the HPCSA's decision to charge me with unprofessional conduct. Unfortunately, the study contained many significant errors which, when cor-rected, reversed its conclusions (see Chapter 6).

When I told my wife, Marilyn, about Volmink's request, she was concerned. But how could I not trust Volmink, dean of medicine at such a prestigious university? If you cannot trust a dean who is also a director at the SAMRC, then whom can you trust in the hallowed research halls?

In my lecture, I decided to cover five separate topics:[8]

1. Economic considerations drove the adoption of the current dietary guidelines without proper scientific evaluation or proof.
2. Within five years of widespread adoption of these guidelines, rates of diabetes and obesity increased explosively.
3. The presence of the genetic predisposing condition known as insulin resistance explains why large numbers of people in predisposed populations become obese and diabetic when exposed to a high-carbohydrate diet.
4. A high-fat diet reverses all known coronary risk factors in people with IR, whereas a high-carbohydrate diet worsens those factors.
5. The 48 836-person Woman's Health Initiative study, of which Rossouw was project director, proves that the 1977 USDA dietary guidelines accelerate disease progression in people with either known heart disease or diabetes. Thus, this landmark study provides definitive evidence disproving the diet-heart hypothesis, which Dr Ancel Keys promoted in the US beginning in the 1950s.

For the first 28 minutes of the lecture, I methodically repeated key pieces of evidence on the first four topics as I had previously presented to the faculty in July and in presentations with Eenfeldt and Forslund. This was evidence that, in my opinion, proved that the diet-heart and lipid hypotheses are just hypotheses. Worse, they are mythical, with no substance in fact.

In my judgement, the killer information that would decide the debate was contained in my fifth point. I would argue that the findings of the $700-million WHIRCDMT were definitive proof that the low-fat diet does not reduce the risk of developing heart disease, T2DM or cancer, and that the low-fat diet has no effect in the prevention or reversal of obesity.

The WHIRCDMT had shown that the health of those who were the sickest, because they already had heart disease when the study began, worsened more rapidly if they were placed on the low-fat diet. This is a classic 'canary in the coal mine' finding, for if a diet is dangerous, who will be the first to provide evidence of that 'danger'? Clearly, those who are at the greatest risk, because they already have underlying pathology. In contrast, those who are initially the healthiest may not show any detrimental effects of a bad diet if the trial is too short for the effects to become apparent. We call this a false negative finding; because of a flaw in its experimental design, a study fails to detect a detrimental outcome that is real.

So this iconic study designed to prove the health benefits of the low-fat diet had, in fact, proved the opposite. And the WHIRCDMT is not the sole RCT to have found this. Two additional studies, which have cost US taxpayers hundreds of millions of dollars more, confirmed this finding.[9]

I was certain that after I had presented this evidence, I would be judged the 'winner' of the debate. Surely, I thought, an unbiased UCT audience would recognise that Rossouw himself had provided evidence that his theory was wrong; and that continuing to defend a theory that his own work had disproved was neither academically nor ethically viable.

As I was about to introduce my killer blow, I got the second surprise. Volmink said that my time was up and I should stop talking. I told him that was censorship and simply carried on. Interestingly, a YouTube video of the debate shows that Volmink interrupted me 28 minutes into my presentation, before the 30-minute time limit was up. Later, I learnt that a cadre of medical professors sitting near the front of the lecture theatre was busily exchanging notes that were eventually passed on to Volmink. Were the professors trying to stop me before I reached my fifth point? Was it their decision that Volmink should use the excuse that I had exceeded my time limit?

I hurriedly presented the final, critical pieces of evidence, which included exposing the missing line in Figure 3 of the original WHIRCDMT publication. (Today, more than a decade after its publication, that error has yet to be corrected, even though I drew attention to it in a scientific article in 2013.[10] Rossouw responded,[11] but still failed to address the substantive issues that I had raised.[12])

I ended my lecture by showing the reluctance of Rossouw and his employer, the NIH, to acknowledge the gravity of their negative finding and to admit that, according to the null hypothesis, the WHIRCDMT disproved the diet-heart hypothesis.* I included reference to what was said at the NIH press conference to announce the (disappointing) results of the trial.

There, cardiologist Dr Elizabeth Nabel, the director of the funding body, the National Heart, Lung, and Blood Institute, had said: 'The results of this study do not change established recommendations on disease prevention. Women should continue to ... work with their doctors to reduce their risks for heart disease including following a diet low in saturated fat, trans fat and cholesterol.'

Her employee, Rossouw, added: 'This study shows that just reducing total fat

---

* The null hypothesis in the WHIRCDMT was that eating a low-fat diet would not produce a different outcome than would eating a higher-fat diet. When this was indeed found, the authors should have concluded that their experiment proved that the low-fat diet does not prevent heart disease. But they did not. Instead, they produced a series of post-hoc modifications to explain why their low-fat diet intervention did not work. One post-hoc revision was to conclude that the subjects did not modify their diets sufficiently and, as a result, their blood cholesterol levels did not drop enough to produce a favourable reduction in adverse heart outcomes. But that supposition can only be true if the authors implicitly believe that cholesterol-lowering reduces heart-attack risk – the very question they were studying. If they were so convinced that their theory was correct, why did they need to spend $700 million to prove their bias? Furthermore, $700 million should have been enough to ensure that the study was properly conducted.

intake does not go far enough to have an impact on heart disease risk. While the participants' overall change in LDL "bad" cholesterol was small, we saw trends towards greater reductions in cholesterol and heart disease risk in women eating less saturated and trans fat.'

In my judgement, I had exposed the key paradox in the Centenary Debate: UCT had chosen the one scientist in the world who had participated in two studies costing hundreds of millions of dollars, and which proved that the low-fat diet is without long-term health benefits and could, in fact, be harmful, to present the opposite argument. How had an institution publicly committed to academic excellence and the search for truth allowed this to happen?

Having exposed the true findings of the WHIRCDMT and the reluctance of both the NIH and Rossouw to report those findings transparently, I was certain that my approach would win the day.

Rossouw began his reply by saying that the error Eenfeldt and I had identified in Figure 3 was clearly a 'printer's error'. He failed to explain why he had yet to direct *JAMA* to correct it. He then started to make his case using the diversionary technique of information overload. My talk, he insinuated, was purely about entertainment; his talk, he promised, would be exclusively about hard science.

The main evidence he presented was secular trends[*] in (declining) heart-disease rates in several countries, including Finland, Poland, northern Sweden, the US, England and Wales. These trends, he implied, proved that the recent adoption of the low-fat diet in those countries was effectively preventing the development of arterial disease in their populations. He believed so strongly in the value of this evidence that after the debate he stated: 'Why mess with success?'

Well, let's consider how other experts without a personal stake in the diet debate interpret the published evidence that Rossouw presented.

One study, quoted by Rossouw in both the debate and a subsequent publication,[13] showed falling heart-attack rates in England and Wales. The authors estimated that about 50 per cent of this reduction was due to smoking avoidance and 40 per cent to improved medical care.[14] At best, dietary change could only explain a maximum of 10 per cent, not the 100 per cent Rossouw implies in his presentations and publications.

The key point is that these secular trends do not constitute definitive proof, because so many variables are changing at the same time; that is why we prefer evidence from RCTs such as the WHIRCDMT, the Multiple Risk Factor Intervention Trial and the Look AHEAD trial, all of which, as Rossouw well knows, disprove absolutely the diet-heart hypothesis.

---

[*] A long-term trend that develops or progresses over many years.

If Rossouw had ever been my student, he would have heard me frequently quote Albert Einstein: 'No amount of experimentation can ever prove me right; a single experiment can prove me wrong.' If you focus on secular trends in heart disease, you cannot ignore the 'Japanese paradox': whereas in Australia, Canada, France, Sweden, the UK and the USA the continuing fall in CHD mortality has been associated with falling blood cholesterol concentrations, the opposite has occurred in Japan. As a result, CHD mortality is 67–75 per cent lower in Japanese men and women than in American men and women, despite higher blood cholesterol concentrations in the Japanese. The authors say that this observation 'may suggest some protective factors unique to Japanese'.[15] What if that factor is nutritional?

This change has occurred as Japanese people of all ages have reduced the amount of carbohydrate in their diets, replacing it with fat, especially from animal sources, but also from vegetables.[16] The point is that for a theory to be true, it must explain *all* observations, not only those that can be cherry-picked to favour one's personal scientific bias.

Rossouw also omitted to mention other evidence from Japan showing that Japanese with low blood cholesterol levels are at increased risk of mortality from stroke, heart disease and cancer.[17] Furthermore, higher intakes of saturated fat appear to be particularly beneficial in the prevention of stroke in East Asians,[18] another finding Rossouw conveniently ignored.

In touting the great successes in reversing CHD in the North Karelia province of Finland – an unusual population that suffered the unimaginable stresses of relocation following the Russo-Finnish Winter War of 1939–1940 – Rossouw conveniently failed to discuss the inconvenient finding from the Finnish province of Kuopio. As Rossouw tells it, Finns living in North Karelia have the highest CHD mortality of all Finns, assumed to be due to their high rates of smoking, hypercholesterolaemia and hypertension. Conveniently ignored is the fact that virtually the entire population of East Finland – 400 000 people, including those living in North Karelia – was displaced in 1940 during the Second World War, when Russia took control of Karelia. It seems rather more likely that the much higher rates of heart disease in East Finland compared to West Finland, despite similar intakes of fat and saturated fat, were a direct result of the Russian invasion during the war, which directly affected those living in the east of Finland, including North Karelia.

In 1972, a community-wide intervention was introduced to reduce these three risk factors – much like CORIS – and the outcome in North Karelia was compared to the neighbouring province of Kuopio, in which CHD mortality rates were equally high, but in which there was no intervention.[19]

Five years later, the decline in total and CHD mortality in both men and women was identical in North Karelia and Kuopio, even though the prevalence of the conventional CHD risk factors had initially fallen much more in North Karelia than in Kuopio.[20] In particular, there was no change in the average number of cigarettes smoked per day, no change in blood cholesterol concentrations and no change in mean blood pressure in those living in Kuopio. Even more difficult to explain was the finding that in both Kuopio and North Karelia, women showed a much greater reduction in CHD mortality than did men, even though the reduction in risk factors in women was generally negligible or non-existent.[21]

Interestingly, as the project continued, the authors combined the results from Kuopio and North Karelia as if both provinces were always part of the original intervention. In that way, an inconvenient truth could be conveniently hidden.

This study, quoted by Rossouw as evidence for the benefits of an intervention that reverses coronary risk factors, like his WHIRCDMT, failed to prove his contention, because CHD and total mortality fell in both men and women in North Karelia and in Kuopio, whether or not coronary risk factors were reduced by an expensive intervention aimed especially at lowering blood cholesterol concentrations.

Nor was Rossouw prepared to discuss the 'Sami paradox'. Specifically, the finding that the Sami reindeer herders living in the northernmost regions of Finland and who, like the Masai and Sambouri, live exclusively on animal products, have exceptionally low rates of CHD, despite blood cholesterol concentrations greater than 6.5 mmol/L, way above values considered to be 'safe'.[22] 'Our current knowledge of cardiovascular risk factors cannot explain the low mortality from IHD [ischaemic heart disease] in the Sami district of Finland,' the authors of one study concluded.[23] Interestingly, reindeer meat is high in the antioxidants selenium and alpha-Tocopherol, and the monounsaturated fat oleic acid.

Rossouw was also not brave enough to mention the Roseto Paradox.[24] Roseto was an exclusively Italian-American town in eastern Pennsylvania with, in the early 1960s, 'a remarkably low rate of coronary heart disease among the living, despite the fact that the conventional risk factors were found to be at least as prevalent in Roseto as in the two control communities'[25] and that 'Rosetans eat at least as much animal fat as the average American'.[26] Thus:

> The oil intake of the Rosetans was relatively low in olive oil. They used a great deal more lard than the wives of the people in this room use. One of their favorite dishes was fried peppers. They would fry the peppers in lard and they are very good. Then you'd take a piece of Italian bread and rub it around in the gravy that is left and eat that and that's delicious! The Rosetans were very poor when they came and they are much more prosperous now. They eat everything. I've had many dinners with Rosetan families. They usually have more than one type of meat. When I eat ham I cut the rim of fat off and don't eat it, same way with roast beef. They cut right through and eat it

all. We were very elaborate in our study of their diet because we had Ancel Keyes [sic] breathing down our necks.[27]

Heart-disease rates and mortality rose over the next 25 years as the population began to move away from its traditional (Mediterranean) 'values of southern Italian villagers'. This included dietary changes that 'occurred ... in the direction of what the American Heart Association calls "prudent". There was less consumption of animal fat.'[28]

The authors made two substantive conclusions. First, that the lower rates of heart disease in Roseto in the 1960s were due to the 'greater social solidarity and homogeneity in Roseto', without any evidence that coronary risk factors were lower than in those living in the neighbouring communities with higher heart-disease mortality rates.[29] Second, that social change over the next 50 years produced the 'sharply increased rates of heart attack amongst men under the age of 65'.[30] This change was not prevented by an increased adoption of the AHA 'prudent' diet with a reduction in saturated-fat intake.

Rossouw's attempt to explain any and all secular changes in heart-disease mortality rates simply on the basis of reduction in saturated-fat intake is simplistic, indeed opportunistic, in the extreme.

He also failed to discuss the other extreme, the 'Israeli paradox'. Israel has replaced dietary saturated fat with higher intakes of omega-6 polyunsaturated fats from vegetable oils so that intakes are 8 per cent higher than in the US and 10–12 per cent higher than in European countries. Israelis suffer from high rates of CHD, hypertension, T2DM and obesity – all markers of IR. Cancer mortality rates are also high, especially in women. The authors of a study looking into the Israeli paradox wondered whether 'rather than being beneficial, high omega-6 polyunsaturated fat diets may have some long-term side effects, within the cluster of hyperinsulinemia, atherosclerosis and tumorigenesis'.[31] I return to this in Chapter 7.

Clearly, proponents of low-fat diets have simply ignored the evidence for the potentially harmful effects of high omega-6 polyunsaturated-fat intake.

Rossouw also ignored a serious concern noted by most of the authors of these studies: that although heart-attack rates may have fallen in some countries since the adoption of his 'heart-healthy' diet, obesity and T2DM rates are rising in those same countries.

This brings us to the bigger paradox, which I had yet to identify in December 2012. In all the countries in which heart-attack rates are (or were) falling, the incidence of T2DM is increasing at an exponential rate, as is obesity. But we know that diabetes (by itself or as part of the metabolic syndrome) is the single best predictor of heart-attack risk. There is also the evidence that life expectancy in the US has now reached its peak and will likely decline by the mid-21st century.[32]

So how can diabetes rates and the prevalence of metabolic syndrome be rising at the same time that heart-attack rates are falling? It makes no sense.

The answer, which may be relatively simple, provides the crucial missing evidence that finally proves just how damaging the low-fat, 'heart-healthy' diet advocated by Rossouw and others is. The key insight comes from understanding how cigarette-smoking causes heart attack.

Rate of cigarette consumption is the single variable that best tracks US heart-attack rates, including the sudden rise after the First World War and the equally dramatic fall beginning in the 1960s (Figure 4.1). This, too, is paradoxical, because we 'know' that arterial disease is a slowly developing disease, occurring over decades.

Figure 4.1

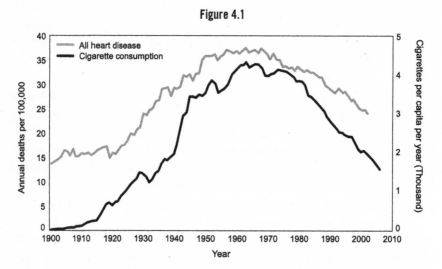

The annual number of deaths from CHD in the US began to rise shortly after the end of the First World War. The rise and subsequent fall in heart disease precisely tracks the rise and fall of cigarette consumption in the US. (Data from US National Vital Statistics)

So how does a change in cigarette consumption produce fairly rapid changes in heart-attack rates if smoking is the direct cause of arterial disease? The answer is that arterial disease – popularly called 'clogging of the coronary arteries', but known medically as the development of arterial plaque – is not the immediate cause of a heart attack. Rather, it is when the plaque itself becomes unstable and suddenly ruptures (acute plaque rupture) that a heart attack (or sudden death) occurs.

Interestingly, the size and extent of any particular arterial plaque does not determine whether or not it will rupture. Small or large arterial plaques seem to have pretty much the same propensity to rupture, which is why coronary bypass grafting or the placement of a stent in a narrowed coronary artery does not guarantee immunity from future heart attacks (see Chapter 3).

So, if heart-attack rates track changes in population smoking rates without a significant time delay (of decades), then smoking must be acting on plaque stability rather than on the long-term development of arterial plaque.

Interestingly, there is one study of the diet-heart hypothesis that showed a dramatic effect in reducing heart-attack rates in those with established heart disease. The effect was so rapid that it can only have been due to plaque stabilisation, not removal of the underlying atherosclerosis.

In the Lyon Diet Heart Study (Figure 4.2), survival was already superior within the first six months in the group fortunate enough to be randomised to eat the 'Mediterranean alpha-linolenic acid-rich diet', compared to the standard low-fat, 'heart-healthy prudent diet' promoted by Rossouw, the NIH and the American Heart Association (AHA).

Figure 4.2

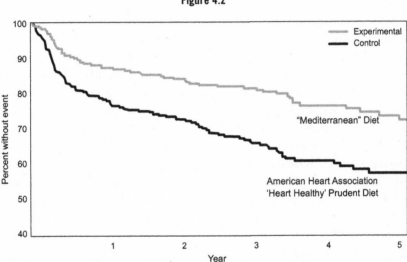

Survival curves after first heart attack in persons randomised to either a 'Mediterranean alpha-linolenic acid-rich diet' or the standard AHA 'heart-healthy prudent diet'. Note that survival is significantly worse in those eating the AHA heart-healthy diet, and that differences in survival on the different diets is already apparent within the first six months on either diet. Redrawn from de Lorgeril *et al.*[33]

There are two reasons why Rossouw and most of his cardiology colleagues must ignore this study.[*] First, it shows that the AHA 'heart-healthy prudent diet' is

---

[*] Incensed by this patronising attitude of scientific denialism, the senior author of the Lyon Diet Heart Study, Dr Michel de Lorgeril, wrote a book, *Cholesterol and Statins: Sham Science and Bad Medicine* (2014; ebook, Thierry Souccar Publishing), expressing his disgust. He is also the author of a number of publications in the scientific literature addressing the absence of proven benefits of statin drugs. Clearly he also qualifies for the title 'Cholesterol Denialist'.

not particularly effective in preventing a second heart attack in those who have survived a first. Second, and much more importantly, the dramatic superiority in survival in those eating the Mediterranean diet could not be explained by lower blood cholesterol concentrations, which were identical in both groups. Superior survival on the Mediterranean diet is, therefore, not due to greater reductions in blood cholesterol concentrations, as Rossouw's model of heart disease demands. So this study provides another paradox that Rossouw seems unwilling to address.

Although T2DM is clearly a major cause of unstable arterial plaque[34] (because it is the best predictor of acute heart-attack risk), the real disease burden of T2DM is the widespread occlusive arterial disease that it causes. This is a progressive, more lethal form of arterial disease that leads to the complete obstruction of flow in the arteries supplying blood to the kidneys (causing kidney failure), the eyes (causing blindness) and the limbs (causing gangrene, requiring amputation), among other organs.

As heart-attack rates have fallen subsequent to the introduction of the low-fat, 'heart-healthy' diet in 1977, low-fat-diet exponents such as Rossouw will have us believe that their diet miraculously prevents *all* arterial disease. To reach this conclusion, they have to ensure that neither doctors, dietitians nor the public notice the elephant in the room: the exponential increase in the incidence of occlusive arterial disease in those with diabetes, the pathology that will ultimately bankrupt all medical services globally.

They are able to do this because the medical profession and pharmaceutical industry present T2DM as a disease principally of abnormal glucose metabolism – causing blood glucose levels that are either too high or too low. In reality, T2DM is a disease of progressive occlusive arterial disease, with catastrophic consequences.

This deception successfully hides the fact that T2DM is by far the worst form of arterial disease. And no one asks: If the low-fat diet prevents arterial disease in the heart vessels, why does it not prevent the form of occlusive arterial disease present at other sites in patients with diabetes? As rates of diabetic arterial disease have increased exponentially since the 1977 low-fat, 'heart-healthy' dietary guidelines were introduced, we must conclude that those guidelines are not preventing this form of arterial disease. In fact, an even more likely conclusion is that the 1977 guidelines are the direct cause of the most prevalent form of arterial disease – that which is present in those with IR and T2DM.

So effective is the industry-directed misinformation campaign that it seems to have become my profession's primary goal to focus obsessively on the risk that our patients will develop heart attacks. What we should really be concerned about is their risk of developing T2DM, the major cause of the most severe form of arterial disease. If we genuinely want to prevent the arterial disease of T2DM, we must understand, as I detail in Chapter 17, that it is the excessive intake of dietary carbohydrates, not dietary fat, in those with IR which causes the progressive, widespread, occlusive arterial disease common in diabetes.

In December 2012, unfortunately, I was still unaware of this key evidence that irrefutably destroys Rossouw's arguments in support of low-fat diets.

Interestingly, in the article he wrote three years after the Centenary Debate, Rossouw seemed to have mellowed on the dangers of LCHF diets:

> It appears that no particular dietary pattern for weight reduction is superior to another. Individual preference determines whether or not to employ a low-fat, high-complex carbohydrate diet; or a low-carbohydrate, high-fat diet, or a diet somewhere in between, provided that the diet also limits energy intake. **There is a general agreement that refined carbohydrates, starches and sugars need to be limited, or even eliminated,** in diets for weight reduction [my emphasis].[35]

The problem with this conclusion is that it conflicts with the evidence from Rossouw's own study, the WHIRCDMT. That study found that postmenopausal women eating Rossouw's favoured low-fat US Dietary Guidelines for Americans 'prudent' diet gained more weight during the study regardless of whether they began the trial with a normal weight, or if they were overweight or obese. The opposite occurred on the low-carbohydrate diet. The authors concluded: 'These findings suggest that a low-fat diet may promote weight gain whereas a reduced-carbohydrate diet may decrease risk of postmenopausal weight gain.'[36]

As a result: 'Consuming a reduced-carbohydrate diet, with moderate fat and high protein intake, may decrease the risk of weight gain in postmenopausal women. **However, prevailing dietary recommendations call for limiting fat intake in order to promote optimal health and prevent chronic disease. Our findings therefore challenge prevailing dietary recommendations, suggesting instead that a low-fat (diet) may promote rather than prevent weight gain after menopause** [my emphasis].'[37]

Can it be that the other authors of the WHIRCDMT may finally be dissociating themselves from the scientifically unsubstantiated opinions of the now retired Rossouw?

His current dietary advice differs from the LCHF eating plan only in that he advises people to eat more wholegrains (whatever those are), fruit, legumes, vegetable oils and low-fat dairy products, and to limit the intake of red meat, especially processed meats.

At the end of the debate and in a speech carefully prepared even before he had heard the debate, Volmink concluded the evening, in the words of one columnist present in the audience, 'by insinuating that Noakes was essentially a "bulls!#&er"'.[38]

To be fair to Volmink, he did not specifically single me out, but some may have interpreted what he said and the way he said it to indicate that I was his target. He suggested that we need reliable research evidence, which the following do not constitute:

- Wild extrapolations from laboratory bench data;
- Reckless claims from observational studies;
- Cherry-picked studies;
- Anecdotal stories; and
- 'Bullshit' provided by people with no interest in the truth and who are simply trying to impress us. They 'make it all up'.

He concluded by saying that he had 'heard nothing this evening that convinces me that we are on the wrong path in terms of these dietary guidelines', and 'at all costs we must not do harm'. Furthermore, Volmink appeared wilfully oblivious to the implications of the fact that Rossouw's WHIRCDMT has provided definitive evidence that a low-fat diet is without benefit and may even be harmful. And that the medical faculty of which he is dean serves a community that is at the epicentre of the South African obesity/T2DM epidemic, caused, in my opinion, by the 'do no harm' low-fat diet that his friend Rossouw continues unrestrainedly to promote.

So if this debate was not about the truth, then what was it really all about? This would become apparent over the next four years, culminating in the HPCSA hearing against me that began in June 2015.

After the debate, I was interviewed by medical science writer Chris Bateman, who also asked Rossouw and two other UCT-linked professors, Krisela Steyn and Naomi Levitt, for their opinions. The responses were published in the February 2013 issue of the *South African Medical Journal* (*SAMJ*).[39] For what was supposed to be an academic debate, the professorial responses seemed remarkably un-academic, and rather too personal, setting the tone for what would become the norm over the next five years.

According to Rossouw, my first error was to overstate the importance of carbohydrate intolerance (insulin resistance), because so few in the world suffer from it. 'The biggest divergence is that Rossouw says he can show that the proportion of truly carbohydrate-intolerant people runs to about six per cent,' wrote Bateman. 'Noakes claims it's at least ten times this.'

But what are the real facts?

In 2012, the American Diabetes Association (ADA) reported that of the US population of 313 million, 9.3 per cent (29.1 million) had T2DM and another 27 per cent (86 million) had pre-diabetes.[40] Thus, in 2012, 34 per cent of the US population had been diagnosed with IR, an incidence nearly six times greater than Rossouw is prepared to acknowledge. Note that this includes only those who were diagnosed because they presented with symptoms caused by their IR.

In fact, the incidence of pre-diabetic US citizens will be much greater than 86 million, because no one has yet performed proper testing for IR in a sizeable proportion of that population. This requires measurement of fasting blood glucose and insulin concentrations, at the very least.

To properly diagnose IR, one needs to measure changes in blood insulin and glucose concentrations for two to five hours after the ingestion of 100 grams of glucose, as first described by Joseph Kraft.[41] He showed that 75 per cent of 4 030 subjects who had normal glucose tolerance by conventional criteria showed an inappropriate hyperinsulinaemic response,[42] indicating that they were insulin resistant, but that their IR was 'hidden' if only their glucose response to glucose ingestion was tested.[*] These included 117 children aged 3–13 years, 45 per cent of whom had normal glucose profiles but who were hyperinsulinaemic, and 651 teenagers aged 14–20 years, 67 per cent of whom had normal glucose tolerance but who were also hyperinsulinaemic.

Other evidence that the rates of IR must be much higher than Rossouw's 6 per cent is provided by US obesity statistics. Currently, more than 69 per cent of US adults are considered to be overweight or obese, with rates continuing to rise precipitously.[43] The majority of those who are overweight or obese will be insulin resistant.[44]

My opinion is that, at the very least, 60 per cent of US citizens are likely to be insulin resistant according to Kraft's definitions.

Rossouw's response reveals that one of the most senior scientists in the NIH – a man in whom the NIH was prepared to entrust $700 million for the WHIRCDMT study – apparently has neither any reasonable knowledge of nor particular interest in the condition of IR. Fifty years of medical education have seemingly not taught him about the single most important global medical condition.

Or is it simply that the omertà prevents him from acknowledging that IR exists? For once he and his colleagues acknowledge its existence, they have to acknowledge the dangers of sugar and carbohydrates, the value of a low-carbohydrate diet and the intellectual poverty of the diet-heart hypothesis. They have to break the omertà.

As they also cannot acknowledge that IR, and not cholesterol, is the underlying

---

[*] If one measures only blood glucose concentrations to identify people with IR, it will be impossible to detect those who require elevated blood insulin concentrations (hyperinsulinaemia) to maintain normal blood glucose concentrations, because they are already insulin resistant. This is stage 1 IR/pre-diabetes. Stage 2 is when both blood glucose and insulin concentrations are elevated both when fasting and after eating. In stage 3, the IR is so severe that blood glucose concentrations rise to 8–9 mmol/L, causing glucose to appear in the urine. This is T2DM as traditionally described.

cause of arterial disease, it is understandable why Rossouw and his colleagues chose to go the personal ad hominem route rather than address the science I had presented. They simply had no valid counter-argument. Instead, they chose to shoot the messenger in a way that even the HPCSA specifically forbids. In fact, the HPCSA's rules on how doctors should interact in public are clear:

Healthcare practitioners should:
- Refrain from speaking ill of colleagues or other healthcare practitioners.
- Not make a patient doubt the knowledge or skills of colleagues by making comments about them that cannot be justified.

What these three colleagues allowed to be published in the *SAMJ* clearly breached that rule. Rossouw told Bateman:

> I think Tim got diabetes because he was obese. God forbid one of these days that he may have to take medicines made by the evil pharmas – he's a good scientist in his field, but he's way outside of his field and comfort zone here. He doesn't understand the science and the whole concept. He's cherry picked and misinterpreted and is going down a very dangerous path. Applying dietetic measures, he's doing harm and flouting the Hippocratic oath.

The article continues:

> [Rossouw] said the debate on lowering cholesterol with statins ... had been 'dead for 20 years'. There was now 'absolute proof' that cholesterol was causal in heart disease. 'Most of the people he cites are zombies from that era and they've been left behind by science. The more Krisela [Steyn] told me about this, the more concerned I became. Noakes' theory had the potential to divert people from diets and treatments that were known to do good. Were I still a faculty member I'd be very concerned about this member undoing a lot of good work done in heart disease prevention. If Noakes came up against anyone in this field he would get the same reception he got at his "faculty meeting" [the Centenary Debate]. His perception is he was set up to be discredited. But he's in the scientific world and his theories have no standing. Any diet that is calorie and energy restricted will reduce weight. They all work ... for some people the approach he advocates may work better. I have no problem with that, but when you generalise and say everyone should be on the diet permanently, eat your fats and no carbs, that's not right, especially when there are no long-term data on that, while there are data on the conventional diet. Why mess with success? I think five years from now we'll be able to stand back and say where we are ... and the public will have stopped

paying attention. I regard this a temporary aberration. Advocating it for wider health promotion will not stand the test of time.'

Yet, in truth, it is Rossouw who is cherry-picking the data, misrepresenting the facts and 'flouting the Hippocratic oath'. Having spent $700 million of US tax-payers' money disproving the diet-heart hypothesis, he still travels the world promoting the opposite of what that study found. I doubt that Hippocrates would have condoned this behaviour.

Particularly interesting is Rossouw's assertion that there is now 'absolute proof' that cholesterol is 'causal in heart disease'. As I show in Chapter 17, this is utterly unfounded. I would also refer Rossouw to the article by Robert DuBroff referenced in Chapter 3, which concludes that the evidence is now overwhelming that lowering blood cholesterol concentrations through diet or drugs 'does not significantly prolong life or consistently prevent coronary heart disease'.[45] All this evidence contradicts Rossouw's reference to the 'zombies' who disagree with the diet-heart hypothesis and his assertion that the diet I promote has no standing in the 'scientific world'. More telling is his opinion that in five years' time, 'the public will have stopped paying attention'.

At the time of this book's publication, exactly five years since Rossouw made his prediction, it is the diet-heart hypothesis that is in terminal decline. The public, at least in South Africa, cannot get enough information about Banting. Five years later, and the 'revolution' Rossouw spent so much effort trying to suppress has exploded into the mainstream,[*] while interest in his low-fat, 'heart-healthy' prudent diet lessens by the day.

Next up in Bateman's article was Professor Krisela Steyn, associate director of a multi-university collaboration called the Chronic Disease Initiative for Africa. Under her watch, the prevalence of chronic diseases, especially T2DM, in her home province of the Western Cape, has increased exponentially. Clearly, whatever research and interventions she has initiated have not produced any positive outcomes. Speaking to Batemen about me, she said: 'Damage is being done here. He's radically oversimplified things.'

Bateman continues:

[Steyn] said it was 'sad' when a good scientist wandered off his area of exper-tise. 'He's lost the plot a little – he's not basing all his public statements on the

---

[*] Prior to the publication of *The Real Meal Revolution* in November 2013, the term Banting was essentially unknown in South Africa. Today the word appears in the South African Afrikaans dictionary. The 'Banting 7 Day Meal Plans' Facebook page, begun in Cape Town in 2014, now has more than 800 000 members and grows by a minimum of 2 000 new members each day. It has more Facebook members than any South African political party. A similar Banting/low-carb Facebook page in Nigeria has more than 1 million members.

best available data. Yes, he's right to question any scientific statement of any type, but please bring the good data.' Steyn said she hoped the charismatic Noakes, whose bona fides she does not question, had a good diabetologist looking after him. 'He's entitled to punt something he totally believes in. But what's scary is that he's damaging patients and the population by insisting on this diet for life, regardless of the cost. My overwhelming emotion is sadness that a person of his stature has made this mistake.' She cited Linus Pauling, the Nobel Prize winner for chemistry, 'going on a tirade about vitamin C curing the common cold', when it was shown that at best it might reduce the duration of the common cold. 'Then we had Mbeki. The question is how does one get there? If you don't deal with the academic data, a person with public standing can do a tremendous amount of harm.' She said the worst time to 'go to the public with health guidelines' was when academics were still debating the truth for a position. 'You go to the public when you have irrefutable evidence that this is the right thing to do.'

Let's dissect her statements, specifically the latter ones. First, both Linus Pauling and former president Thabo Mbeki promoted hypotheses for which there was no firm evidence or plausible biological explanation. For all we know, Pauling may still turn out to be right. If we have yet to grasp the reasoning behind his hypothesis, it is perhaps because we lack the double Nobel Prize winner's extraordinary grasp of biochemistry and molecular biology. I have learnt not to dismiss the ideas of genius simply because there is not yet a plausible explanation.

In contrast, there is a large body of peer-reviewed evidence, including Rossouw's WHIRCDMT, that actually disproves the diet-heart hypothesis. There is also a wealth of evidence showing the value of low-carbohydrate diets. If Steyn is unaware of the evidence, it is because of her unwillingness to break the omertà and to engage with the published literature. This is allied, perhaps, with a reluctance to acknowledge that what she believes and has taught two generations of students is wrong.

Second, Steyn herself has repeatedly over the past four decades 'gone to the public' with her 'irrefutable evidence' allegedly proving the diet-heart hypothesis, the alleged value of substituting polyunsaturated vegetable oils for dietary saturated fat, and her belief that a low salt intake is essential to prevent high blood pressure. Unfortunately, there is no such 'irrefutable evidence' for any of these claims.

For example, a recent analysis concludes that whereas a high sodium intake is associated with increased risk of cardiovascular events (heart attack and stroke) and death in people with hypertension,[46] there is no such association in those with normal blood pressures. Furthermore, the same study found that low sodium intakes are associated with increased risk for cardiovascular events and death; a finding also reported in five other studies.[47] In other words, advocating a low-salt diet could be causing harm.[48]

Then there is a new study showing that almost everything we understand about human salt metabolism is wrong. This research was stimulated by the observation that increased dietary salt intake reduced fluid intake, the precise opposite of what we have been taught for decades. Instead, this study found that the 'kidneys, liver and skeletal muscle form a physiological-regulatory network' to control the amount of fluid the body retains.[49] The point is that a high salt intake produces metabolic changes in the liver and skeletal muscles that no one ever predicted; these changes do not cause body water content to increase – the popular explanation of how a high salt diet supposedly causes blood pressure to rise.

Since this is to some extent the opposite of what we predicted, and if salt does not raise the blood pressure causing hypertension, perhaps now is the time to begin a proper evaluation of whether we need to either reduce or increase our dietary salt intakes. For example, there is more than enough evidence to show that hypertension is a condition caused by diets high in sugar and carbohydrates in those with IR,[50] so that by targeting salt rather than sugar we have focused on the wrong 'white crystals'.[51]

Will these latest findings lead Steyn to question the wisdom of her decades-long crusade advocating low salt intakes by all South Africans according to the principle of 'first do no harm'?[52] Or will she continue to support what appears to be an industry-directed omertà?*

I invited US science journalist Nina Teicholz and UK obesity researcher Dr Zoë Harcombe – the two people who have provided the most complete bodies of evidence disproving the diet-heart dogma – to provide expert witness on my behalf at my HPCSA hearing in October 2016 (see Chapter 13). Steyn did not avail herself of the opportunity to hear these two world authorities in person, but I hope that she is now aware that her 'irrefutable evidence' for the diet-heart hypothesis is nonsense and that she will reconsider her statements. She should ask herself whether the diet she promotes could actually be the cause of the growing ill health of the communities she is employed to serve.

The last to invoke the omertà for Bateman's report was Professor Naomi 'Dinky' Levitt, head of endocrinology and diabetic medicine at UCT and co-director with Steyn of the Chronic Disease Initiative for Africa. I graduated

---

* The Salt Watch, which drives the low-salt movement in South Africa, lists the following as its funders and partners: HSFSA, North-West University, Nutrition Society of South Africa (NSSA), ADSA, Consumer Goods Council of South Africa, SAMRC, University of Pretoria, Unilever, PepsiCo, Tiger Brands, and 'retailers and other industry partners'. Among the latter, perhaps too shy to acknowledge their support, are Kellogg's and the South African Sugar Association (SASA). Focusing on salt as the cause of hypertension is especially attractive if it removes any potential inquiry into the effects of sugar as the far more likely cause of hypertension, especially in those with IR.

from UCT as a doctor a year ahead of Levitt, and we received our subsequent MD degrees at the same graduation ceremony in 1981.

I often wonder if Levitt thinks back to those years when T2DM was relatively uncommon in the Western Cape. Today, it is the most common cause of mortality in the province. I also wonder if she ever asks herself whether she played any part in this human disaster and if she could have done things differently. Could she, the professor of endocrinology and diabetes at a premier medical institution in the Western Cape, have slowed the growth of the T2DM epidemic in the province, then in South Africa and, perhaps, even the world?

Or is T2DM, as she teaches her students, a disease of inevitability from which there is no escape; that will require patients to inject insulin or take drugs for the rest of their lives; and which progresses inevitably to death from disseminated obstructive arterial disease, as was my father's experience, regardless of our best medical efforts? Given this 'inevitability', what is a professor meant to do other than criticise anyone who ignores the omertà and proposes that perhaps T2DM does not have to be an 'inevitable' disease with unavoidable, fatal consequences.

In the article, Levitt[*] described me as 'irresponsible', saying:

> I think Rossouw showed him up based on science and Tim's rather super-ficial understanding of epidemiology. [The debate] highlighted his lack of appreciation of the complexities of fat metabolism. You'd expect better of Tim. He has a good reputation, so this is extremely dangerous.

Perhaps unsurprisingly, Levitt, like Rossouw and Steyn, failed to address the evidence I had presented and the manner in which it disproves cherished dogmas. Clearly, she had not listened to a single word I had said.

Bateman's *SAMJ* report ended with the statement that, according to Steyn and Levitt, the Cochrane Centre, under the direction of Volmink, would be releasing a review of all existing data on the subject by the end of February 2013. Eventually published in July 2014, this meta-analysis of 'low-carbohydrate' RCTs would become known as the Stellenbosch or Naudé review, which would play a central role in the HPCSA's September 2014 decision to prosecute me.

As will become apparent, the Naudé review and Volmink's confident statement concluding the Centenary Debate are evidence linking these four professors (Rossouw, Volmink, Steyn and Levitt), the debate, and senior colleagues in the UCT and Stellenbosch medical faculties to the sequence of actions that culminated in the HPCSA hearing against me.

---

[*] In 2004, the College of Physicians granted Levitt fellowship of the college by 'peer review', which is highly unusual, and in what appears to have been an exclusive arrangement for the college. Acceptance into the college is usually achieved only after an onerous training and examination process.

Surprisingly, on 24 January 2013, I received a personally signed letter from Levitt and Steyn thanking me for making the debate 'a very good evening of academia'. They continued: 'The standard you set was very high and extremely important in South Africa at this point in time.' However, these words were contradicted a week later with the publication of Bateman's *SAMJ* report on the debate. I still had much to learn about the spiritual and ethical darkness into which my profession had descended in the past four decades.

'Experts warn against the Noakes diet'. Under this headline, published within 10 weeks of the Centenary Debate, *Health24* carried an article in which UCT Faculty of Health Sciences professor of medicine (now dean) and Volmink's long-time friend Bongani Mayosi stated: 'There will be no change in how students at UCT are taught about the risk factors for heart disease. It is clear to me that the diet-heart hypothesis is alive and well and we do not see any reason to change what we teach our students about the link between an unhealthy diet, high blood cholesterol and heart disease.'[53]

Importantly, in a 2012 scientific publication, Mayosi had written that 'Ancel Keys proved unequivocally that cholesterol causes heart disease'.[54] Actually, Keys never proved anything of the sort. He could not, since most of his best-known studies are simple associational studies (see Chapter 17) that cannot prove causation. Worse, it appears that Keys may have resorted to dubious methods to 'prove' his associations.[55] To provide definitive proof that cholesterol causes heart disease requires, as Mayosi should know, rather more complex science. So complex, in fact, that a causal link between cholesterol and heart disease has never been proven.

In fact, Keys should have announced in 1973 already that his diet-heart hypothesis was false. But when he realised that the data from his first proper RCT to test the diet-heart hypothesis – the Minnesota Coronary Experiment (1968–1973), involving 9 423 Minnesotan mental patients[56] – actually disproved it,[57] he may simply have buried the data.[58]

Speaking in 2016, the son of Dr Ivan Frantz, who headed up the Minnesota Coronary Experiment, recalled: 'My father definitely believed in reducing saturated fats, and I grew up that way. We followed a relatively low-fat diet at home, and on Sundays or special occasions, we'd have bacon and eggs ... When it turned out that it [a diet low in saturated fat] didn't reduce risk, it was quite puzzling. And since it was effective in lowering cholesterol, it was weird.'[59]

Steven Broste, who, as a student at the University of Minnesota at the time, had access to all the data for his 1981 master's thesis, suggested to the *Washington Post* that

at least part of the reason for the incomplete publication of the data might have been human nature. The Minnesota investigators had a theory that they believed in – that reducing blood cholesterol would make people healthier … So when the data they collected from the mental patients conflicted with this theory, the scientists may have been reluctant to believe what their experiment had turned up.

'The results flew in the face of what people believed at the time,' said Broste. 'Everyone thought cholesterol was the culprit. This theory was so widely held and so firmly believed – and then it wasn't borne out by the data. The question then became: Was it a bad theory? Or was it bad data? … My perception was they were hung up trying to understand the results.'[60]

Perhaps, like Rossouw, Frantz and Keys also failed to grasp the significance of the null hypothesis.

The truth about the Minnesota study was only exposed in 2016, when the original data was recovered and properly analysed.[61] One of the lead authors of the re-analysis, Daisy Zamora, subsequently stated: 'Had this research been published 40 years ago, it might have changed the trajectory of diet-heart research and recommendations.'[62] Had that happened, it is probable that the 1977 USDA dietary guidelines might never have come into being and the subsequent obesity and diabetes epidemics would have been avoided.

But Mayosi's ringing endorsement of the diet-heart hypothesis in February 2013 would have provided welcome reassurance to the South African pharmaceutical industry. It confirmed that the UCT Faculty of Health Sciences would not be questioning the scientific basis for one of that industry's most lucrative businesses, specifically the prescription of (largely ineffective) statin drugs to lower blood cholesterol concentrations in those believed to be at risk of developing heart disease or stroke.

The same *Health24* article outlined how, in the Centenary Debate, Rossouw had 'presented extensive data collected over many decades that supports the current consensus that blood cholesterol occurs as "good" HDL cholesterol, which protects arteries by removing cholesterol from artery walls, and "bad" LDL cholesterol that carries cholesterol molecules into the artery walls'. Many of us continue to wonder how the same compound can be both good and bad. After all, cholesterol is simply a chemical; it lacks the character to be both good and bad, or indeed either.[*]

The article quotes Rossouw: 'This is true for men and women, people of all

---

[*] Cholesterol is insoluble in water. Thus it does not exist in the bloodstream as cholesterol, but travels within water-soluble fat–protein particles called lipoproteins. Certain of these lipoproteins are associated with CHD, in particular large numbers of small, dense LDL particles, especially when they become oxidised. Using the terms 'good' and 'bad' cholesterol is dated and unhelpful, and fails to explain what is currently known about the true relationship between cholesterol, lipoproteins and CHD.

ages and those with diabetes and after suffering a heart attack. High levels of "bad" cholesterol can be treated with a group of drugs called statins, which reduce heart attacks in people using them.'

I have to ask why Rossouw, who has spent his life studying the non-medical prevention of heart disease and heart attacks, felt compelled to mention the role of statins in lowering blood cholesterol concentrations. If he has spent his life studying the effects of a low-fat diet in preventing heart disease, why not use the example of dietary interventions to prevent heart attack? The obvious answer is that he knows there is no evidence, at least for the low-fat diet he tested in the WHIRCDMT. There is still no published evidence showing that lowering cholesterol with a low-fat diet reduces heart-attack risk, or anything else for that matter. Instead, replacing dietary saturated fat with manufactured polyunsaturated fat either has no effect or impairs health and may even increase the risk for developing cancer (see Chapter 7).

Rossouw is further quoted by *Health24* as saying: 'The science is clear that if one follows an unhealthy diet high in fat, one increases one's "bad" cholesterol levels causing heart attacks and angina.'

This statement is also false. There is no RCT showing that people placed on high-fat diets develop more heart disease as a result. And there is no evidence that those with established heart disease eat more fat or saturated fat than those without the disease. Instead, it is more likely that they eat more sugar, refined carbohydrates and vegetable oils.

The article continues to give an account of Rossouw's presentation in the debate:

> Rossouw explained that the trend of increasing obesity could be attributed to factors like poor diet, lack of physical activity and the environment in which people live. 'The association between overweight and diabetes,' he said, 'is clearly illustrated, as is the benefit of losing weight to prevent diabetes. The data shows that reduced calorie diets result in clinically meaningful weight loss, regardless of which foods are present in low calorie diets.'

Again, why would he stray onto the topic of weight control and specifically mention the (failed) CICO model of weight control? Is it because this is the model favoured by those who teach dietetics in South Africa under the auspices of ADSA, the HPCSA and the International Life Sciences Institute, a known Coca-Cola front organisation?

The article concludes its account of Rossouw's argument with the following:

> Rossouw warns, 'Noakes maintains that diabetics do not have higher blood cholesterol levels than other people, that half of all heart attacks occur in

people with normal blood cholesterol, that glucose is the single most important predictor of risk and a high-fat diet reverses almost all coronary risk
factors. Except for a very few close followers, the scientific evidence is clear
and he's flying against it. There is now absolute proof that high blood cholesterol is causal in heart disease.'

The problem is that Rossouw is unable to move on; he continues to present the
disproved beliefs of the 1950s as if they are still current, and despite his own
$700-million WHIRCDMT disproving them. There is simply no 'absolute proof
that high blood cholesterol is causal in heart disease'. It is lipoproteins, not cholesterol, that are weakly linked, by association, to heart disease in those with IR
and NAFLD, and who persist in eating high-carbohydrate diets loaded with
polyunsaturated vegetable oils (see Chapter 17). The published scientific literature
already supports this fact.

In sticking to a belief that even his own research has disproved, Rossouw
reminds me of what German theoretical physicist Max Planck once wrote: 'A new
scientific truth does not triumph by convincing its opponents and making them
see the light, but rather because its opponents eventually die, and a new generation grows up that is familiar with it.'[63] Or, as sometimes paraphrased: 'Truth
never triumphs – its opponents just die out.' In other words, as Planck also said,
'Science advances one funeral at a time.'

Perhaps Rossouw should heed the words of American physicist and Nobel
Prize laureate Dr Richard Feynman, who said: 'It doesn't matter how beautiful
your theory is, it doesn't matter how smart you are. If it doesn't agree with
experiment, it's wrong.' And: 'The first principle is that you must not fool yourself
– and you are the easiest person to fool.'

The *Health24* article also quoted endocrinologist Dr Vash Mungal-Singh,
then chief executive officer of the HSFSA:

> Any diet that is calorie and energy restricted will reduce weight. But caution
> should be used when generalising and saying that everyone should eat fats,
> no sugar and no carbs, especially when there is no long-term data on this,
> while there is extensive data on the conventional diet.

Predictably, Mungal-Singh forgot to mention that the 'extensive data on the
conventional diet' had proved it to be not only hopelessly ineffective, but also
the direct cause of the global obesity/T2DM epidemic that is the principal
contributor to heart attacks and strokes in South Africa and elsewhere. Or that
Rossouw, the then president of the organisation that paid her salary, was one of
the key drivers of the WHIRCDMT, which definitively disproved the diet-heart
hypothesis.

One wonders what continues to drive this cognitive dissonance in the HSFSA. In Mungal-Singh's case, could it have been the sponsors of the HSFSA who effectively paid her salary? (The HSFSA receives funding and support from a wide range of organisations, as listed in Chapter 7, Table 7.1.) Or was it her misguided sense of loyalty to the ILSI, on whose board of directors she also serves?

One of the great ironies of my journey is that in 1976 I was one of a group of five people, including two cardiologists, who started the Cape Heart Foundation, which would ultimately become the Heart and Stroke Foundation of South Africa. Naturally, we innovators were the first personally to adopt the 1977 USDA Dietary Guidelines for Americans that promoted LFHC diets based on '7–11 servings a day of cereals and grains'. It is my opinion that because of my genetic predisposition – my father suffered all the worst complications of T2DM, ultimately dying from it, while specialists advised him to eat a high-carbohydrate diet – it was this diet that caused my T2DM, even though I was (reasonably) active all my life and never obese (although my body mass index did increase gradually to reach an undesirable, overweight 28 kg/m^2 in December 2010).

Today, the HSFSA continues to promote low-fat diets as the cornerstone for the prevention of heart disease. It also fails to warn of the heart dangers of ingesting partially hydrogenated vegetable oils, especially those found in the margarines produced by one of the HSFSA's most dedicated funders. The advice to follow the low-fat diet is a direct cause of the explosion of the most severe form of arterial disease, T2DM. Thus, far from preventing arterial disease (of the heart), the low-fat diet that the HSFSA promotes is the direct cause of the horrendous increase in diabetic arterial disease that will swamp global medical services within the next decade.

In retrospect, I could not then appreciate the extent to which the Centenary Debate was the opening salvo of what I believe to have been a much wider campaign, the ultimate goal of which was to silence me through public humiliation. It is a well-known technique called refutation by denigration. My perception is that if the actions of my colleagues meant that my status as an A1-rated scientist, who had contributed greatly to the scientific and financial efforts of UCT's Faculty of Health Sciences over 35 years, was destroyed, well, in their opinion, that was just too bad. According to their worldview, I was the architect of my own downfall.

Only later, when I read Alice Dreger's *Galileo's Middle Finger: Heretics, Activists, and One Scholar's Search for Justice*, did I begin to appreciate what I was really up against. Dreger's book explores the unrelenting battle between scholars who put the pursuit of hard truths ahead of personal comfort and the social activists determined to silence them. She uses the voice of the social activist to explain what drives activists in their battles with empirical science and scientists:

We have to use our privilege to advance the rights of the marginalized. We can't let [scientists] say what is true about the world. We have to give voice and power to the oppressed and let *them* say what is true about the world. Science is as biased as all human endeavors, and so we have to empower the disempowered, and speak always with them.[64]

The difference, of course, is that the activists I was facing, in my view, were not motivated to advance the voices of the oppressed and disempowered, but, either wittingly or by proxy, rather the opposite.

In the face of this, what is the responsibility of those scientists who see their role as the pursuit of 'truth'? Dreger's answer is this:

To scholars I want to say more: Our fellow human beings can't afford to have us act like cattle in an industrial farming system. If we take seriously the importance of truth to justice and recognize the many factors now acting against the pursuit of knowledge – *if we really get why our role in democracy is like no other* – then we really ought to feel that we must do more to protect each other and the public from misinformation and disinformation ...[65]

We scholars had to put the search for evidence before everything else, even when the evidence pointed to facts we did not want to see. The world needed that of us, to maintain – by our example, by our very existence – a world that would keep learning and questioning, that would remain free in thought, inquiry, and word.[66]

In the end, she concludes: 'Justice cannot be determined merely by social position. Justice cannot be advanced by letting "truth" be determined by political goals.'[67] Nor, I might add, can commercial interests be allowed to determine what is the 'truth'.

Dreger's final message is this: 'Evidence really is an ethical issue, the most important ethical issue in a modern democracy. If you want justice, you must work for truth. And if you want to work for truth, you must do a little more than wish for justice.'[68]

As the media onslaught began, I did not understand that these academic activists seemingly did not care about the science. Neither did the tabloid journalists or Twitter trolls, including some medical colleagues, who at about the same time began to target me on social media. Were they also willing co-conspirators in the rush to silence my voice?

5

The UCT Professors' Letter

'The paradox is that medicine is supposedly more enlightened, but
it has never been more tyrannical, hierarchical, controlled, intolerant,
and dogmatic. Working doctors who dissent are cowed because failure to
comply with the medical orthodoxy threatens livelihood and registration.
Much of modern medicine is an intellectual void.'
– Dr Des Spence, Scottish GP[1]

I have written many books and most have taken years, even decades, to complete. *The Real Meal Revolution*, however, which I co-wrote with nutritional therapist Sally-Ann Creed, adventure runner and chef David Grier, and chef and aspiring endurance athlete Jonno Proudfoot, took just five weeks in July/August 2013. It is the book that has caused me both the greatest pleasure and the worst pain. For while the book would sell in excess of 250 000 copies in South Africa, and set off the Banting Revolution in this country, it would be the direct cause of the worst moment in my entire academic career: the publication of the letter signed by four University of Cape Town professors, three of whom were long-standing colleagues of mine at the time.

In retrospect I now realise how inconvenient the publication of *The Real Meal Revolution* in November 2013 was for those who, behind the scenes, were busily sharpening their knives in anticipation of my early elimination. They were waiting for the Naudé meta-analysis, which would play a pivotal role in the HPCSA's decision to charge me. The study, which should have been published in February 2013, was now already nine months overdue.

During that time, I, their intended quarry, had published an article in the *SAMJ* that would become one of the journal's most-read articles of all time. I wrote it after receiving letters from people who had changed their diets to LCHF. Some of the letters contained stories that were nothing short of miraculous, so I decided to collate and analyse the best 100 or so for a scientific publication in the *SAMJ*.

I was careful to make the point that this was an 'occasional survey', not definitive evidence, and that it had significant limitations. Thus, I began the discussion acknowledging that:

The study has several potential limitations. First, all data are self-reported and were not verified but it is unlikely that all participants would fabricate this information. Second, there is no record of exactly what each person ate. Third, all reports describe only short-term outcomes. To collect this information as part of an RCT involving 254 subjects would have been very costly.[2]

It was probably the next sentence that really caused the trouble. 'Despite these substantive limitations, this information challenges current conventional wisdom (widely taught at medical schools),' I wrote. I was perhaps still too naive to appreciate that, in the educational climate of today, one does not challenge what is taught at medical schools.

Further, to indicate that I at least understood that this was not conventional research, I concluded the abstract with the sentence: 'A randomised controlled clinical trial is urgently required to disprove the hypothesis that the LCHF eating plan can reverse cases of T2DM, metabolic syndrome and hypertension without pharmacotherapy.'

The high point of the paper for me was the chance to describe five 'miracle' cases that at the time challenged what I had been taught about medical care for patients with T2DM.

Billy Tosh lost 83 kilograms in 28 weeks (see Figure 5.1) and reversed his hypertension and T2DM. The solution was simple, he said: absolutely no sugar, no processed foods and less than 25 grams of carbohydrates per day. He concluded that the LCHF diet had 'saved' his life and that 'label reading has opened my eyes to the almost criminal levels of carbs in everyday processed foods and the propensity of these foods to cause weight gain'.

Brian Berkman also reversed his T2DM and lost 73 kilograms over 18 months by adopting the LCHF eating plan, limiting his carbohydrates to less than 25 grams per day and avoiding all sugar. He concluded: 'I totally subscribe to the view that sugar and carbohydrates are drugs to the body. I was an addict.'

Dr Gerhard Schoonbee, a 57-year-old rural general practitioner, had warned his wife that he did not expect to reach his 65th birthday because of the effects of his T2DM. He also had hypertension, a high blood cholesterol concentration, sleep apnoea and constant fatigue. In May 2012, he read about the LCHF diet, adopted it, lost 25 kilograms in eight months and cured himself of all his afflictions so that he no longer needed any medications. He now prescribes the LCHF diet for his patients of all social classes.

Figure 5.1

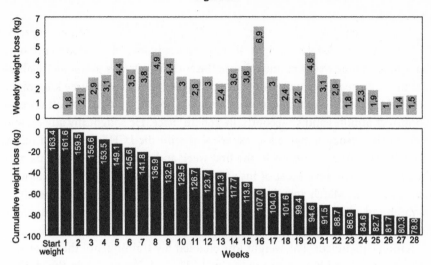

Weekly weights of Billy Tosh following adoption of the LCHF diet. Note that in 28 weeks, Tosh lost 83 kilograms and put his hypertension and T2DM into remission

Figure 5.2

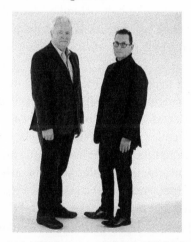

Two of the three Capetonians who lost a total of 181 kilograms by adopting the LCHF diet. None now requires medications to treat their T2DM and only one continues to use medication to control hypertension. Markers of blood glucose control are now normal in all three without medication use. This picture was taken in September 2017, more than four years after each had begun the diet. These individuals taught me that, at least in some, the LCHF diet can 'reverse' T2DM, the disease that killed my father

A 23-year-old mother began to eat addictively after the birth of her first child. Her weight ballooned to 120 kilograms and she developed T2DM. She adopted the LCHF diet, lost 45 kilograms and reversed all diabetic symptoms. She concluded: 'for the life of me I don't know why I struggled so much [to control my weight] since it really isn't that difficult. It was more of a lifestyle change for me than a diet.'

Thirty-seven-year-old Simon Gear, a lifelong runner, was finding it increasingly difficult to control his weight. To activate weight loss, he decided to run nine marathons in nine weeks, culminating in the 2012 Two Oceans 56-kilometre ultra-marathon. Instead, his marathon running caused him to gain three kilograms. He finished the ultra-marathon two minutes short of the official cut-off time, in 6 hours 57 minutes and 57 seconds, in 7 668th place. He sought my advice, and after much persuasion agreed to experiment with the LCHF diet for an initial 100 days. He lost 2 kilograms in the first week and a total of 15 kilograms over the next seven months. Most of his weight loss occurred when he was running the least. On 16 March 2013, he completed the Two Oceans 56-kilometre ultra-marathon in 3 hours 59 minutes and 42 seconds, in 208th position, nearly three hours and 7 460 positions better than his performance 12 months earlier.

Simon concluded: 'The weight loss enabled my training, not the other way around. I feel like I have won my life back.' He had discovered, in the clearest possible way, that it is not possible to outrun a bad diet.

When my father battled with T2DM, dying a diminished man as a result of the complications of disseminated obstructive diabetic arterial disease, my medical training allowed me to hide behind a false reality. I believed that some outcomes in medicine are just inevitable: that people with T2DM are predestined to become progressively sicker until they die an awful death. That is just the way it is.

But here were four people with T2DM telling me that it does not have to be this way. By just changing their diets, they had managed to reverse all their symptoms. It seemed a reasonable assumption that as long as they continued to follow the LCHF eating plan and their new lifestyle, they would not necessarily die from the arterial complications that had claimed my father. As someone with T2DM, I found this information profoundly liberating and hopeful. That we might finally have an intervention that could truly help patients with T2DM was a revelation. I assumed that my colleagues and peers would embrace the article as an exciting opportunity to try something new to address a problem for which we did not have a solution.

After all, there was nothing to lose, as current treatment methods are pretty ineffective. Imagine, I thought, how much good we could do if we offered this simple, cheap intervention to the millions of South Africans suffering from these harmful chronic diseases. Finally, we could offer hope to our patients with T2DM.

I was underestimating the power of the omertà.

The response was immediate and, in retrospect, predictable. Within a day or two of the article's publication, then editor of the *Mail & Guardian* Nic Dawes tweeted to the effect that it was a disgrace for the *SAMJ* to publish this type of article in the guise of 'science'.

Others joined in. The theme of their collective message was 'Noakes has lost it'. Perhaps he was once a good scientist, they said, but if he thinks this is 'science', then he is clearly senile. We need to warn the world of his mental decline. No longer can anything he says be trusted.

My conclusion now is that these attacks were not random events.

Yet in writing *The Real Meal Revolution*, we had also begun to attract our strongest ally – the general public – although we did not know it at the time. I also did not then appreciate that it would be the public support generated by *The Real Meal Revolution* that would ultimately save my scientific credibility.

However, it was the introduction of *The Real Meal Revolution* to a group of South African parliamentarians and their support staffs that produced the most ferocious response from my academic colleagues at UCT.

On two previous occasions, I had spoken to different groups at Parliament about the role of IR and high-carbohydrate diets in many of our nation's health problems. I spoke about how restricting the intake of sugar and refined carbohydrates, and increasing the intake of 'healthy' fats, could reverse our nation's progressive slide into ill health.

On the basis of those two talks, I was invited to speak to a larger group of perhaps 150 people in one of the luxurious chambers at Parliament on another of their regular Wellness Days. Importantly, I did not seek out the invitation. In no way was I taking my crusade to Parliament, as my colleagues would later claim. I was asked to speak and, out of courtesy, I accepted the invitation. As is usually the case for such public talks to wellness groups, my foundation was not paid for my time.

Shorty after I began my talk to Parliament's Wellness Unit on 18 August 2014, the data projector failed. I was reduced to speaking without the prepared script provided by the slides, but managed to give a selection of the most important ideas from the 120 lectures on nutrition that I had given around the country since December 2013. During the talk I did not mention *The Real Meal Revolution*, but I did say that the solution to the South African obesity/diabetes epidemic was the promotion of the LCHF diet. I could tell that the organisers and the audience were receptive to my lecture. They also treated me with respect and consideration.

The next morning, I awoke to find my picture on the front page of the *Cape Times*, presenting a copy of *The Real Meal Revolution* to the Deputy Speaker, Lechesa Tsenoli. He had requested this picture and had possibly innocently encouraged the newspaper to publish it. The lead story was about my presentation to the Wellness Unit.[3]

The article quoted me accurately enough, saying that South Africa was sitting on a disease 'time bomb', and that we ran the risk of becoming the 'fattest' country in the world (note, we are currently the world's third fattest). 'Noakes said one way to address the problem would be through his high-fat, high-protein diet (including meat, full-cream milk, cheese and butter) and by consuming less sugar and processed food, and fewer carbohydrates,' the journalist wrote. That statement was not altogether correct: I had, and always have, made it clear that the evidence is for a moderate-protein, not high-protein, diet.

The article further quoted me as saying that 'if we don't reverse [the] obesity and diabetes epidemic, our nation disappears ... because we will go financially bankrupt because we don't have the money to provide medical services in the near future'.

I also said:

> We (South Africa) are sitting on a time bomb if we don't do anything about it. It is not rocket science what I'm going to tell you. The obesity and diabetes epidemic has one cause and we can sort it out. We are told that it's our fault, we're lazy, we eat too much, we don't exercise. That is nonsense. It does not say exactly what is the cause of the obesity and diabetes epidemic and we either accept it, address it and cure the nation. Or ... we will become the fattest nation in the world.

The article included my suggestion that we should feed children in poorer communities protein, such as offal from animals, and that we should all 'eat animals from nose to tail'. It concluded with a comment I have made frequently over the years:

> I was born in 1949 and when I went to school everyone looked like me, everyone. We had one kid who was a bit fat and we thought he had cancer because it was so uncommon. When I go and speak to the young girls of South Africa across every grouping and every social class, I'm astonished and frightened at the obesity that I see.

Tsenoli was quoted as saying that my message was 'very powerful' and that it must be 'translated and communicated in all languages'. He continued: 'It's interesting stuff. What I like about it is that the guy is being scientific. There are some who would like to portray him as someone who is talking bullsh*t, yet what he's saying makes sense and he's nuanced. He's not articulating anything in absolute terms.' He said that my talk had exposed the risks of the 'commodification' of things like sugar and what that did to our general health.

Only in time did I realise that this newspaper report posed a massive threat to those I believe were busily plotting the HPCSA actions against me. They were, at that very moment, about to convene a preliminary inquiry committee of senior medical and legal colleagues to decide whether or not I should be charged. If some members of Parliament and, worse, the minister of health supported me, that would seriously jeopardise their actions and case against me.

Willem 'Slim Wim' de Villiers had recently been appointed dean of the UCT Faculty of Health Sciences, but was already eyeing the vacated post of rector of the University of Stellenbosch. I did not know it then, but De Villiers was flexing his muscles as head of the medical 'herd'.

Dr Jay Wortman, one of the speakers at the Cape Town low-carb summit in February 2015, has explained the dynamics and dangers of the herd mentality and the key role of the alpha male in directing the actions of the herd. Wortman is an associate professor of medicine at the University of British Columbia. He is a First Nation, Métis Canadian, born in the small northern Alberta village of Fort Vermilion, an early settlement in the network of fur-trading posts developed by the Hudson's Bay Company in Canada's formative years. Wortman relates the story of the American Plains Indians and their relationship to their vital food source, the American bison. Each bison herd has only one male leader. Without their leader, herds have no idea what to do when threatened. The Plains Indians learnt an important lesson: to control a Bison herd successfully, the first step is to remove its alpha-male leader.

Medicine, Wortman says, is a bit like that. Our herd mentality forces us to follow the single powerful Anointed, typically the professor of medicine or, even better, the dean of the medical faculty. That Anointed alpha male knows that if he wishes to depose a hostile opinion that threatens his position, all he need do is oust the leader of the competing herd. He knows that his own loyal medical herd will never threaten his status.

So it was that at the height of the LCHF debate in South Africa, a new alpha male was introduced into the herd of those controlling medical education in the Western Cape. The threat had been identified for De Villiers: the LCHF/Banting position already gaining traction throughout South Africa as a result of the publication of *The Real Meal Revolution*. And he had his mandate: neutralise the leaders of any and all competing opinions to conventional medical care.

A number of factors jumped out at me as I read the CV[4] of UCT's newest, and soon to be shortest-reigning, dean of medicine. De Villiers had matriculated as the top student in the then Cape Province, hence the nickname Slim Wim. He had trained at the universities of Stellenbosch, Oxford and Harvard before ending up at the University of Kentucky Medical Center in 1996. In 2016, the University of Kentucky Medical Center was ranked 67th best in research and 74th best in primary care among US institutions. Harvard, Stanford, Johns Hopkins, the University of California, San Francisco and the University of Pennsylvania were ranked the top five medical institutions. Why, I wondered, had Slim Wim not pursued his academic career at one of these more academically challenging medical institutions?

Perhaps it was because academic research was not De Villiers's real passion. In the two decades since receiving his PhD in 1995, De Villiers had supervised and co-supervised a total of just four successful doctoral candidates. During the same period, he had found time to work as a consultant to 18 pharmaceutical companies, nine of which have been fee-paying affiliates of the ILSI.*

De Villiers's CV also records that during his career he was the principal investigator in '35 Inflammatory Bowel Disease industry sponsored studies'. I would guess that none addressed the possible role of specific dietary factors such as gluten tim the causation of inflammatory bowel conditions.

Before she went home on Friday 22 August 2014, Linda Rhoda, head of marketing and communications for the UCT Faculty of Health Sciences, completed a last action: she sent an email to the *Cape Times* titled 'Noakes' diet and health implications', cc'ing me, National Assembly Speaker Baleka Mbete, minister of health Dr Aaron Motsoaledi, Western Cape MEC of health Dr Theuns Botha, and members of the South African Committee of Medical Deans. The latter would have included the deans of all the South African universities charged with the responsibility of training medical doctors.

At the time, I was en route to the Western Cape nature reserve Bartholomeus Klip, near the village of Hermon. Early the next morning, I opened my email and read the attached letter with growing incredulity. It carried the names (but not signatures) of four UCT academics, as well as – importantly – the logos of UCT and the UCT Faculty of Health Sciences. It therefore, in effect, signalled my ultimate academic rejection by all members of the university, and especially the medical faculty that I had served with distinction for 35 years. Only the deaths of my parents, Bob Woolmer and a few other close friends surpassed the emotional devastation this email caused me. It is published here in full on pages 90–91.

---

* Under 'Consultative Service' on his CV, De Villiers declares that he worked with the following 18 pharmaceutical companies: Abbott, Abbvie, AstraZeneca, Axcan-Scandipharm, Berlex, Centocor, Elan, Genentech, Johnson & Johnson, Novartis, Santarus, Prometheus, Proctor & Gamble, Protein Design Labs, Shire, UCB, UCG and Wyeth. Of these, nine – Abbott, Abbvie, AstraZeneca, Berlex, Johnson & Johnson, Novartis, Procter & Gamble, UCB and Wyeth – have been dues-paying members of the ILSI. In addition, four of these companies – Abbott ($1.5 billion), AstraZeneca ($520 million), Johnson & Johnson ($1.1 billion) and Novartis ($423 million) – feature among the top 10 pharmacuetical companies that paid the largest fines for research misconduct and fraud between 2007 and 2012 (Gøtzsche, *Deadly Medicines and Organised Crime*). De Villiers also declares that from July 1999 to June 2000 he was the recipient of the Atorvastatin Research Award. Marketed under the trade name Lipitor, atorvastatin (a cholesterol-lowering statin drug) became the world's bestselling drug with more than $125 billion in sales over approximately 14 years, from 1996 to 2012.

As I read it, I pondered all the lessons I had learnt from the great coaches with whom I had worked, such as Bob Woolmer, Jake White, John Dobson and Kevin Musikanth. They all taught me that team success begins with developing personal relationships.

As the exceptional football coach Carlo Ancelotti explains:

> First you have to build good relationships, good chemistry with the group you're working with. After that, you can add the strategy. I think that the most important thing is the relationship with the people, and the relationship with the people makes a better organization. I'm sure of this. I speak with my players but I know that first of all they are people. So you have to treat them with respect. It's important to have a good relationship on the same level, not them looking up to me or me looking down on them.[5]

How could my senior medical colleagues not understand these fundamental truths? Why, despite their education, were they so lacking in these basic human skills? Did they not understand that to build successful teams, you begin by respecting those with whom you work? Why, instead, had they resorted to the lowest forms of academic discourse – bigotry and harmful academic bullying?

My initial response when reading the email was that, besides its poverty of honesty and intellectual content, it was wholly inappropriate. If this were purely an academic disagreement, then the correct forum for its resolution lay within the moderating halls of UCT, not in the columns of a local 'tabloid' newspaper.

Why, I wondered, had these academics not called me in for a discussion first? That would have given me the opportunity to explain my views and answer their criticisms directly. The fact that De Villiers and his colleagues had chosen this bizarre route indicated that this was not a matter simply of academics and science. It had become much more. I believe that these professors were dancing to someone else's tune, and that this letter and De Villiers's subsequent actions were essential drivers for the HPCSA charges against me. Without this letter, the HPCSA hearing might never have happened.

In the first place, I found it difficult to believe that Lionel Opie, a man of honour and integrity, as I believed him to be, would dignify what I see as scurrilous drivel with his signature. Just three months earlier, at a Franschhoek Literary Festival debate with me on 17 May 2014, Opie had confirmed to my wife that, while he was happy to participate in that event, he did not wish to do anything to damage the special relationship we had enjoyed since 1972.

FACULTY OF HEALTH SCIENCES
UNIVERSITY OF CAPE TOWN

The Editor
Cape Times
22 August 2014

Noakes' diet and health implications

The apparent endorsement by Members of Parliament of South Africa of the latest fashionable diet, 'Banting' ('SA's Ticking Time-bomb', Cape Times, 19 August 2014), and the message it sends out to the public about healthy eating, is cause for deep concern - not only regarding Parliament's support for it as an evidenced-based 'diet revolution', but sadly, the long-term impact this may have on the health of the very people they have been elected to serve.

Any diet for weight loss and maintenance should be safe and promote health in the long-term. Currently the long term safety and health benefits of low carbohydrate, high fat diets – such as Atkins, Paleo and South Beach, and in which Banting falls - are unproven, and in particular whether it is safe in pregnancy and childhood.

Importantly, while the consumption of a low carbohydrate, high fat diet may lead to initial weight loss and associated health benefits - as indeed would a balanced weight loss diet - there is good reason for concern that this diet may rather result in nutritional deficiencies, increased risk for heart disease, diabetes mellitus, kidney problems, constipation, certain cancers and excessive iron stores in some individuals in the long term. Research leaves no doubt that healthy balanced eating is very important in reducing disease risk (see web page below dedicated to this debate).

It is therefore a serious concern that Professor Timothy Noakes, a colleague respected for his research in Sports Science, is aggressively promoting this diet as a 'revolution', making outrageous unproven claims about disease prevention, and maligning the integrity and credibility of peers who criticise his diet for being evidence-deficient and not conforming to the tenets of good and responsible science. This goes against the University of Cape Town's commitment to academic freedom as the prerequisite to fostering responsible and respectful intellectual debate and free enquiry.

This is not the forum to debate details of diets, but to draw attention to the need for us to be pragmatic. Research in this field has proven time and again that the quest for lean and healthy bodies cannot be a quick-fix , 'one- size-fits-all' solution. The major challenge lies in establishing sustainable and healthy dietary and physical activity patterns to promote long term weight maintenance and health after weight loss, and includes addressing psychosocial, environmental and physiological factors.

1

Our bodies need a range of nutrients sourced from a variety of food groups to survive. Diets like the Banting are, however, typically 'one dimensional' in focus. They promote increased intake of protein and fat containing foods at the expense of healthy carbohydrate containing foods, and focus on adherence to a limited food plan. Ignored are the other important factors impacting on health - like physical activity (the importance of which we cannot emphasise enough), environmental factors, and individual health profiles.

UCT's Faculty of Health Sciences, a leading research institution in Africa, has a reputation for research excellence to uphold. Above all, our research must be socially responsible. We have therefore taken the unusual step of distancing ourselves from the proponents of this diet. To foster informed engagement of the issues related to the Diet debate, the Faculty has established a web page with material on this: http://www.health.uct.ac.za/fhs/news/high-fat-diet-debate.

Sincerely

Prof Wim de Villiers (Dean: Faculty of Health Sciences, University of Cape Town)

Prof Bongani Mayosi (Head: Department of Medicine, UCT)

Emeritus Prof Lionel Opie (Hatter Institute of Cardiology, Department of Medicine)

Associate Professor Marjanne Senekal: Assoc Prof (Head: Division of Human Nutrition)

Copied to:

Prof Timothy Noakes (University of Cape Town)

Hon Baleka Mbete, Speaker of Parliament

Minister of Health, Dr Aaron Motsaeledi

MEC for Health, Western Cape Government, Dr Theuns Botha

Members of the South African Committee of Medical Deans

ENDS

Issued by:

COMMUNICATIONS AND MARKETING
Linda Rhoda, Manager
tel. +27 21 406 6685 fax: +27 21 447 8955 or +27 86 612 6390
Faculty of Health Sciences, University of Cape Town, P/Bag X3 Observatory 7935
linda.rhoda@uct.ac.za www.health.uct.ac.za

Opie had also written a letter to the *Sunday Times* on 27 July, in which he sought to clarify some attributed statements in an article published by the paper the previous week. In this letter, he expressed opinions quite different from those that would appear in the UCT professors' email, and included a partial endorsement of the Banting diet:

I regard the New Atkins low-carbohydrate diet as a good starting point for weight reduction because it has a two-year placebo-controlled study to its credit. I will not propose that Noakes is 'dangerously wrong', as stated in your subheading, as his diet also induces weight loss. But we must face facts. The Noakes diet, although related to the Atkins diet, crucially differs by emphasising the high-fat diet that has no supportive trial data. Note a long-term danger after short-term weight loss, namely the increased risk of breast cancer.[6]

Crucially, Opie was refusing to state publicly that I was 'dangerously wrong'; instead he endorsed LCHF as a reasonable initial diet for weight loss. He limits any further endorsement only because of concerns about a lack of long-term trials. This was essentially what he had said at our debate at the Franschhoek Literary Festival: begin your weight-loss journey on the LCHF diet and then switch to the 'Mediterranean diet' (whatever that is) for long-term health.

How could he have changed his opinion so drastically in the space of a few weeks? How could our relationship of more than 42 years suddenly mean so little to him? Would he really add his name to an email that was so intellectually and ethically deficient and so professionally degrading for all involved? My instinct told me no, this is not what Professor Lionel Opie stands for.

I did not know quite what to make of it, but I knew I had to at least try.

What struck me most about the letter was its cruelty and inhumanity, and that the authors showed not the slightest hint of conscience in publicly shaming me. Medicine is meant to be a caring profession in which we are concerned with the emotional health and needs of not just our patients, but also our colleagues and students. De Villiers appears to understand this. When he was eventually appointed rector and vice chancellor of the University of Stellenbosch in December 2014, his university profile stated: 'He believes the University should offer an experience that is pleasant, welcoming and hospitable – in an inclusive environment.'[7] Those admirable sentiments were remarkable for their absence from the *Cape Times* professors' letter.

Instead, the letter is a textbook example of academic bullying, a topic recently reviewed by Dr Fleur Howells, senior lecturer in psychiatry at UCT. Howells writes that there are three forms of academic bullying. The third, 'social bullying, also known as relational aggression, is the deliberate or active exclusion or damage to the social standing of the victim through, for example, publicly undermining a junior academic's viewpoint'.[8] The four key components of bullying are intent to harm, experience of harm, exploitation of power and aggression. The professors' letter thus neatly fulfils all the diagnostic criteria for academic bullying.

Jacqui Hoepner is currently completing her PhD thesis at the Australian National University, studying the use of these bullying tactics to suppress or silence dissenting scientific opinions.[9] In a discussion with Daryl Ilbury, author of *Tim Noakes: The Quiet Maverick*, Hoepner disclosed her original assumption that most cases of academic suppression or silencing arise from outside academic circles. To her surprise, she discovered the opposite – 'the bulk of suppression or silencing came from within academia, from colleagues and competitors', she told Ilbury. 'This suggests that the assumed model of respect and disagreement between academics is inaccurate.'

Hoepner was astonished to uncover 43 different 'silencing behaviours' that fly in the face of the concept of academic freedom: 'Every policy and university guideline I looked at suggested that academic freedom was absolutely central to what academics do and their place in society ... [But] there's a real disconnect between what academics think they are guaranteed under academic freedom and what the reality is for the life of an academic.'

She also discovered that the nature of these silencing attacks was 'more of a personal gut response: that someone has crossed a boundary and we need to punish them. The exact motivation differed from case to case, but it seemed very much a visceral response.'

Typically, attacks are ad hominem, with accusations of conflicts of interest 'to undermine credibility ... without any attempt by the claimant of the accusations to provide any evidence'; and with allegations such as 'You're doing real harm', 'You're causing confusion' or you're undermining the public's faith in science; and ending with summons that the researcher be 'fired or disciplined in some way'.

Perhaps with direct relevance to my experience, Hoepner said: 'If a scientist discovers evidence that contradicts decades of public health messaging and says that data doesn't support the messaging, and that person is attacked, and publicly ... that's insane!'

Returning to the professors' letter, it is also blatantly defamatory because it implies that I, as a medical practitioner: promote a diet that may cause harm ('heart disease, diabetes mellitus, kidney problems ... certain cancers'); make 'outrageous unproven claims'; malign the integrity and credibility of peers who disagree with me; and undertake research that is not 'socially responsible' in the judgement of UCT.

The letter also breaches the HPCSA's own ethical guidelines. Professor Bongani Mayosi, another signatory to the letter, was involved at that time in a review of the HPCSA management and functioning, and therefore should have been well versed in the ethical guidelines of the organisation he was investigating. According to section 6 of the HPCSA 'General Ethical Guidelines for the Health Care Professions':

Health care professionals should:
6.2.1 Work with and respect other health care professionals in pursuit of the best health care possible for all patients ...

6.2.3 Refrain from speaking ill of colleagues or other health care practitioners.

6.3.4 Not make a patient doubt the knowledge or skills of colleagues by making comments about them that cannot be fully justified.[10]

The four UCT academics therefore had an ethical responsibility, mandated by the HPCSA, to treat me with respect and dignity. In addition, the medical profession provides specific strategies for how medical colleagues are expected to communicate with one another when there are disagreements. These include:

- Respectfully raising your concerns with your colleague.
- Framing your words around achieving the best result for the patient.
- Attempting to negotiate a mutually agreeable resolution.
- Taking action until you are satisfied that the patient's best interest is being served.

Thus, the initial responsibility of the four UCT academics was to negotiate with me directly to find a 'mutually agreeable resolution'. They chose not to do this. Instead, they took their disagreement public in the pages of a local newspaper, and it subsequently spread via social media and radio to the rest of the world. And what of my ethical responsibilities? I believe one of my responsibilities is to provide patients with information that, as a result of my medical and scientific training, I believe will improve their health. This, too, falls within the requirements of the HPCSA, specifically that the medical practitioner shall at all times:

27A (d) provide ... any other pertinent information to enable the patient to exercise a choice in terms of treatment and informed decision-making pertaining to his or her health and that of others.[11]

And how does the UCT Faculty of Health Sciences expect their graduates to act? At graduation, my colleagues and I, including the co-signatories of the *Cape Times* letter, made the following declaration:

I solemnly pledge to serve humanity.

My most important considerations will be the health of patients and the health of their communities.

I will not permit considerations of age, gender, race, religion, ethnic origin, sexual orientation, disease, disability or any other factor to adversely affect the care I give to patients.

I will uphold human rights and civil liberties to advance health, even under threat.

I will engage patients and colleagues as partners in healthcare.

I will practise my profession with conscience and dignity.

I will respect the confidentiality of patients, present or past, living or deceased.

I will value research and will be guided in its conduct by the highest ethical standards.

I commit myself to lifelong learning.

I make these promises solemnly, freely and upon my honour.[12]

It seemed the four UCT professors might have forgotten some aspects of their solemn oath.

Besides failing to treat me, their colleague, with respect and dignity, they clearly wished to restrict my ability to 'value research' and to provide patients with 'any other pertinent information' that would enable informed decisions. They also appeared to want to prevent me from fulfilling my most important professional responsibility, which is to the health of patients and communities, not to other special interests, including personal ego and the pharmaceutical and food industries.

In the 43 years since I first graduated as a medical doctor from the UCT Faculty of Health Sciences, I have observed a steady decline in the health of the communities that UCT serves. Surely my duty is to ask why this is so. And if I think I have a scientifically based answer, my responsibility – according to the UCT graduands' declaration – is to do all in my power to promote whatever change may be necessary.

My concern, which I expressed to Parliament's wellness group, is the imminent diabetes tsunami that will bankrupt South Africa's medical services within the next 10 to 15 years. This is especially important for the Western Cape, which is the diabetes capital of South Africa. My message is that we cannot reverse this epidemic unless we change our national eating patterns by consuming more fat and less sugar, processed foods and carbohydrates, a point which now even the HSFSA fully endorses.

Interestingly, not once in my presentation to Parliament's wellness group had I mentioned LCHF/Banting and *The Real Meal Revolution*, as the four professors clearly assumed I had done. My talk was about the biology of IR, the causes of the obesity/diabetes epidemic, the role of the processed-food industry and its addictive foods, and the evidence for the role of nutrition in fighting life-threatening diseases.

If the four UCT professors really believed that my message to Parliament's wellness group was 'dangerous', they needed to explain why. Why did they find my main message that South Africans should eat less sugar, less processed foods and fewer carbohydrates so threatening? It cannot be because replacing sugar, refined carbohydrates and excess carbohydrates with real foods will lead to an epidemic of other diseases, as there is no evidence that this will happen. Why, then, were these academics so desperately concerned by this revolutionary advice, which millions of people in South Africa and globally had already come to accept as mere common sense?

Let's return first to the 'academic' issues in the letter and all the errors it contains.

Their first error is to label LCHF/Banting 'the latest fashionable diet'; in other words, a fad. This is wrong. The Banting diet takes its name from an obese 19th-century undertaker, William Banting. First described in 1863, Banting is the oldest diet included in medical texts. Perhaps the most iconic medical text of all time, Sir William Osler's *The Principles and Practice of Medicine*, published in 1892, includes the Banting/Ebstein diet as the diet for the treatment of obesity (on page 1020 of that edition).[13] The reality is that the only non-fad diet is the Banting diet; all subsequent diets, and most especially the low-fat diet that the UCT academics promote, are 'the latest fashionable diets'. Opie, who has such a grasp of the history of medicine, would never, in my opinion, attach his signature to a letter that included such an obvious misrepresentation.

The authors write with the certainty of dogmatic arrogance that they are deeply concerned about this 'diet revolution' and 'the long-term impact this may have on the health of the very people they [parliamentarians] have been elected to serve'. They conveniently ignore the fact that the low-fat dietary guidelines they promote were adopted in the absence of any robust evidence for either safety or efficacy. And since the adoption of those dietary guidelines, there has been an unprecedented pandemic of obesity and T2DM, most especially in their area of influence, the Western Cape.

Surely these academics should be asking themselves why this has happened and what they should be doing about it. Surely they should be excited at the prospect of Parliament finally taking this issue seriously enough to ask me to address members on this topic.

The next point the authors reiterate is that 'the long term safety and health benefits of low carbohydrate, high fat diets … are unproven'. This ignores two facts. Firstly, there is no long-term data showing the safety of the LFHC diet, which the UCT Faculty of Health Sciences has promoted for the past 50 years. Yet the professors demand scientific proof for a diet that modern humans have eaten safely for more than 150 years, and our ancestors for millions of years. Secondly, they fail to acknowledge that if a diet is 'dangerous', it must show that 'danger' within a reasonable period of time. The LCHF/Banting diet has consistently outperformed all other diets in the correction of the metabolic risk factors for arterial disease.[14] This makes sense biologically, because arterial disease is caused by high-carbohydrate diets in those with IR and NAFLD, what I have termed the diet-liver-heart hypothesis. Furthermore, it is a general rule that two years is sufficient to determine whether or not an intervention is likely to be healthy or harmful. For how can an eating plan that corrects the metabolic abnormalities causing arterial disease suddenly become dangerous after two years and one day? There are at least four studies of this diet that have run for two years[15] and another seven for one year without even a hint of harm.[16]

The authors reveal their petticoats of bias when they claim that the benefits of LCHF diets 'are unproven, and in particular whether it is safe in pregnancy and childhood'. *The Real Meal Revolution* makes no mention of using this diet in pregnancy and childhood. At the time, I had never even spoken about pregnancy nutrition, and there was nothing in the *Cape Times* report saying that I had mentioned pregnancy and childhood nutrition to the parliamentarians.

The reason for the inclusion of this sentence in the letter would only become apparent during the HPCSA hearing in 2016. The UCT professors' letter turned out to be a crucial part of the evidence trail that the HPCSA needed to create in order to charge me with unprofessional conduct. It is why I conclude that De Villiers felt it essential to copy the letter to the minister of health and the South African Committee of Medical Deans. The letter would be the final piece of evidence the HPCSA preliminary inquiry committee required as proof that all of South African academic medicine was united in its disapproval of Professor Timothy Noakes's unprofessional conduct in questioning current medical orthodoxy.

In this context, having Opie's signature on the letter was vitally important for the herd. Like me, he is an A1-rated scientist, and perhaps the most decorated UCT medical scientist of all time. It is widely known that he was my MD supervisor, that I wrote a glowing foreword for his nutrition book, *Living Longer, Living Better*, and that I have the highest regard for him, as I unreservedly expressed in my biography, *Challenging Beliefs.*[*] To have Opie's signature on the letter would be a massive coup for De Villiers and his team. It would be the final repudiation of me, my ultimate outing as a devilish, 'dietary quack'.

Next, the authors' acknowledgement that the LCHF diet 'may lead to initial weight loss and associated health benefits – as indeed would a balanced weight loss diet', indicates their limited understanding of how different diets produce weight loss.

Standard teaching at the UCT Faculty of Health Sciences is that fat is the most energy-dense macronutrient. So people just need to remove fat from the diet if they want to lose weight. That is according to the uber-simplistic CICO model of obesity discussed in detail in *The Real Meal Revolution*. Importantly,

---

* In the acknowledgements to *Challenging Beliefs*, I wrote the following: 'Four of my tutors – Lionel Opie, the late Ralph Paffenbarger, George Brooks and the late George Sheehan – are (or were) utterly extraordinary individuals: the best of the very best. It is said that a guru gives himself and then his system, whereas a teacher gives us his subject and then ourselves. From these gurus I learnt the methods of scientific inquiry, of scientific and popular writing, and of public speaking; through their personalities and their teachings, these icons gave me myself.' (pp. viii–ix)

this is the model that the food industry advances, because it allows nutrition scientists to promote the false idea that the sole impact different foods have on our human physiology can be predicted from their varying calorie contents. We can therefore eat junk food, including, importantly, sugary soda drinks, as long as we burn off any excess with plenty of vigorous exercise.

In their letter, the four UCT experts now seem to be acknowledging that their model must be wrong, since they agree that it is possible to lose weight on a high-fat diet. What forced them to acknowledge their error? Quite simply, the effects of *The Real Meal Revolution*. They would have been exposed daily to stories of South Africans who had lost substantial amounts of weight. They may even have read my article in the *SAMJ* detailing patient-reported experiences with the LCHF diet, including the stories of Billy Tosh, Brian Berkman and Dr Gerhard Schoonbee (see Figure 5.2).

The 'associated health benefits' of the LCHF diet that the UCT professors admit to are, in their view, simply because weight loss itself is 'healthy'. But how do they know that the improvements in health of those on the LCHF diet are due simply to weight loss? What if they are due, instead, to the removal of the toxic effects of excess dietary carbohydrates in those who are insulin resistant, and the accompanying reversal of persistent hyperinsulinaemia and NAFLD, improvements that are not produced to the same extent by their calorie-restricted, hunger-generating, low-fat diet?

Then they add the great non sequitur: if weight loss always produces beneficial health outcomes, how are those health benefits suddenly reversed in patients who have managed to keep the weight off by continuing to eat the hunger-busting LCHF diet?

The faculty experts have chosen not to explain this anomaly. Instead, they have stayed loyal to the omertà, slipping into the standard dogma that 'this diet may rather result in nutritional deficiencies, increased risk of heart disease, diabetes mellitus, kidney problems, constipation, certain cancers and excessive iron stores in some individuals in the long term. Research leaves no doubt that healthy balanced eating is very important in reducing disease risk.'

I am always intrigued by my profession's casual use of the words 'may' and 'could'. One day during the course of the HPCSA hearing, I asked my legal expert and friend Advocate Dr Rocky Ramdass, a practising medical doctor who trained to become an advocate: 'Rocky, what is the difference between medicine and law?'

'Simple,' he responded. 'Medicine is what might or could be. The law is what is.'

Certainly, until the possibility is disproven, any diet 'might' cause anything. But our scientific responsibility is to back up our contentions with hard science. And there is no data or any definitive evidence (from appropriate RCTs) that the LCHF diet increases the risk of heart disease, T2DM, kidney problems, constipation, cancer and/or excessive iron storage. Instead, heart disease, obesity, dementia and probably cancer have all been shown to be symptoms of the same underlying abnormality – insulin resistance. And it is a high-carbohydrate diet that turns the benign condition of IR into the killer condition that is destroying global health. The irrefutable evidence for this is presented in Chapter 17.

It is the next paragraph in the letter ('It is therefore a serious concern that Professor Timothy Noakes ...') that constitutes defamation.

The professors start by saying that I am respected for research in sports science, ignoring my A1 rating in both exercise science *and* sports nutrition. (It goes without saying that it is not possible to be an expert in sports nutrition if you do not understand nutrition in general.)

Their first complaint is that I was 'aggressively' promoting the diet as a 'revolution', whereas all I did was provide a 25 000-word chapter to a recipe book and to suggest that the title should include the word 'revolution'. What happened afterwards – my subsequent lectures on the biology of IR and obesity, and how to treat both, delivered to about 30 000 South Africans during the book's promotion – was not of my doing. I did not force any of those 30 000 to come and listen, and I certainly did not force them to believe what I said or to follow an LCHF diet. If they did so, it was because they had weighed the evidence and chosen to change. After that, it was the South African public who drove the 'revolution', not Tim Noakes. I was perhaps the spark that lit the flame, but those who have benefited are the ones carrying forward the ensuing conflagration.

South African Rita Venter has a Banting support group on Facebook, 'Banting 7 Day Meal Plans', which she launched in September 2014. As of September 2017, she had more than 800 000 followers, growing by around 2 000 a day. Many people have written to say they have lost as much as 50 kilograms, 'reversed' their diabetes and hypertension, and have more energy. Any one of these achievements in hundreds of thousands of South Africans would be enough to spark an aggressive revolution. My continuing contribution has become unnecessary.

We are now dealing with a 'viral' phenomenon in which South Africans are taking control of their own health and using social media particularly to drive the diet revolution. They are increasingly ignoring the advice of professionals constrained by the omertà. The four UCT professors need to understand what is happening here; in choosing to blame me, they will not turn back the revolutionary tide.

Their second complaint is that I was 'making outrageous unproven claims about disease prevention'. I presume they are referring to the case reports I included in my *SAMJ* article and subsequently in *The Real Meal Revolution*. But these were not my claims; these were the claims of the individuals involved. Of course, they are 'outrageous' to colleagues who believe and lecture daily to doctors, medical students and dietitians that all these conditions – including obesity, T2DM, metabolic syndrome and hypertension – are the fault of slothful and gluttonous patients, and are irreversible and degenerative.

My view that conventional medical training does not address the real causes – IR and a high-carbohydrate diet – must be deeply disturbing to these anointed professors. For, if it is true, what I and many others are saying strikes at the very core of the current practice of clinical medicine. It is much easier to simply demonise Tim Noakes as a quack making outrageous claims than to consider the possible truth in what many South Africans and others around the globe are now saying.

In a final irony, the professors accuse me of trying to prevent intellectual debate. In reality, it is they who have tried to stifle the debate that I ignited with the publication of *Challenging Beliefs* and *The Real Meal Revolution*. They are the ones who ensure that UCT medical and dietetics students are not taught the LCHF diet. It is UCT's Division of Human Nutrition that decrees that no doctor at Groote Schuur Hospital may prescribe any diet other than one low in fat and high in carbohydrate. It is the students in that division who are warned never to mention the words LCHF or Banting within earshot of their professors and lecturers.

In the next paragraph, the professors say that the letter 'is not the forum to debate details of diets', and then list all the aspects of the LCHF diet that require investigation. Yet three years after their letter's publication, I am not aware that any of these professors have produced any evidence against LCHF. I, however, have contributed to an intervention trial showing the remarkable effects of a high-fat diet in reversing metabolic syndrome.[17]

I am not sure what the authors mean when they say that the Banting diet is '"one dimensional" in focus'. I also do not know exactly what constitutes 'healthy carbohydrate containing foods'. And their accusation that I ignore physical activity is ironic, given that I wrote one of the most famous running books of all time and introduced the science of sport to an extremely reluctant Faculty of Health Sciences in the 1970s. Of course I promote physical activity, but, as an expert in nutrition, I understand that nutrition is more important than physical activity when it comes to weight loss. I understand that you cannot out-exercise (or out-medicate or out-monitor) the effects of a bad diet.[18]

In a final personal insult, the authors distance themselves from me, one of the very few A1 scientists in their faculty. They omit that, through my efforts over 40 years, I personally have contributed in no small measure to the development of the faculty's 'reputation for research excellence'.

I spent much of that weekend at Bartholomeus Klip responding to the UCT professors' letter. I emailed a four-page private response, addressed to Wim de Villiers, to Linda Rhoda and the *Cape Times* on the evening of Sunday 24 August.

The letter includes information that is private, and so I will not reproduce it here in full. It will, however, be housed in the UCT archives, along with other relevant material, for posterity. Instead, this is a summary of the key points I made:

1. The UCT professors' letter is defamatory.
2. The letter is littered with errors of fact and interpretation that are an embarrassment to the authors.
3. The insinuation is that I have no credibility in studying or talking about low-carbohydrate diets, but the facts speak differently.

I gave an account of my credentials, saying that I had published my first paper on low-carbohydrate eating in 1980 in the *Journal of Physiology*.[19] My most recent publication at the time was an editorial in the *British Journal of Sports Medicine*, which I had written with two of the world's established leaders in the field, American professors Jeff Volek and Stephen Phinney.[20]

I outlined my involvement in *The Real Meal Revolution*, describing the 32 pages of text and four pages of references that I personally wrote on the science supporting the low-carbohydrate eating plan. These pages were, I said, an extension and refinement of what I initially wrote in *Challenging Beliefs*. All the evidence I presented to support the book's claims was fully referenced and most of the articles were peer-reviewed. That evidence refutes the claim in the UCT professors' letter that there is no evidence for the beneficial effects of low-carbohydrate diets in the management of IR, the one condition for which I promote such an eating plan. I suggested that 'it behoves you and your colleagues to go through all those references and to explain why the conclusions I have reached in that book are invalid'. I continued: 'I was trained by Professor Lionel Opie between 1976 and 1981 to ensure that I knew ALL the evidence before I came to any hypotheses/conclusions. It appears that this dictum may no longer apply in the new teaching philosophy in your Faculty.'

I drew attention to a study that I and my colleagues in Canada had just completed, which showed that a large percentage of obese rural Canadians had reduced their prevalence of metabolic syndrome from 60 to 20 per cent within three to eight months of adopting a rigorous low-carbohydrate diet without any exercise. Those who had reversed their metabolic syndrome would no longer need to use pharmaceutical products. (This paper has since been published.[21]) The problem for these four UCT academics, I said in my letter, is that they and all who practise conventional medicine teach that metabolic syndrome is irreversible. They also fail to ask why the prevalence of metabolic syndrome has increased exponentially since the introduction of the 1977 US dietary guidelines, which promote the ingestion of 'healthy carbohydrates'. Those clinicians who do understand that high-carbohydrate diets produce metabolic syndrome in people with IR will easily appreciate the importance of this study, I said.

I also described how I had invested the R500 000 prize I received for my 2012 NRF Lifetime Achievement Award in a study of 14 subjects habitually adapted to either a high-fat or a high-carbohydrate diet. This study was the first in the world to measure liver glucose production at rest and during exercise in athletes adapted to the LCHF diet. (The subsequently published paper proved that we have the ability to measure liver glucose production accurately, and that we can now use this technique to study the response of patients with T2DM to the LCHF diet.[22])

I also drew attention to the fact that I had raised funds for a study of obesity and IR in marathon runners, directed and subsequently completed by MSc student David Leith. We had also raised a grant of R1.6 million from an overseas donor to study the biology of the reversal of T2DM. When completed, this study, I said, will no doubt bring further credit to the UCT Faculty of Health Sciences. (We have since raised a further R4 million from the same donor.)

I concluded my letter with the following:

> Fortunately, neither of my parents is still alive so that neither will be subjected to the humiliation of reading you and your colleagues' letter in tomorrow morning's *Cape Times*.
>
> Unfortunately, my wife, myself and my family do not have that option.

Predictably, and in line with my initial assessment, at the time of writing in September 2017 I have received a response solely from Professor Lionel Opie. No word yet from De Villiers, Mayosi or Senekal. Not that I am expecting one.

Over the course of the weekend, Francesca Villette of the *Cape Times* corresponded with me at length. When the UCT letter was subsequently featured on the front page of the newspaper on Monday 25 August, she included significant input from me – something I would discover was usual for her, but unusual for many other South African journalists with whom I interacted. She quoted me as saying: 'If that message [that a high-carbohydrate diet is detrimental to the health of people with IR] is without scientific support, then the faculty has every right to cross the civil divide as it has now chosen – an action which, I suspect, is unprecedented in the history of the faculty and perhaps also in the history of UCT.' I added:

> Carbohydrate restriction in this group can be profoundly beneficial as it can reverse obesity and in some cases type 2 diabetes mellitus – the two conditions that will ultimately bankrupt South African medical services unless we take appropriate preventive actions.
>
> If there is evidence for my position, then the faculty is guilty of failing fully to inform its past and present science, medical and dietetics graduates

in a manner that should be appropriate for a faculty that considers itself a world leader.[23]

As Marilyn and I drove back to Cape Town from Bartholomeus Klip, we wondered how Lionel Opie could have allowed his name to be attached to this unscientific personal attack. For as long as I had known him, he'd had one overriding dictum: 'No data, no paper.' In other words, opinions are worthless unless supported by data. But where was the data in the *Cape Times* letter? Could his name have been added without his consent? Marilyn and I both knew that I would have to confront my lifelong mentor to hear his side of the story.

The response in the media to this personal onslaught reflected the individual biases of the respondents. The anti-Banters were delighted that the hierarchy had finally put me in my place; those who supported me suggested that De Villiers and his herd needed to provide scientific evidence for their position. Others wrote about how the Banting diet had improved their health in ways that the 'balanced' diet had never done and, in their opinion, never could.

A Somerset West doctor, Jacques Breitenbach, was typical of those who believe that, as the leader of supposedly the most scientifically rigorous health-science faculty in Africa, De Villiers should stick to the science. In a letter to the *Cape Times* on 26 August 2014, under the heading 'Produce evidence', Breitenbach wrote:

> Dr Wim de Villiers and others claim Noakes is making 'outrageous, unproven claims about disease prevention'. I have read Dr Tim Noakes' books and he provides some compelling arguments to back up his diet.
>
> De Villiers and the naysayers went on to state that 'there is good reason to believe it could result in nutritional deficiencies and increase the risk of heart disease, diabetes, kidney problems, constipation and some cancers'.
>
> On what evidence do you make those outrageous statements? You and your fellow doctors at the Faculty of Health Sciences will have to do a lot better than that.

Another general practitioner who trained at UCT, Dr Rosalind Adlard, also suggested that De Villiers and his colleagues 'read the evidence'. In her letter to the *Cape Times* on 29 August, Adlard wrote:

> As a graduate of UCT medical school myself, I owe Professor Noakes an inordinate debt of gratitude for opening my eyes to an alternative explanation for obesity which I was not taught at medical school.
>
> However, one thing I consistently find is that most people who criticize

the Banting diet don't know much about it and have not read any of the books Professor Noakes recommends.

I would thus like to challenge all doctors – and indeed anyone interested in the debate – to read Gary Taubes's book, *Why We Get Fat (and what to do about it)*. It's easy to read, inexpensive and readily available, in both print and electronic format.

At worst, you'll understand some of the theory and evidence behind the Banting diet, even if you disagree with it. At best you may, like me, also reap benefits for yourself and/or your patients.

Less than two weeks later, the publication of another scientific study in the *Annals of Internal Medicine* dealt a blow to the official UCT position by showing the superiority of the LCHF diet over the so-called heart-healthy, prudent, balanced diet when it came to weight loss and coronary risk factors.[24] 'This is now the 24th such study showing these outcomes,' I was quoted as saying in the press. 'The other 23 have been ignored but it seems this one might not be so easy to ignore.'[25] At the time, Linda Rhoda responded to the media saying that the professors were 'working on a response'. By September 2017, they had still not responded.

One retired Cape Town medical practitioner, Dr Jack Slabbert, did respond. Under the heading 'Work with Noakes', his letter to the *Cape Times* on 6 September read:

A month ago, a letter from professors in the faculty of medicine at the University of Cape Town appeared in your paper. They were highly critical of the views held by Professor Tim Noakes regarding a low-fat/high-carbohydrate diet versus a high-fat/low-carbohydrate diet, the latter being advocated by Noakes.

The story 'New study supports Noakes's low-carb, high-fat diet' (*Cape Times*, September 4) states that a study supporting Noakes' views has been published in the *Annals of Internal Medicine*, a publication held in very high regard by the medical profession.

Noakes has told your reporter that this is the 24th study stating support for his views, but 'the other 23 have been ignored'. Now I find this statement most disturbing because, if true, the reputation of UCT's medical faculty will suffer a significant blow.

Sixty years ago, I graduated with an MBChB degree from UCT and now, long retired from medical practice, it hurts me to see an internal strife in the medical faculty becoming front page news, probably all over the world.

What clinical research had the professors undertaken to statistically prove Noakes to be wrong, and also to make 'outrageous, unproven claims about disease prevention'?

Noakes has been well-known and well-regarded in medical sports circles for many years. I do not know him personally but he has earned my respect in being honest and forthright in dealing with difficult medical problems in sport. As far as I am concerned, he has served UCT well, and I just cannot see him acting as a doctor who has no regard for the welfare of his patients.

This dispute has some significant practical consequences for UCT. Are the medical students now being told that Noakes is a charlatan? The *Annals of Internal Medicine* would appear to negate such a belief.

There is a way out of this impasse. It should be possible to do research together, although it will require a willingness to let 'bygones be bygones'.

The dietary treatment for coronary and stroke recovering patients, followed-up for a long-term period, needs to be done. There is an epidemic of obesity, particularly severe in South Africa. UCT must lead the way. A dietary solution is urgently required.

Be the leader in this research in Africa! Appoint Noakes as a consultant to the Department of Medicine. All parties working together is what UCT needs. The rewards will be great.

Dr Slabbert raised an interesting point. How active is the UCT Faculty of Health Sciences in researching dietary solutions for the diabetes/obesity epidemic that has swamped the Western Cape in the past 40 years? Indeed, what is the quality and relevance of the research being undertaken at UCT's Division of Human Nutrition, the then head of which (Marjanne Senekal) was a co-signatory of the *Cape Times* letter?

One particularly challenging response came from a senior colleague, UCT emeritus professor Max Klein, who sent an email to De Villiers on 4 September, cc'ing me. Sadly, Klein passed away suddenly in early 2015, without ever receiving a response, or even an acknowledgement, from De Villiers.

Bias and distasteful villification of Noakes

Max Klein [mklein01@gmail.com]
Sent: Thursday, September 04, 2014 9:21 AM
To: Wim De Villiers
Cc: Timothy Noakes

Professor Willem de Villiers
Dean Faculty of Health Sciences

Dear Professor de Villiers

I protest in the strongest terms the biased presentation of "facts" on your web-page which in the guise of informing debate is aimed at discrediting Professor Noakes.

> The Big Fat Debate
> http://www.health.uct.ac.za/fhs/news/high-fat-diet-debate

Instead of presenting facts in a manner which gives a literate person the opportunity to form their own opinion, the web page presents confusing verbiage in a torrent which plays to parochial prejudice. Opinions, newspaper articles and performance before TV cameras are used as substitute for a clear delineation of the issues and the intelligible presentation of the facts. A propaganda onslaught is presented in the guise of an effort to inform discussion and help the public to make rational choices on an important health matter.

A model of how facts should be be presented for perusal is this article by Gunnars:

> 23 Studies on Low-Carb and Low-Fat Diets – Time to Retire The Fad
> By Kris Gunnars
> **http://authoritynutrition.com/23-studies-on-low-carb-and-low-fat-diets/**

Please, could you give Gunnars' article prominence on the web-page together with the following article published 2 days ago in the New York Times and almost simultaneously in the National Post, which is the latest, if not the last word on the subject? They should act as a corrective to the current hysteria.

> New York Times, Sept 1, 2014
> A Call for a Low-Carb Diet That Embraces Fat
> http://www.nytimes.com/2014/09/02/health/low-carb-vs-low-fat-diet.html?_r=0

> National Post
> Low-carb, high-fat diet is best for weight loss, heart health, U.S. study says
> http://news.nationalpost.com/2014/09/02/low-carb-high-fat-diet-is-best-for-weight-loss-heart-health-u-s-study-says/

I also wish to protest protest strenuously the unprecedented criticism and vilification of Professor Noakes in your letter to the Cape Times.

> The Editor
> Cape Times
> 22 August 2014
>   ...
>
> "It is therefore a serious concern that Professor Timothy Noakes, a colleague respected for his
> research in Sports Science, is aggressively promoting this diet as a 'revolution', making
> outrageous unproven claims about disease prevention, and maligning the integrity and credibility of peers who criticise his diet for being evidence-deficient and not conforming to the
> tenets of good and responsible science. This goes against the University of Cape Town's
> commitment to academic freedom as the prerequisite to fostering responsible and respectful
> intellectual debate and free enquiry."

I find the letter distasteful. It diminishes the the Faculty's stature and credibility. That letter was ostensibly sent on behalf of the Faculty but in fact it merely expresses the personal views of the authors. Your signature gives it a deceptive cloak of authority.

As I understand it, only the Faculty Board can speak for the Health Sciences Faculty. I am open to correction but to my knowledge the Faculty Board has not expressed itself on the Banting diet and to my mind it would have be foolhardy for it to take sides on such a contentious matter.

Based on the facts available, the only responsible advice anyone can give the public at present is this:

> **If Banting works for you, go for it**
>   but
> **Tell your doctor**
>   and
> **Ask your doctor to monitor your progress**

What I admire is Tim Noakes' integrity and courage in the face of such a hostility to keep going. He's a controversialist by nature and in this case as in others he had strong opinions about he seems to have found the right track.

UCT has a long "investment" in the fat hypothesis - set in ideas dating back over 50 years to the studies of Dr Brian Bronte-Stewart - in whose memory one of the Faculty's most prestigious awards is named. Some ego's have obviously been badly bruised by the fact that an A-Graded Sports Scientist ("*nogal*") has had the temerity to seize the initiative in a field others see as their private reserve. However, one of the important lessons from the history of science is that advances often come from people in parallel fields rather from the "experts" in a particular field. Experts have their status on the basis of past knowledge and achievement and are are often too set in their ways of thinking about a problem to be able to see it in a different light.

The late physicist and Nobel Prize winner Dr Richard Feynman - the subject also of Glieck's brilliant biography GENIUS - had a succinct definition of Science:

> **"Science is the belief in the ignorance of experts. "**
> Link to a source

What is abundantly clear is that Professor Noakes is not alone on the international stage, nor is he very original in holding the views he does about carbohydrates, fat and health, nor does he claim to be the only responsible scientist who holds them. He is unfairly represented as an irresponsible loose cannon.

His approach to promoting his ideas by means of a brilliant cookery book is certainly novel and perhaps his unprecedented success is what galls?

The vociferous backlash reminds me of the criticisms by the grumpy-guts who were pushed into the shadows following Chris Barnard's successful Heart Transplant. Noakes' & co-authors' reputed donation of over R300,000* from sales of the cookery book towards cleft-palate repairs in children reminds me also of Barnard's generous endowment to the University.

The Faculty's approach in this "discussion" focusses only on over-nutrition. Noakes has a broader appreciation. Under-nutrition is also a serious problem in our country. Noakes has identified offal (almost pure protein) as an affordable but wasted nutrient source for poor people and especially for farm-workers and their families. That is a highly original insight with profound implications for the health of our communities which stems directly from his interpretation of the data on nutrition.

Instead of wasting its time and credibility on attempts to rubbish Noakes' ideas *in toto*, the Faculty should celebrate at least this important insight as another *First for UCT* and give the idea its whole-hearted support.

I would prefer that the Faculty take corrective measures than for me to have to air these views in public media. Unfortunately the SAMJ's has closed discussion on one of the most important health issues to hit its columns in a long time

Sincerely

Max Klein
Emeritus Assoc Prof Paediatrics

Cc: Professor TD Noakes
Bcc:'d recipients: Please maintain confidentiality and do not distribute - thank you

* In fact, sales of *The Real Mal Revolution* would generate in excess of R1 million for Operation Smile, allowing surgical correction for more than 200 children with cleft-lip deformities. This was never acknowledged by any of the four professors, the Faculty of Health Sciences or UCT. One wonders why not.

The key point that I learnt from Klein's email was that De Villiers had sent the letter to the *Cape Times* on behalf of the board of the Faculty of Health Sciences without even consulting the board for its approval. Yet readers would have assumed that the letter carried the full support of the faculty as well as that of UCT. At the time it was unclear to me whether or not the university had been consulted. If it had not, UCT's senior management should have called De Villiers in to explain to Vice Chancellor Max Price why he had written such a defamatory letter with the apparent backing of UCT and its Faculty of Health Sciences without consulting either.

Price should then have informed De Villiers that UCT defends and treasures academic freedom, and that academic debate should always be respectful and free of public vilification and humiliation of anyone with whom those in power do not agree.

That the university's senior management failed to respond in this way indicates, sadly, that they were complicit in the entire affair.

But were De Villiers and UCT complicit in a much larger action against me? And what of Lionel Opie's involvement in the drafting of the letter?

Over the course of the next two years, Marilyn and I pondered how Opie had become involved. At a meeting I requested with De Villiers and Mayosi at UCT in December 2014, De Villiers was adamant that not only had Opie signed the letter, but he had also been the person most responsible for its writing. Opie, he assured me, had also suggested that the letter be sent to the minister of health. I was incredulous because, at the time, Opie had assured both Marilyn and I that this was not the case. As that meeting broke up, I presented De Villiers and Mayosi with copies of Nina Teicholz's book, *The Big Fat Surprise*, and an editorial published the previous week in the *British Medical Journal* (*BMJ*). The editorial was a review of Teicholz's book written by a former *BMJ* editor, Dr Richard Smith.[26] In it, he wrote the following:

> By far the best of the books I've read to write this article is Nina Teicholz's *The Big Fat Surprise*, whose subtitle is 'Why butter, meat, and cheese belong in a healthy diet.' The title, the subtitle, and the cover of the book are all demeaning, but the forensic demotion of the hypothesis that saturated fat is the cause of cardiovascular disease is impressive. Indeed, the book is deeply disturbing in showing how overenthusiastic scientists, poor science, massive conflicts of interest, and politically driven policy makers can make deeply damaging mistakes. Over 40 years I've come to recognize what I might have known from the beginning that science is a human activity with the error, self deception, grandiosity, bias, self interest, cruelty, fraud and theft that is inherent in all human activities (together with some saintliness), but this book shook me.

After describing the bad science underlying all aspects of Ancel Keys's diet-heart hypothesis, Smith concluded:

> Reading these books and consulting some of the original studies has been a sobering experience. The successful attempt to reduce fat in the diet of Americans and others around the world has been a global, uncontrolled experiment, which like all experiments may well have led to bad outcomes. What's more, it has initiated a further set of uncontrolled global experiments that are continuing. Teicholz has done a remarkable job in analyzing how weak science, strong personalities, vested interests, and political expediency have initiated this series of experiments. She quotes Nancy Harmon Jenkins, author of the *Mediterranean Diet Cookbook* and one of the founders of Oldways, as saying, 'The food world is particularly prey to consumption, because so much money is made on food and so much depends on talk and especially the opinions of experts.' It's surely time for better science and for humility among experts.

In 2017, the other great British medical journal, *The Lancet*, published a similar review, concluding: 'This is a disquieting book about scientific incompetence, evangelical ambition, and ruthless silencing of dissent that shaped our lives for decades … Researchers, clinicians, and health policy advisers should read this provocative book that reminds us about the importance of good science and the need to challenge dogma.'[27]

My hope was that Teicholz's book would be well read, especially by Mayosi, a long-time defender of Keys and the diet-heart hypothesis, who has since been appointed, in September 2016, as UCT's dean of health sciences, succeeding De Villiers.

More than two years after that meeting, in early 2017, my legal team gained access to an email chain describing at least some of the events leading up to the writing of the UCT professors' letter. The emails revealed, rather surprisingly, that the person driving the letter was the Faculty of Health Sciences' marketing and communications manager, Linda Rhoda. In her original email, Rhoda referred to my 'crusade' that seemed 'to have reached Parliament'.

It is interesting that the head of marketing and communications has the power to decide how the faculty should respond to what she calls my 'crusade'. I would have thought her job was to project the faculty in a positive light, not to try to bring the career of a devoted faculty member into disrepute by protesting about his actions to the minister of health. It smacks of kindergarten politics.

Unfortunately, within 10 minutes Opie had responded, indicating his support for the initiative. By the same time the next day, a draft letter of 208 words, apparently crafted by Rhoda, was circulating. By Thursday afternoon, Opie and Senekal had added their comments, bringing the word count to 647.

Rhoda responded by asking that De Villiers and Mayosi complete the article in time to get it into 'Monday's Papers'. She also indicated that the article would need to be sent timeously to 'Max Price's office and the UCT Director of Communications and Marketing'.

This email seems to confirm that, at the very highest level – the office of the vice chancellor, Dr Max Price – UCT was complicit in this action against me.

The university chose not to provide any further emails to my legal team, so it is not clear exactly how much of the letter-writing was undertaken by De Villiers and Mayosi. It seems that Rhoda and Opie concocted the core, with inputs from Senekal.

I suspect the reason why Opie did not recall any of these events was that he was extremely unwell at the time. Already on the afternoon of Tuesday 19 August, the same day that the *Cape Times* carried the story about my speech, Opie was ill enough to consult a medical practitioner. His condition worsened over the following days, culminating in his admission to hospital on Friday 22 August. He underwent emergency surgery the next day and was only released from hospital on 8 September. Thus, on the Friday that the letter that would humiliate me and damage my reputation was being finalised under Rhoda's stewardship, Opie was battling a potentially fatal condition.

Do I think that Professor Opie was in any condition on that Friday to properly add his intellectual support to the final draft of the letter that would appear in the *Cape Times* three days later? My answer is no. Having worked with Opie for five years in the late 1970s, and having observed him ever since, I learnt much about the way he conducts himself. He is meticulous and would only ever submit work when he considered it to be perfect. I learnt that his process of finalising a manuscript could last days, if not weeks, as he carefully read and reread and re-corrected the work until finally he would say: 'Yes, Tim, this paper is now ready for submission. We can do no more.'

The UCT professors' letter was not perfect – far from it. Its use of language lacked the elegance and attention to scientific detail and integrity that has always characterised Opie's thoughts and ideas. Worse, it had no basis in science. Over more than 40 years, Opie had taught me that science must be the sole basis for anything I might choose to profess.

So I can only conclude that if he did read the final draft of the letter and if he did support its publication, then Opie was acting completely out of character. Indeed, when we subsequently discussed the matter, Opie gave me a copy of another letter he had sent to De Villiers in November 2014. It included the following:

The fact is I strongly disassociate myself from certain statements and particularly with the aggressive tone of 4th paragraph starting: 'It is therefore a serious concern that Professor Noakes ...'

Any disagreement with the views of Professor Noakes could have been expressed in a way appropriate to academic discourse and healthy debate which should be devoid of hostility and aggression. Incidentally, no reference was made in the letter to Professor Noakes' fine achievement in initiating and building up the Sports Science Centre as the Director over many years, to the credit of UCT. He funded the construction entirely from 5 major donors listed in the entrance. No one can dispute the fact that due to his very considerable personal efforts SA and UCT in particular have appeared as world-class players in the area of exercise physiology.

Accordingly, I would like to have the opportunity of sending a letter of disagreement and correction as based on the details of my objections as given above.

I would appreciate your personal views on this matter.

I suspect that Opie is still awaiting a reply to his request.

He is correct to recoil from the aggressive tone of the email because he understands that it represents nothing more than academic bullying and the silencing of a dissenting opinion. In our most recent correspondence, in early 2017, I put it to my long-term sage that associating himself with the *Cape Times* letter and its three authors had perhaps been an 'error of judgement' on his part.

To which he instantly agreed.

6

The Naudé Review

'It is difficult to get a man to understand something,
when his salary depends on his not understanding it.'
– Upton Sinclair, American writer

I suspect that in writing their defamatory letter to the *Cape Times*, the four UCT professors had been emboldened by the publication, a month earlier, of a meta-analysis that would become known as the Naudé/Stellenbosch/UCT review comparing the effects of LFHC and (allegedly) LCHF diets on weight loss and other health markers.[1] I would later learn that the Naudé review was also decisive in directing the decision of the HPCSA preliminary inquiry committee to charge me with 'disgraceful conduct' in September 2014.

During my HPCSA trial in November 2015, the complainant, dietitian Claire Julsing Strydom, stated under oath:

Because everyone was going on what the evidence was saying. Everybody was waiting for this publication [the Naudé review] because we could not simply go ahead and make [a] statement about Prof. Noakes's hypothesis or diet without looking at the evidence. So everybody, *all these big organisations* were waiting on the publication of this information before we could make any kind of media statement ...

In any science ... expert opinions is [*sic*] your lowest level of evidence and a systematic review and meta-analysis would be the highest level. So before any media statements could be made we had to get that information and *all these associations* were waiting on that. It is not like you are saying it. It is not like everybody joined together to now make a statement against Prof. Noakes. We were all waiting for the evidence to be published ... We would not just want to say oh, we do not agree with it [Noakes's opinion] just because of nothing. We had to wait for that research to be complete. So the, *all these associations* were waiting for this information, and that is what it was [all emphasis my own].

Who these 'big organisations' and 'associations' were and why they had expressed such an interest in the Naudé review became clear in press statements they issued immediately after its publication. They were the HSFSA, ADSA and HPCSA, among others.

I first became aware of the existence of the Naudé review in the report of the Centenary Debate published in the *SAMJ* in February 2013.[2] There, UCT professors Naomi 'Dinky' Levitt and Krisela Steyn had stated that the SAMRC would soon be releasing its own paper on the LCHF diet. A former student then working for a leading medical insurance company subsequently confirmed in 2014 that a meta-analysis was indeed being prepared.

I was mildly surprised, as a meta-analysis of the effects of true LCHF diets had already been published the previous year. In the *British Journal of Nutrition* in May 2013, Nassib Bezerra Bueno and his colleagues showed that people eating less than 50 grams of carbs per day (the diet I was promoting) lost more weight than those eating higher-carb diets. What is more, important health markers showed greater improvement in those eating the low-carb diet.[3] I could not understand why we would need another meta-analysis of the same data.

Unless, of course, the study was motivated by something other than the advancement of truth and science.

On 9 July 2014 I received a phone call from journalist Wilma Stassen, who informed me that she had received a press release from the HSFSA about a new University of Stellenbosch meta-analysis that was relevant to the Banting diet. At the time I was unaware that Stassen is employed as a journalist by Stellenbosch's Faculty of Medicine and Health Sciences, and that she is, in effect, an embedded journalist within the faculty.

In her article, published the following day, titled 'Noakes's low-carb diet not healthier', Stassen referred to me as a 'celebrity professor' and described the Banting diet as a 'fad'. She quoted the study's lead author, Dr Celeste Naudé of the Centre for Evidence-based Health Care at Stellenbosch University: 'This study shows that when the amount of energy consumed by people following the low carbohydrate and balanced diets was similar, there was no difference in weight loss.'[4]

This finding would not have come as a surprise to the authors, especially Dr (now Associate Professor) Naudé, who teaches that all food calories are created equal and that, for weight loss, 'calories in' must always be less than 'calories out'. Based on this belief system, how could Naudé ever have expected a difference in weight loss between two diets providing the same number of daily calories? So even before they began their analysis, Naudé and her colleagues had biased the study to ensure a predictable outcome, specifically that there would be no difference in weight loss between the LFHC and LCHF diets.

Then, to make certain that the Banting/LCHF/'Noakes' diet had absolutely no hope of coming out on top, they did not even look at the diet that I advocate.

Instead, they studied diets with an average carbohydrate content of 35 per cent, knowing full well that the upper limit of the LCHF diet that I prescribe is between 5 and 10 per cent, providing between 25 and 50 grams of carbohydrate per day. For Stassen then to describe the studied (relatively high-carbohydrate) diet as 'Noakes's low-carb diet' was doubly questionable. As an embedded journalist, was she writing what she had been told to report by the Faculty of Medicine and Health Sciences at the University of Stellenbosch?

Designing a study, the result of which is predictable before the study even begins, is not science. Rather, it is the scientific equivalent of match-fixing in sport. And, as in sport, if science is fixed, the question is, who is the ultimate beneficiary? Someone or some organisation/s is benefiting financially.

Stassen's article continued: 'Based on these findings the Heart and Stroke Foundation of South Africa, the Association for Dietetics in South Africa and other health groups are warning the public about the possible health risks associated with banting.'

On behalf of the HSFSA, its then chief executive, endocrinologist Dr Vash Mungal-Singh, who had recently stated that heart disease is a carbohydrate-driven disease (see Chapter 7), seemed suddenly to have changed her opinion to suit the changed circumstances: 'Decades of research have shown the balanced diet to be safe and healthy in the long term, and along with a healthy lifestyle, is associated with a lower risk of heart disease, stroke, diabetes and certain cancers.'

Unconstrained by any real facts, she continued:

> We do not have similar proof that a low-carbohydrate diet is safe and healthy in the long term, and some studies already point towards an increased risk of heart disease and death with low carbohydrate diets. Chronic diseases like heart disease, stroke, cancer and diabetes develop over many years of exposure to risk factors.
>
> The follow-up of the trials included in the review is no longer than two years, which is too short to provide an adequate picture of the long-term risk of following a low carbohydrate diet. Based on the current evidence we cannot recommend a low carbohydrate diet to the public.

Instead, in the absence of any long-term RCT studies showing the value of a low-fat diet, and despite the findings of the WHIRCDMT, which once and for all disproved the safety and efficacy of the low-fat diet (Chapters 4 and 17), Mungal-Singh continues to burden South Africans with this false information.

ADSA spokesperson and soon-to-be-president Maryke Gallagher also gave comment for Stassen's article, linking her and her organisation to the collective effort by individuals from the University of Stellenbosch's Faculty of Medicine and Health Sciences, the SAMRC and the HSFSA to discredit me and the Banting diet.

The standout problem with the Naudé review, which all these expert commentators ignored, is that it was clearly designed to produce a predetermined out-come. Its design was then skilfully hidden from all but the most inquisitive readers.

The authors manipulated the analysis by including only those studies in which the energy intakes of subjects eating either the LCHF or low-fat diets were 'isoenergetic', i.e. the diets contained the same number of calories. For those like Naudé, who believe unequivocally in the CICO model of obesity and weight con-trol, there can obviously be only one outcome: there should not be any difference in the amount of weight lost by people eating either LCHF or LFHC if the diets are isoenergetic.

The isoenergetic research design is devious because it negates the key advan-tage of the LCHF diet, which is to reduce hunger, thereby allowing one to eat fewer calories without being constantly hungry and grumpy – or 'hangry', as US adult and child psychiatrist Dr Ann Childers calls it. That is how I lost 20 kilo-grams. By not binge-eating because I was continuously hungry, I was able to cut my daily calorie intake by roughly 1 000 calories without any hunger or food cravings – indeed, without any conscious effort whatsoever. In contrast, the only way that many people are able to lose weight on the conventional LFHC diet is because they have the discipline to ignore the sensations of hunger and to eat fewer calories than their brains and bodies desire. Research during the Second World War showed just how difficult it is to sustain this popular 'semi-starvation' dietary approach to weight loss. In fact, Ancel Keys, the diet activist who intro-duced the world to the low-fat dogma in the 1950s, is almost as famous – or notorious – for his semi-starvation studies in the 1940s.[5]

In one experiment, 36 US military conscientious objectors were placed on a 1 600 calories per day diet that included only those foods that were still available to European civilians during the period of famine at the end of the war – namely, 'whole-wheat bread, potatoes, cereals and considerable amounts of turnips and cabbage', with only 'token amounts' of meat and dairy. According to modern dietetics, this prescription would be considered ideal for weight loss, as it is low in calories and very low in fat, with just 17 per cent of calories coming from fat. As US science writer and author Gary Taubes noted: 'What happened to these men is a lesson in our ability to deal with caloric deprivation, which means, as well, a lesson in any expectation we might have about most current weight-loss advice, and perhaps particularly the kind that begins with "eat less" and "restrict fat."'[6]

Over the six months of the experiment, in addition to a multitude of adverse physiological effects, these men developed what Keys labelled 'semi-starvation neurosis', characterised by 'weakness and lack of energy (which are somewhat but not adequately covered by the item "tiredness"), general slowing down, sen-sitivity to cold, concerns with thoughts about food, and decrease in sociability'.[7] After six months of semi-starvation, almost all subjects reported that they tired quickly, felt unsteady when walking and had sensations of being 'weak all over'.

In addition, a majority found it hard 'to keep their mind on the job at hand', felt 'down-hearted frequently' and were 'frequently bored with people' so that 50 per cent 'preferred to be left alone'.[8]

I do not believe that it was the low-calorie content alone of the semi-starvation diet that caused these effects. I know of many people eating low-calorie LCHF diets who have not experienced these changes. Quite the opposite, they have been energised. Instead, I suggest that it was the extremely low fat content of the diet that caused these psychological effects. My point is that it is possible to eat fewer calories and not be hungry, provided the calorie-restricted diet is also high in fat.

A result of this unique, hunger-satisfying effect of the low-calorie LCHF diet – as described by Anne Stock and John Yudkin,[9] Atkins[10] and Westman, Phinney and Volek[11] – is that when LFHC and LCHF diets are used in isoenergetic weight-loss studies, those eating the LCHF diet must ingest more calories than are required to satisfy their hunger. In other words, the design of the experiment forces them to eat more calories than they need. As a result, they will lose less weight than they would have had they ingested the fewer calories that their satiated brains now found acceptable. Alternatively, if those on LCHF eat only the number of calories their brains direct them to eat, then to make the diets isoenergetic, those on LFHC must eat fewer calories than their brains desire, with the result that they would be perpetually hungry, experiencing a measure of the semi-starvation neurosis described by Keys.

Typically, the authors of isoenergetic studies do not appreciate this critical difference between the LFHC and LCHF diets. And why should they? They 'know' that hunger is driven by calories. Therefore, if both groups are eating the same number of calories, then both will be equally hungry or equally satiated. Unfortunately for them, science and experimentation with LFHC and LCHF diets show their theory to be incorrect. Furthermore, LFHC proponents never consider that their balanced isoenergetic diets, containing at least 45 per cent carbohydrate, might actually be driving hunger. Hence, they needlessly drive calorie consumption beyond what is necessary, thereby preventing weight loss and promoting weight gain and obesity.

Stassen did at least have the decency to quote my opinion on this in her article:

> But Noakes argues that a high fat and protein diet has been known to reduce hunger, leading to less food intake and thus less energy intake. He argues this diet is the easiest to follow. 'Unless the diet takes away hunger it will not produce the change in lifestyle necessary to sustain weight loss,' Noakes told Health-e News. 'Low-carb (diets) take away hunger in a way that no other diet does, that's why it is the easiest diet to follow and the most effective.'
>
> Noakes says that particularly favourable results are achieved on the low-carbohydrate diet in people with insulin resistance (pre-diabetes) ...

Another way in which the Naudé review was designed to produce a predictable outcome unfavourable to those of us promoting the LCHF/Banting diet was that it conveniently failed to investigate true low-carbohydrate diets. Instead, the range of carbohydrate intakes in the 'low-carbohydrate' interventions was 90 to 200 grams per day, comprising an average of 35 per cent of ingested calories. According to the LCHF/Banting definition, these constitute high-carbohydrate diets, because the carbohydrate content is way in excess of the range of 20 to 50 grams carbohydrate per day that we prescribe for people with significant weight problems and higher levels of IR.

Indeed, a key point that few people, other than those of us who have lost significant weight on the LCHF diet, understand is the exquisite sensitivity of weight loss to the level of carbohydrate intake in people with varying degrees of IR or appestat (the region of the brain that is believed to control appetite) malfunction. Figure 6.1 shows that those who are insulin sensitive (bottom line) can probably ingest carbohydrates over a wide range (0 to 500 grams per day) without gaining weight. But as they become progressively more insulin resistant, so increasingly fewer carbohydrates ingested daily will cause them to become overweight (second line from the bottom), obese (third line) or morbidly obese (top line).

Figure 6.1

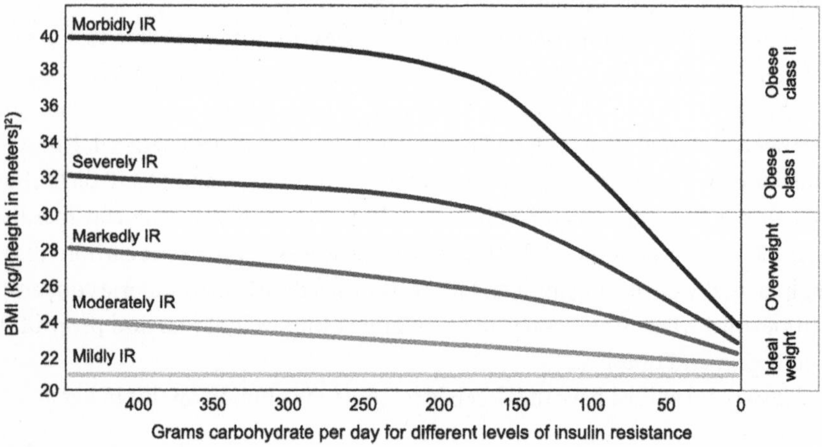

A theoretical model to project changes in body mass index (kg/m²) with changes in daily carbohydrate intake (grams/day) in people with different degrees of IR

The notable feature of this graph is the response to changes in dietary carbohydrate intake for a person with severe IR and appestat malfunction (top line). Should that individual decide to reduce her daily carbohydrate intake from over 400 to about 200 grams per day (horizontal axis), her body weight (vertical axis) will stubbornly refuse to change. She will be as morbidly obese eating 200 grams carbohydrate per day as she was when she ate 400 grams per day. But should she reduce her carbohydrate intake to less than 50 grams per day, the miracle occurs and dramatic weight loss begins.

Our current explanation is that a dramatic reduction in carbohydrate intake reduces blood insulin concentrations, reversing the persistent hyperinsulinaemia that is the defining characteristic of IR. But there are probably other factors as well. For example, the LCHF diet removes hunger, so the desire to eat excess calories is reduced, and this effect might be independent of the insulin effect. Removal of sugar and grains may also reduce the addictive drive to eat. Furthermore, the dramatic change in the nature of the foods eaten on LCHF may beneficially alter the gut microbiome in such a way that it increases weight loss, for we now know that the bacteria in our gut 'talk' to our brains!

Recall how Billy Tosh lost 83 kilograms in 28 weeks the moment he reduced his carbohydrate intake to about 25 grams per day and removed all sugar from his diet (see Chapter 5, Figure 5.1). He ascribed at least some of the effect to the removal of addictive foods from his diet.

From this we can infer that daily carbohydrate intakes well above 50 grams per day – the studies included by Naudé and her colleagues in their meta-analysis – are unlikely to have any real effect, particularly in those who are seriously overweight as a result of significant IR or appestat malfunction or, more usually, both.

Design flaws aside, it was the sweeping statements made by the representatives of the various health associations in Stassen's article that really made me despair of the authors' intentions. The implication that the Naudé review proved that the LCHF diet was dangerous and could cause increased rates of heart disease and other dread diseases was misleading. As Stassen should have pointed out, the Naudé meta-analysis did not ever set out to measure whether the LCHF diet was 'dangerous'. Instead, it measured changes in surrogate biological markers, such as blood LDL cholesterol concentrations, none of which can quantify danger. Also, the study found no difference in any of the surrogate markers that might have been interpreted as indicators of danger in people eating either 'low-carbohydrate' (according to their definition) or LFHC diets. Most interestingly, there were no differences in LDL cholesterol concentrations between those eating 'low-carbohydrate' and those eating LFHC diets.

The scientific conclusion should have been that, because there was no increase in LDL cholesterol concentrations (their marker of danger) in those on the 'low-carbohydrate' diets, according to their diet-heart hypothesis, the 'low-carbohydrate' diet could not possibly be considered dangerous. This is not how real science is meant to work. If there is no difference, there is no difference, however much you may personally wish that there was one.

On the same day, 10 July 2014, what appeared to be a second version of Stassen's article was published on *SA Breaking News* under the sensational headline 'New research shows Noakes diet no more than dangerous fad'.[12] According to this report, 3 200 participants in 19 international trials were placed on either the Banting diet or a balanced weight-loss diet for a period of between three months and two years. Because the review found that weight loss was the same on both diets, the writer concluded: 'This means Noakes' diet, which drastically reduces the intake of carbohydrates in favour of fats, resulted in weight loss by limiting the amount of calories (kilojoules) the body took in. In effect, a person lost weight because they reduced their caloric intake rather than restricting the amount of carbohydrates.'

The point, of course, is that not one of the 3 200 participants was ever put on the so-called Noakes diet. Furthermore, the review did not prove that the Noakes diet is dangerous because, in the first place, it did not study the Noakes diet. And, in the second place, there was no difference in any measured outcome between the different dietary interventions. The articles in the press could just as easily have stated that the popular LFHC diet promoted by ADSA and the HSFSA to lose weight and to prevent heart disease is no better than the 'Noakes diet' and therefore 'no more than a dangerous fad'.

When I read the Naudé review and the accompanying press releases from the embedded journalist, my faith in South African nutritional science was shaken. Was this science with an agenda? The agenda being to discredit Tim Noakes and 'his' diet so that no one would give any credence to anything he said or any inconvenient questions he raised?

As time went by, I began to wonder if perhaps the Naudé review might also be bogus. My suspicions of foul play only really began to surface in July 2016, when I reread Chris Bateman's review of the UCT Centenary Debate, published in the *SAMJ* in February 2013. Now one sentence in particular attracted my attention: 'According to Steyn and Levitt, the Cochrane Collaboration at the Medical Research Council is due to release a formal review of all existing data on the subject by the end of February 2013.'

If my opponents had been so keen to silence me, and if they believed they had definitive proof that I was wrong in the form of the Naudé review already in February 2013, why was that paper only published in July 2014? Why had they given me those 17 months to further advance my argument, and to publish *The Real Meal Revolution*? What could possibly have delayed the publication of such a politically charged paper?

Could it be that the paper had originally produced a result that was the opposite of what the authors (and their backers) had desired? If that had indeed happened, then the authors faced an appalling choice: either they publish the truth, which would essentially terminate the attacks on me and the Banting diet, or they modify the paper in ways that would show Banting to be either no better or significantly worse than the 'balanced' LFHC diet. The latter could then be spun to the South African public by compliant, embedded journalists as evidence that Banting is a 'dangerous fad'.

If the Naudé meta-analysis had actually shown that even a poor imitation of a real LCHF diet produced superior weight loss, the campaign to discredit me and Banting would have imploded. Would the HPCSA, who used the paper as the final piece of evidence vindicating their decision to prosecute me, still have been able to justify their actions? And what would have been the response if the media had announced that the 'balanced' LFHC diet advocated by ADSA and the HPCSA, and which forms the basis for essentially all government dietary interventions across the globe, is nothing better than a 'dangerous fad'?

This finding would have been utterly unacceptable to all involved in the study. Too many people, especially dietitians, were already aware that the study was proceeding for it to be shelved. And they were all expecting the Naudé review to finally discredit the Banting diet, and me, once and for all. The only way to save the day would have been to modify the analysis in ways that hopefully would not be detected by the expert referees appointed to review the paper when it was eventually submitted for publication. The authors would require just enough modifications to make the LFHC diet appear to be at least as effective as the 'low-carbohydrate' diet, particularly in terms of weight loss. With the assistance of a compliant media and organisations such as the HPCSA, ADSA and the HSFSA, Noakes and his diet would be appropriately discredited and the manipulations would lie undetected. The complicit scientists would all stay loyal to the omertà.

For the next two days, I wondered how I could test my hypothesis that the original analysis of the data in the Naudé review had shown that the 'low-carbohydrate' diet outperformed the 'balanced' LFHC diet. I realised that I needed to invite an expert in meta-analysis to perform a forensic analysis of the Naudé review. But who in South Africa could be trusted to do such a study without informing on me? Then it occurred to me that one of the world's leading health statisticians, Dr Zoë Harcombe, was coming to Cape Town in October to serve as one of my three expert witnesses in the HPCSA hearing. She had been one of the most impressive speakers at the February 2015 low-carb summit in Cape Town and had recently completed her PhD thesis, which was based on a series of meta-analyses of all the available evidence in the 1970s and 1980s that might have justified the adoption of the LFHC diet for the prevention of heart disease.[13] (As she would testify at the hearing, there was no such evidence. See Chapter 13.)

I emailed Harcombe to ask for her help, and within a few hours she had confirmed her enthusiasm for the task. At her request, I sent her PDF copies of the 14 studies that Naudé and her colleagues had used in their meta-analysis. And then I waited. Within a few days, Harcombe emailed to say that there were 'problems' with the paper; within a week she had sent me a draft of a potential article that she suggested we write for submission to the *SAMJ*.

For the rest of July and August we worked on the paper, submitting it for the first time in early September. After significant corrections at the suggestion of two expert referees, our manuscript was accepted for publication on 29 September 2016. 'The universities of Stellenbosch/Cape Town low-carbohydrate diet review: Mistake or mischief?' was published in the December 2016 issue of the *SAMJ*.[14]

We identified the following 15 material errors in the Naudé review:

Material errors 1–6

Naudé and her colleagues selected 14 studies[15] for inclusion in their meta-analysis; however, four of these should have been excluded: (1) and (2) reported the same data, and so only one should have been included; (3) and (4) failed Naudé and her colleagues' own inclusion criteria, as the fat content of the 'balanced' diet was less than their stipulated 25 to 35 per cent; and (5) did not report results in a manner that could be used in a meta-analysis looking at average weight loss. This particular paper, along with the other by De Luis (6), used the weight of participants at the end of the trial when the rest used average (mean) weight loss. This meant that, on a list of average weight losses ranging between 2.65 and 10.2 kilograms, Naudé and her colleagues tried to put end weight loss (of 88 to 91 kilograms) as the data to be used for the two De Luis studies. There was no reference to starting weight – only the participants' final body weights at the end of the trial were given. Harcombe and I called this 'absurd' – not a word to be used lightly in an academic paper, but we could think of no other. Anyone reading the Naudé review should easily have detected these fifth and sixth material errors.

Material errors 7–12

The strength of the meta-analysis method is that it assigns different weightings to different studies on the basis, among other criteria, of the number of subjects studied, the duration of the trial and, of course, in this study, the magnitude of the weight lost during the trial. Thus studies with more subjects, which continue for longer and whose subjects lose more weight, attract more 'weighting' in the meta-analysis than do shorter trials with fewer subjects who lose less weight.

For four of the studies (7–10), Naudé and her colleagues reported the number of subjects who completed the trial at a time later than that at which the weight-loss data they included had been recorded. Because fewer subjects completed these trials than had their weights measured at interim stages during the trials, in the meta-analysis these trials would appear to include fewer participants than was the case, and hence would receive a less-favourable rating. In all these studies, weight loss was greater in the 'low-carbohydrate' diet groups. As a result, this method of analysis disadvantaged the overall pooled effect for the 'low-carbohydrate' diets.

In addition, in the case of the Wycherley study (10), Naudé and her colleagues claimed that they had used weight-loss data for 52 weeks of the trial, but they had not. Instead, they had used data from 12 weeks of the trial. Using the 52-week data would have favoured the 'low-carbohydrate' intervention.

The Keogh study (3) also reported higher weight loss in the 'low-carbohydrate' group. However, while the data for the number of completers was taken at the end of the trial, the weight loss was taken from an earlier stage of the trial. In the subsequent meta-analysis, this mitigated the superiority of the 'low-carbohydrate' diet.

Material errors 13–15
The Naudé review reported weight loss in the control group in the Farnsworth study (2) as 7.95 kilograms, whereas the actual value given in the paper is 7.9 kilograms. This change favoured the 'balanced' LFHC diet.

Naudé and her colleagues reported that the weight losses in the two diet interventions in the Krauss study (11) were the same, specifically minus 2.65 kilograms. We were unable to locate this data in the original manuscript. Instead, in Table 2 of their paper, Krauss *et al.* reported weight losses of 5.4 and 5.3 kilograms for the 'low-carbohydrate' and 'balanced' LFHC diets respectively. Again, this change favoured the LFHC diet.

The slightly greater weight loss in the 'low-carbohydrate' group in the Sacks study (4) was wrongly assigned to the 'balanced' LFHC group in the Naudé review, and the lesser weight loss in that group was allotted to the 'low-carbohydrate' group, a modification that once again favoured the LFHC diet.

Despite the facts – that the Naudé meta-analysis did not review genuinely low-carbohydrate diets of the type that we promote; that the inclusion of isoenergetic studies negated the key benefit of the LCHF diet in reducing calorie consumption by reducing hunger; and that few of the studies used were actually designed to evaluate weight loss as their primary objective – Harcombe and I decided to repeat the meta-analysis using the 10 studies that fulfilled Naudé and her colleagues' inclusion criteria, and after correcting the 15 material errors.

Despite everything being apparently stacked against the 'low-carbohydrate' diet, our finding was absolutely clear: 'In conclusion, when meta-analysis was performed on the 10 studies that qualified for the inclusion in the study of Naudé *et al.* using their own criteria, the data confirmed that the lower-CHO [carbohydrate] diet produced significantly greater weight loss than did the balanced diet.'[16]

Perhaps unsurprisingly, our paper was met with silence. No embedded scientists published articles stating that our re-analysis of the Naudé review had established that the 'balanced' LFHC diet is inferior to a low-carbohydrate diet for weight loss. The only journalist to suggest that our re-analysis showed that the low-fat 'balanced' diet is a dangerous fad that South Africans should avoid at all costs was the co-author of this book, Marika Sboros. She was also the only one to address the core issue: that the Naudé review might possibly contain evidence of scientific fraud.

Even more disturbingly, at the time of writing in September 2017, neither the universities involved (Stellenbosch, Cape Town and Liverpool) nor the SAMRC have taken any definitive actions to determine whether or not the paper is fraudulent. The editors of the journal in which the original meta-analysis was published, *PLoS One*, have taken more than nine months to decide if they will act on our request to decide whether the paper should be withdrawn, as it appears to be fraudulent.

On Tuesday 20 December 2016, I was waiting in line at a local coffee shop when the person in front of me pointed to a newspaper and said, 'I see you are in the news again.' He was referring to an article in the *Cape Times* titled 'Noakes disputes diet study'.[17]

It was a report of my and Harcombe's *SAMJ* analysis of the Naudé review. For the most part, the journalist quoted directly from our paper. But the final two paragraphs attracted my attention:

> In a statement, authors of the original study – Celeste Naude, Anel Schoonees, Taryn Young and Jimmy Volmink of Stellenbosch, and Marjanne Senekal of UCT and Paul Garner of the Liverpool School of Tropical Medicine – said that Harcombe and Noakes' paper was submitted as evidence in the recent HPCSA hearing into the professional conduct of Noakes.
>
> 'The numerous criticisms of the review in the Harcombe paper were addressed in the hearing during the cross-examination of Dr Harcombe. Dr Harcombe conceded more than seven times that the "errors" she had pointed out in her paper were in fact not material to the findings of the review. Some "errors" were in fact found to be sound statistical methods,' they said.

For those of us who were actually present at the HPCSA hearing, this was certainly an unusual interpretation. Rechecking the transcripts of Harcombe's testimony told us that their statement had no basis in fact.

This was the first response from Naudé and her colleagues to our analysis that I had seen. If this was the best they could do, then they clearly had no answers to counter the obvious implication of our detective work.

Harcombe and I spent a few hours the next day preparing a response, which was published in the *Cape Times* on Friday 23 December.[18] 'The defence [of

Naudé *et al.*] is as poor as the original article,' we began. 'The authors have made no attempt to address the 14 [*sic*] material errors we identified, all but part of one in their favour.' We pointed out that their use of a duplicate study was sufficient to warrant retraction of the paper by *PLoS One*, and that the authors had made no attempt to defend their conclusions or the tens of errors 'sloppy and unworthy of the esteemed organisations they represent'.

We next pointed out that their claims that our criticisms were addressed during Harcombe's cross-examination, and that Harcombe conceded that the errors were not material, were simply not true:

> Dr Harcombe conceded nothing. She was the one who presented faithfully to the panel which errors were material, which were not, and the consequences of each.
>
> The hearing transcripts confirm that while giving testimony Dr Harcombe used the term 'material error' 16 times. While under cross-examination, Dr Harcombe twice dismissed questions by volunteering 'I did not report this/that as a material error'. The authors' errors thus remain unaddressed and unexplained. As a consequence, our question remains unaddressed and unexplained. Was this mistake or mischief?

A few weeks later, a *News24* article quoted Stellenbosch University as saying: 'The researchers rigorously applied the international gold standard of research synthesis, namely the Cochrane review process, which lends the greatest level of credibility to their results.'[19]

The same article quoted Harcombe's response: 'Cochrane is a methodology. It needs to be used accurately and honestly and in good faith to achieve the results it can produce. Cochrane methodology should enhance the reputation of a paper. This paper has managed to impair the reputation of Cochrane.' (Privately, Harcombe was of the opinion that Stellenbosch was really saying: 'We used Cochrane and we are very experienced, so we cannot have erred.' This is not, of course, a credible answer for a university that wishes to be taken seriously.)

The article ended with the following promise: 'Stellenbosch University said a formal response to the points of contention Noakes and Harcombe had raised would be submitted to the *South African Medical Journal.*'

Two months later, Naudé *et al.*'s response appeared in the *SAMJ* in the form of a letter, imposingly titled 'Reliable systematic review of low-carbohydrate diets shows similar weight-loss effects compared with balanced diets and no cardiovascular risk benefits: Response to methodological criticisms'.[20] Unfortunately, once again, the authors failed miserably to address our concerns. They admitted to just one of the 15 material errors – the use of duplicate publications – and ignored the rest. Perhaps they believe that if they do not address them, they will somehow magically disappear. 'We welcome scrutiny and comments,' they concluded. 'Having considered these carefully, we stand by our analysis and results.'

The letter was signed by all six authors, indicating that they are each equally responsible for any errors in the original paper. It is noteworthy that their conflict-of-interest statement indicated that five of the authors 'work for a charity committed to using scientifically defensible methods to prepare and update systematic reviews of the effects of health interventions'. None was bold enough to name the charity. It is, in fact, the Liverpool School of Tropical Medicine's Effective Health Care Research Consortium. One wonders why they didn't just say so.

Our response was written within a week and appeared in the May issue of the *SAMJ*.[21] We began by stating that it is common cause that the Naudé meta-analysis played a decisive role in my prosecution by the HPCSA, and that in her testimony under oath on 24 November 2015, Claire Julsing Strydom had said: 'So before any media statements could be made we had to get that information and all these associations were waiting on that ... We were all waiting for the evidence to be published.' We continued:

> Another prosecution witness, Prof. H Vorster, referred to the Naude *et al.* meta-analysis five times and quoted from it verbatim once. A third prosecution witness, Prof. A Dhansay, referenced the meta-analysis twice, using the term 'Cochrane' to ensure that it was afforded the appropriate esteem. Without the 'correct conclusion' from this meta-analysis, it is possible that the HPCSA trial against Noakes might never have happened. Therefore, the importance of the Naude *et al.* meta-analysis extends far beyond any role purely as a neutral scientific publication.

We then wrote that if we had realised that disproportionate consideration would be given to this ostensibly innocuous publication in the HPCSA hearing, we would have examined it sooner. Having now submitted it to careful analysis, we found it to be 'replete with errors'.

Next we traced the tardy response of the authors to our detailed re-analysis, before launching into more ferocious criticisms:

> The authors cheaply suggest that we show a 'lack of understanding' of their protocol. We understand the Naude *et al.* protocol only too well. Indeed, we appear to understand it rather better than do its authors:
> - We understand that the authors set isolcaloric as a criterion, which would mitigate the satiety advantage of low(er)-carbohydrate (CHO) diets.
> - We understand that the authors selected studies with an average CHO intake of 35% (35% fat, 30% protein) to represent 'low CHO' diets, which is substantially different from the 5% CHO (<50 g/day), moderate-

protein and high-fat diet that is used for the therapeutic management of obesity and type 2 diabetes mellitus.

- We understand that they set an inclusion criterion of 25–35% fat in the so-called balanced diet. This criterion was reiterated in Tables 2 and 3 and yet ignored by the authors, as they included two studies that failed their own criterion. These errors remain unaddressed by the authors in any of their responses.
- We understand that they set the key outcome measure as 'total weight change'. They then used end weight, with no reference to start weight, in two studies, which was in breach of their own protocol and absurd. These errors remain unaddressed by the authors.

In their response to the *SAMJ*, the authors have accepted only one of the numerous errors that we documented in their article – their admission that they included a duplicate study. This alone is grounds for retraction of the article.

The authors have not addressed any of the other numerous errors, material or otherwise, which we documented.

We then once more went through each of the material errors that the authors continued to ignore, at the same time addressing a set of red herrings that they had introduced in their response, and which only indicated that there were additional material errors that we had not originally identified.

It is understandable that the authors chose rather to raise new issues (ITT, standard mean difference and significance) and to ignore the numerous errors that we identified in our critique, presumably because they have no cogent answers. As a result, those material errors have remained unanswered since October 2016 and unless addressed, they render the article worthless, other than of retraction.

Given that only one error has been addressed and accepted (the duplication), we may never receive an answer to our research question: was this mistake or mischief? We may also never know if Prof. Noakes would have suffered for years in the way he has, had this article not made competence or conspiratorial errors.

Especially because 'our repeat of the authors' meta-analysis, using their methodology, but without the errors, produced a different result – a result that would *not* have given those keen to prosecute Prof. Noakes the ammunition they were "waiting for"' – namely, that the 'low-carbohydrate' diet, even as inappropriately described by Naudé and her colleagues, outperformed the 'balanced' diet. Which was exactly what I had suspected might be the case when Harcombe and I began our re-analysis in July 2016.

This undignified academic tussle raises a number of tough questions. First, because Naudé *et al.* are so reluctant to explain the origin of the material errors in their paper, we may never know whether they were simple mistakes or part of something more sinister. Second, and related, if the meta-analysis had been performed properly and had shown that the 'low-carbohydrate' diet outperformed the low-fat 'balanced' diet, it would have been extraordinarily difficult for the HPCSA preliminary inquiry committee to initiate their action against me. These six authors therefore played a material role in bringing about most of what we describe in this book. Was this by design?

Third, the reluctance of the editors of *PLoS One* to properly investigate the nature of the material errors raises questions of who the journal is protecting, and why. If the journal wanted to make a statement but did not wish to investigate the authors for data manipulation, it could simply have withdrawn the paper on the basis that the analysis included duplicate publications. Fourth, the failure of the universities and the SAMRC to take action raises similar questions. The credibility of Cochrane organisations worldwide has also been tarnished, yet they, too, have done nothing.

So what effects did the publication of this paper have on me and the six authors?

I was saddled with a multimillion-rand hearing that lasted more than three years. Celeste Naudé, however, was appointed co-director of the newly established Cochrane Nutrition Field (CNF) on 23 August 2016. A Stellenbosch University Faculty of Medicine and Health Sciences press release stated:

> The CNF will be under the leadership of Cochrane South Africa, the South African Medical Research Council, and the Centre for Evidence-based Health Care (CEBHC) at the FMHS [Faculty of Medicine and Health Sciences], along with international partners.
>
> The field will be led by Co-Directors Solange Durão of Cochrane SA and Celeste Naude of the CEBHC, with guidance from an international advisory board comprising representatives from multiple stakeholder and partner groups.
>
> 'The vision of Cochrane Nutrition is that Cochrane will be the independent, globally recognised go-to place for nutrition systematic reviews,' said Solange Durão. 'Cochrane Nutrition will support and enable evidence-informed decision-making for nutrition policy and practice by advancing the production and use of high-quality, globally relevant nutrition-related Cochrane reviews,' she continued ...

'Cochrane Nutrition will aim to coordinate activities related to nutrition reviews within Cochrane; to ensure that priority nutrition reviews are conducted with rigorous methodological approaches; and, to promote the use of evidence from nutrition systematic reviews to inform healthcare decision-making,' said Celeste Naudé.

'An exploratory meeting with interested stakeholders held in Cape Town in 2015 established that there is broad-based support for such a field from both Cochrane and external stakeholders,' she continued.[22]

We can be certain of the exact nature of the nutrition advice that the public will be receiving from the CNF. My guess is that the South African food industry, in particular, would have been especially pleased by Naudé's appointment.

For example, in another meta-analysis, Naudé proposes that 'increasing vegetable and fruit intake in South Africa could potentially contribute to reducing the burden of nutrition-related conditions in this country. Increasing vegetable and fruit intake in preschool children could improve their vitamin A nutriture.'[23]

She is prepared to make this suggestion even though (a) the optimum sources of vitamin A are animal or fish, not plant, sources, and (b) she acknowledges that: 'It should be kept in mind that the quality of the included systematic reviews ranged from low to high (AMSTAR), and most reviews did not assess the scientific quality of the studies.'[24]

If Naudé honestly wished to improve the vitamin A 'nutriture' of South African children, she did not need to undertake this meta-analysis of low-quality 'evidence'. Rather, she could simply have studied a textbook of human nutrition. Or read the publication of one of the HPCSA's expert witness, Muhammad Ali Dhansay, whose study found that the prevalence of vitamin A deficiency in undernourished South African schoolchildren was only 6 per cent in those who ate liver at least once a month, compared to the national deficiency prevalence of 64 per cent.[25]

But this would require that Naudé promote the eating of animal produce, a suggestion which, in my opinion, probably conflicts with her own dietary inclinations. So her final conclusion remains: 'This evidence supports the need to promote greater vegetable and fruit intake in South Africa.'

It appears that according to Naudé's logic, provided one acknowledges that the evidence is weak, once can still draw exactly the same definitive conclusion that one wished to derive, even before the meta-analysis has begun. This is known as confirmation bias and is unscientific.

When I was being trained in medicine in the 1970s, the standard joke was that orthopaedic surgeons use science in the same way that a drunk uses a lamp post: for support, not for illumination. Now I would argue, as perhaps does

Professor John Ioannidis, discussed shortly, that nutritional epidemiologists are the modern drunkards of medical science.

I am sure many more similar meta-analyses will be forthcoming from the Centre for Evidence-based Health Care over the next years and decades, and these will continue to promote the essentiality of 'balanced, prudent, heart-healthy diets, in moderation', the value of plant-based diets, the dangers of animal produce and the absolute innocence of sugar. So do we really need a CEBHC if we already know what they will conclude?

The sole UCT representative on the Naudé review, Marjanne Senekal, was promoted to full professor at the university's Faculty of Health Sciences on 9 May 2017.

In November 2016, the dean of medicine at Stellenbosch University, Jimmy Volmink (who had moderated the Centenary Debate), received an SAMRC recognition award for 'outstanding achievements in contributions to evidence-based healthcare in Africa'. The Faculty of Medicine and Health Sciences press release stated:

> The African region's 'father of evidence-based healthcare' is what the South African Medical Research Council (MRC) called Prof Jimmy Volmink …
>
> 'Volmink is an internationally renowned researcher, leader, mentor, critic and teacher in clinical epidemiology and evidence-based healthcare,' the MRC said in their commendation statement …
>
> 'Volmink was never afraid to challenge the accepted norms and doctrines. For example, his systematic reviews of the evidence regarding Directly Observed Therapy for Tuberculosis and Prevention of Mother to Child Transmission of HIV directly contradicted South Africa health policy at the time, and highlighted the complexity of policymaking in spite of available best evidence,' the statement continued.
>
> 'His work was underscored by the mission of Cochrane South Africa which stated that health care decision-making on the African continent should be informed by best-available evidence.'[26]

Given his stated position at the end of the Centenary Debate, specifically that he had 'heard nothing this evening that convinces me that we are on the wrong path in terms of these dietary guidelines' and that 'at all costs we must not do harm', I am sure Volmink can be trusted not to challenge 'the accepted norms and doctrines' of our current dietary guidelines. This despite the fact that, as dean of the medical faculty at the epicentre of the South African diabetes epidemic, he must be exposed to the tragic personal and other costs of this plague daily.

I wonder if South African medical science should really be investing so much effort in developing its capacity to undertake yet more meta-analyses. Professor

Figure 6.2

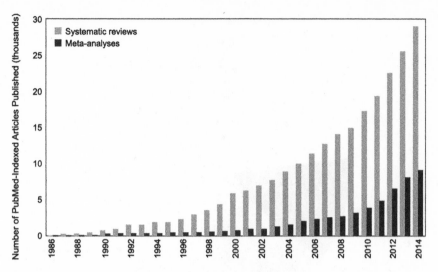

Number of 'systematic reviews' or meta-analyses published between 1986 and 2014. Reproduced from Ioannidis, 'The mass production of redundant, misleading, and conflicted systematic reviews and meta-analyses', *The Milbank Quarterly*

John Ioannidis of Stanford University thinks not. The title of his article on the topic signals his unconventional position: 'The mass production of redundant, misleading, and conflicted systematic reviews and meta-analyses'.[27] Figure 6.2 shows the massive increase in the number of systematic reviews and meta-analyses since 1986. If ever there was a growth industry in science, this is it.

His conclusions about the real value of such an explosion are not so sanguine:

> Currently, there is massive production of unnecessary, misleading, and con-flicted systematic reviews and meta-analyses. Instead of promoting evidence-based medicine and health care, these instruments often serve mostly as easily produced publishable units or marketing tools. Suboptimal systematic reviews and meta-analyses can be harmful given the major prestige and influence these types of studies have acquired. The publication of systematic reviews and meta-analyses should be realigned to remove biases and vested interests and to integrate them better with the primary production of evidence.

Figure 6.3 on page 132 shows Ioannidis's analysis of the value of all those system-atic reviews and meta-analyses. His conclusion is that only 3 per cent are decent and clinically useful; 17 per cent are decent, but not useful; 20 per cent are flawed beyond repair; and 27 per cent are redundant and unnecessary. Of the rest, 13 per cent were misleading and 20 per cent went unpublished.

Figure 6.3

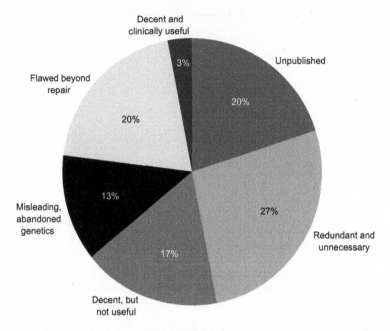

A summary of the usefulness of currently produced meta-analyses. Reproduced from Ioannidis, 'The mass production of redundant, misleading, and conflicted systematic reviews and meta-analyses', *The Milbank Quarterly*

Will the CNF under the co-direction of Naudé really make any difference to the future nutritional health of South Africans? When will nutritional epidemiologists acknowledge that memory-based dietary assessment methods – their key measurement tools – are 'fundamentally flawed owing to well-established scientific facts and analytic truths'?[28] So, should we not perhaps rather focus on human biology and how it is influenced by what we eat? In my opinion, this is the only way we are ever going to return the majority of South Africans to some measure of improved health.

The overriding message of the Naudé affair is that, while you have a responsibility to report what you think is scientific fraud, never expect anyone to thank you for your troubles.

7

Responses of Official Bodies

'The most difficult subjects can be explained to the most slow-witted man
if he has not formed any idea of them already; but the simplest thing
cannot be made clear to the most intelligent man if he is firmly persuaded
that he knows already, without a shadow of doubt, what is laid before him.'
– Leo Tolstoy, Russian author[1]

Although most of the attacks on me and the Banting/LCHF/Noakes diet originated from within South African academic institutions, a number were instigated
by official bodies interested in maintaining the status quo. Indeed, the very first
public attack came from the Centre for Diabetes and Endocrinology (CDE) in
Johannesburg.

Following the publication of my article in the *Discovery* magazine in 2011 and
the updated edition of *Challenging Beliefs* a few months later, the CDE released
a position statement on 4 April 2012 to counter what I was saying. They claimed
that '"carb-free", "low-carb", "high-protein" and other such diets have shown no
long-term benefit over conventionally balanced healthy eating plans'. The public,
they warned, 'should receive their guidance from practitioners trained in diabetes
rather than from the media'.[2]

The CDE encourages a uniform approach to the management of diabetes
in South Africa. It does this by training and certifying physicians in 280 centres
across the country in a standard, CDE-certified method for managing diabetes.
To its credit, the CDE monitors patient outcomes in an attempt to promote
what it believes are best practices for the management of T2DM in South Africa.
The problem is that, when looking at patient outcomes, the CDE sees what it has
become programmed to see.

The CDE promotes high-carbohydrate diets and the liberal use of insulin
to 'control' the predictably high blood glucose concentrations that occur in
diabetic patients whenever they eat carbohydrates.[3] In Chapter 17, I present
evidence that long-term studies have not found that the prescription of insulin
to patients with either type-1 diabetes mellitus (T1DM) or T2DM is the optimal
form of management.

The CDE position statement makes three key points:

- 'Diabetes UK recommends that for a 2000 kcal (8400 kJ) diet, 45%–60% of the total energy [for patients with either form of diabetes] should be supplied by carbohydrates (225–300 g per day).'
- 'Not only would a low-carbohydrate diet not be recommended for those with type 1 diabetes, but also it could be considered to be absolutely contra-indicated.'
- 'The use of a low-carbohydrate diet in individuals with type 1 diabetes may well promote ketosis and predispose these individuals to either ketoacidosis or to severe hypoglycaemia following exercise.'

Predictably, because South African–trained dietitians are prohibited from pre-scribing LCHF diets, CDE-certified dietitians cannot understand the cardinal features of the pathophysiology of diabetes, or why prescribing high-carbohydrate diets to people with diabetes is, in my opinion, medically negligent.

My advice that those with either form of diabetes should eat carbohydrate-restricted diets is based on a number of scientific studies, which have established the benefits of this approach.[4] In addition, the most basic understanding of human carbohydrate metabolism supports this position. Here is my counter-argument to the CDE position statement:

1. Carbohydrates are not an essential component of the human diet. There is no known medical condition that is caused by a deficiency of dietary carbohydrate. As a result, the influential US National Academy of Medicine, formerly called the Institute of Medicine, concludes: 'The lower limit of dietary carbohydrate com-patible with life apparently is zero, provided that adequate amounts of protein and fat are consumed.'[5] Hence, no human, and especially not anyone with an impaired capacity to metabolise carbohydrate, needs to eat carbohydrate.

2. This is to be expected, because, until the Neolithic period, which began with the agricultural revolution about 12 000 years ago, carbohydrates provided a minority of the food energy ingested by humans and human ancestors; most of the energy came from fat and protein.[6] Only in the last 40 years has carbo-hydrate become the major source of food energy in Europe and North America, as is now the case in all countries swamped by the obesity/T2DM epidemic.[7]

3. It is conventionally argued that people with diabetes must eat carbohydrates in order to ensure that their brains receive sufficient glucose for optimal function. While the human brain does have an obligatory glucose requirement of about 25 grams per day, this can be adequately supplied by the liver, which produces glucose from fat and protein in the process known as hepatic gluconeogenesis. We see this in the traditional Arctic Inuit and the Masai of East Africa, who eat essentially no carbohydrate, other than that present in milk.

Importantly, but often overlooked, the key biological feature of T2DM is the uncontrolled overproduction of glucose by the liver. Logically, if diabetic patients are already in a state of glucose overproduction, then their brains, as well as all their bodily tissues, must already be wallowing in an excess of carbohydrate. Why would they need more? How will the excess carbohydrates they are commanded to eat reverse their biological abnormality? Logically, it will only increase their already too high blood glucose concentrations.

4. Patients with T2DM do not die because of an inadequate supply of glucose to their brains. They die as a result of widespread obstructive disease in all their arteries (and capillaries), including those supplying blood to the heart and brain, causing heart attacks, strokes and blindness; to the kidneys, causing kidney failure, the treatment of which requires expensive but life-saving renal dialysis; and to the limbs, especially legs, leading to infection and gangrene, treatable only by amputation. The incidence of all these conditions is rising exponentially across the globe, like a disease tsunami that is completely out of control.[8] But because the certain cause was the misguided adoption of the 1977 Dietary Guidelines for Americans, no one involved in developing those guidelines is keen to acknowledge their contribution to this mounting global catastrophe. And until those responsible own up to their mistake, this global calamity will grow progressively worse.

5. When humans ingest carbohydrate, their blood glucose concentrations rise (see Figure 7.1 on page 136). To limit this rise, the body secretes the hormone insulin to switch off liver glucose production and to remove excess glucose from the bloodstream. However, as I explain more fully in Chapter 17, the rise in blood glucose and insulin concentrations is greatest in those with T2DM (because their tissues, including their livers, are insulin resistant, meaning that insulin is less effective in slowing down the liver's excessive glucose production and diverting glucose out of the bloodstream for storage in the muscles and liver).

What should be of real concern is that insulin is probably the key driver of most of the pathological changes that occur in those with IR who persist in eating high-carbohydrate diets. I discuss this in detail in Chapter 17.

If the ingested food includes fat and carbohydrate, the response is essentially the same – the blood glucose response is reduced, but insulin secretion is again increased.[9] Ingestion of fat alone does not induce an insulin response.[10] Interestingly, fat ingestion uniquely produces very large increases in secretion of gastric inhibitory polypeptide, the hormone whose key functions remain partially uncertain.

Figure 7.1

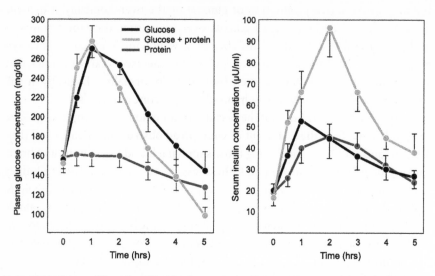

Changes in blood glucose (left panel) and blood insulin concentrations (right panel) in response to ingestion of protein, glucose, and glucose and protein at time 0 in persons with T2DM. Note that whereas protein ingestion did not cause the blood glucose concentration to rise, it did cause a moderate increase in blood insulin concentration (right panel). The co-ingestion of glucose and protein increased insulin secretion substantially, which reduced the blood glucose response (left panel). Reproduced from Nuttall *et al*.[11]

Figure 7.1 shows the response of blood glucose and insulin concentrations to a single meal. However, when food is ingested repeatedly during the day, these effects become additive, producing more frequent periods of hyperglycaemia (raised blood glucose concentration) and hyperinsulinaemia (raised blood insulin concentration), as shown in Figure 7.2 on page 137. These biological effects produced every few hours for decades are the cause of the explosion of chronic disease in people eating modern, highly processed, high-carbohydrate, high-sugar diets.

These findings show very clearly why high-fat diets with low-carbohydrate and low-protein contents produce the least insulin secretion and should, therefore, be the logical dietary choice for those with IR and diabetes of either type. Indeed, before the discovery of insulin in 1921/22 by Frederick Banting (no relation to William Banting) and colleagues at the University of Toronto, a diet very low in calories and carbohydrates was the only diet that could prolong the lives of children with type-1 (insulin deficient) diabetes.[12]

In the 1870s, William Morgan wrote that the aim of treatment of T1DM was 'avoiding feeding the disease, by selecting a diet devoid of saccharine matter [carbohydrates]'.[13] In 1848, the work of Claude Bernard had shown that the 'HUMAN RACE, like SUGAR-CANES, possess a sugar-manufacturing organ – the liver. In fact, that marvellous gland is as busily and actively engaged, both hourly and daily, in fabricating sugar, as it is in manufacturing and secreting

Figure 7.2

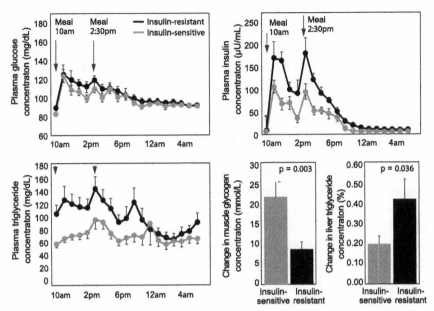

Changes in plasma glucose, insulin, triglyceride, and liver and muscle glycogen concentrations in response to the ingestion of two high-carbohydrate mixed meals in insulin-sensitive and insulin-resistant young men. Note that in response to carbohydrate ingestion, those with IR show similar changes in blood glucose concentrations when compared to insulin-sensitive young men, but larger increases in blood insulin, blood triglyceride and liver triglyceride concentrations, and smaller increases in muscle glycogen concentrations. Reproduced from Petersen *et al.*[14]

bile.'[15] So to clear the urine of glucose, Morgan wrote, 'a diabetic should exclude all saccharine and farinaceous materials from his diet'.[16] He concluded: 'Theoretically, the Diabetic should be supplied pretty largely with FAT; and practically it is found that its effect is highly beneficial.'[17]

This advice persisted through the early 1900s: 'there should be absolute avoidance of carbohydrates and accordingly a diet composed exclusively of fat and meat';[18] '10–25gm carbohydrate per 24 hours';[19] 'the total carbohydrate in the diet of diabetic patients is almost invariably restricted, and seldom exceeds 100 grams [per day]';[20] and, perhaps over-optimistically, 'If the [diabetic] patient stops overeating and eats less sugar and starch, most of the symptoms of diabetes will vanish.'[21] The Michigan Diet for Diabetes[22] also restricted carbohydrate intake to about 20 grams per day, and re-analysis of the Allen Diet for Type-1 Diabetes reveals that it typically contained approximately 39 grams carbohydrate per day (8 per cent of calories).[23] All this advice was based on the knowledge that it was dietary carbohydrate that raised blood glucose concentrations.

Unfortunately, with the discovery of insulin in the 1920s, physicians caring for patients with T1DM allowed dietary carbohydrate content to increase progressively, decade by decade. Whereas in 1915 the prescribed diet contained only

25 grams carbohydrate per day, by the 1940s this had increased to 172 grams per day.[24]

6. There are just 5 grams of glucose in 5 litres of human blood. Yet few portions of carbohydrate-rich foods contain less than 25 to 50 grams carbohydrate. This means that every time we eat a reasonable serving of carbohydrates, glucose in amounts of 5 to 10 times greater than the entire glucose-carrying capacity of our blood circulation is suddenly entering our system. This is a metabolic crisis for which humans, as a result of our evolution from an original primate ancestor, are simply not designed (see Chapter 16).

Considered together, these facts do not suggest that carbohydrates should be the primary source of energy in the diabetic's diet, as the CDE proposes.

Because of significant errors in their understanding of the biology of IR and T2DM, the CDE uses erroneous logic to explain how people with these conditions can and should ingest carbohydrates. The global model of diabetes management currently taught holds that diabetics have the right to eat all the foods found in the 'heart-healthy' LFHC diet. This diet is based on an intake of predominantly carbohydrates in the form of cereals and grains, starchy vegetables, fruits and sugar-sweetened beverages. Since the diet allows processed foods, including cakes, biscuits and desserts, it is also sugar-rich and rich in hydrogenated vegetable oils and trans fats. There is no need, we are assured, for those with sugar sickness and IR, and thus with an inability to properly metabolise carbohydrate, to restrict their sugar and carbohydrate intakes any more than those with a normal ability to metabolise carbohydrate.

All this makes the management of diabetes unique. The medical profession has never encouraged people with lactose intolerance to ingest milk; those with gluten or peanut intolerance to ingest wheat or peanuts; or those with alcoholism to keep drinking alcohol. Yet somehow this common-sense rule seemingly does not apply to the treatment of diabetes.

The result is that, when eating these high-carbohydrate/sugar combinations, those with T2DM develop persistently elevated blood glucose and insulin concentrations. But because patients with T2DM are insulin resistant, even this excess insulin production will not be sufficient to maintain normal blood glucose concentrations (because their livers are insulin resistant and will therefore continue to overproduce glucose regardless of how much carbohydrate is ingested and insulin secreted). So patients with T2DM are told that to lower these (unnecessary) carbohydrate-induced increases in blood glucose concentrations, all they need do is inject more insulin, a hormone that those who are insulin resistant are already secreting in excess and to which their bodies are already resistant (and becoming progressively more so with each passing day). We now understand that insulin, whether self-secreted or injected, further worsens IR (see Chapter 17).[25]

So the current diabetes advice is simple: Be 'normal'. Eat carbohydrates, because that is your constitutional right. Inject insulin. And ignore the risk of long-term consequences, because we all know that people with T2DM will die prematurely from their disease anyway.

The long-term consequences of following this advice are well documented. A recent analysis of systematic reviews and meta-analyses of contemporary RCTs concluded that ideal care, which maximises tight glycaemic control, produces no better outcomes than less-good care in patients with T2DM.[26] With regards specifically to insulin therapy, another meta-analysis concluded: 'There is no significant evidence of long term efficacy of insulin on any clinical outcome in T2D. However, there is a trend to clinically harmful adverse effects such as hypoglycaemia and weight gain. The only benefit could be limited to short term hyperglycemia.'[27]

In fact, the most expensive and intensive prospective study of the management of patients with T2DM – the Look AHEAD trial – was terminated prematurely when the researchers realised there was no prospect of a favourable outcome.[28] In all, T2DM patients who received what the American Diabetes Association believes to be the absolute optimum treatment did no better than those who received inferior care. I doubt whether the authors of these studies ever questioned if their failure to show any beneficial effects of this management approach was because patients on the trial were encouraged to eat LFHC diets. As we will learn, you cannot out-medicate the effects of a bad (high-carbohydrate) diet in those with IR.

Such disappointing outcomes only reinforce the belief that diabetes is an irreversible condition that must inevitably worsen with age. Of course, the pharmaceutical industry is only too pleased by my profession's promotion of this pessimistic prospect, because each year this gloomy disease model generates millions of new customers for its diabetic products. And with the promise that every customer will, over time, become more dependent on Big Pharma's increasingly expensive wares, profits for companies specialising in diabetes care are predicted to rise by about 20 per cent per year, essentially forever.

And even if the disease is perhaps not quite as lethal as the pessimists propose, we can still always blame the patient for any failed outcomes. So treatment failures occur because patients do not fully comply – they fail to take their medications as prescribed, they do not exercise enough, they become too stressed and do not get sufficient sleep, and they eat too much fat and not enough 'heart-healthy' carbohydrates.

The reason why the CDE's advice is wrong is because people with T2DM or IR cannot metabolise carbohydrates normally; they are carbohydrate intolerant. As a result, if they persist in eating high-carbohydrate diets, they become progressively sicker and more insulin resistant, requiring more medications, and ultimately die from the effects of widespread obstructive arterial disease caused by the continuous over-secretion (or self-injection) of insulin.

Therefore, logically, the first line of treatment must be to restrict the intake of carbohydrates in those with IR.

Fortunately, failed medical treatments based on fictitious biology cannot succeed forever. The power of social media will in time force change, as patients with IR learn that there is a better and simpler way to ensure their future health.

That same day, 4 April 2012, *The Times* picked up the story. In an article titled 'Experts refute Noakes's diabetes diet claims', Dr Stan Landau, a senior physician at the CDE, 'said there is no evidence that low-carbohydrate diets are good for people with type 1 or type 2 diabetes or people at risk. In fact, a low-carbohydrate diet can be harmful to them … Landau also said that Noakes has spoken out about diabetes like it is [a] "sinister and malignant" condition when in fact [it] is a "chronically manageable condition".'[29]

Had my opinion been sought, I would have shown that the published scientific evidence does not support Landau's statements. First, as I have described, the low-calorie, low-carbohydrate diet was the original diet for the management of T1DM before insulin was discovered in 1921/22. The diet was prescribed specifically because it delayed death in insulin-deficient children with T1DM. It was used in the hope that these children could be kept alive long enough for a life-saving 'cure' to be discovered.

For example, *Diabetic Cookery*, a famous cookbook of the day written for diabetics by Rebecca W. Oppenheimer, included lists of the ideal foods for diabetics, as well as lists of foods that should be avoided.

Included in her list of 'especially valuable' foods 'owing to their great nutritive qualities' are butter, olive oil, cream cheeses, meat, poultry, fish and eggs. In contrast, 29 foods high in carbohydrate are listed as 'strictly forbidden'. William Morgan provided similar lists in his 1877 publication, *Diabetes Mellitus: Its History, Chemistry, Anatomy, Pathology, Physiology, and Treatment*. The green list in *The Real Meal Revolution* includes only those foods Oppenheimer prescribed, while those she prohibited are on the orange and red lists, which include foods to be eaten only occasionally or not at all.

Second, there is no evidence that it is dangerous for modern diabetics to eat LCHF; in fact, quite the opposite. In 2014, Dr Osama Hamdy, medical director at the famous Joslin Diabetes Center, wrote:

It is clear that we made a major mistake in recommending the increase of carbohydrate load to >40% of total caloric intake. This era should come to an end if we seriously want to reduce the obesity and diabetes epidemics. Such a move may also improve diabetes control and reduce the risk for

Figure 7.3

12	DIABETIC COOKERY		13

DIABETIC COOKERY 12

CHEESES

1. Chester	3. Roquefort
2. Edam	4. Swiss

TABLE III

The following foods, owing to their great nutritive qualities, are especially valuable.

1. Butter	3. Cream
2. Olive Oil	4. Devonshire Cream

CREAM CHEESES

1. Gervais	5. Brie
2. Neufchâtel	6. Camembert
3. Stilton	7. Pot-cheese
4. Cheddar	8. Philadelphia Cream Cheese

MEAT AND POULTRY

1. Bacon	5. Beef
2. Ham	6. Mutton
3. Pork	7. Goose
4. Tongue	8. Duck

FISH AND EGGS

1. Mackerel	3. Caviar
2. Salmon	4. Eggs

DIABETIC COOKERY 13

TABLE IV

FOODS STRICTLY FORBIDDEN

1. Sugars	15. Beets (on doctor's order)
2. All Farinaceous Foods and Starches	16. Large Onions
3. Pies	17. All Sweet and Dried Fruits
4. Puddings	18. Honey
5. Flour	19. Levulose
6. Bread	20. All Sweet Wines
7. Biscuits	21. Liqueurs
8. Rice (by permission only)	22. Cordials
9. Sago	23. Syrups
10. Arrowroot	24. Beer
11. Barley	25. Ale
12. Oatmeal (by permission only)	26. Stout
13. Tapioca	27. Porter
14. Macaroni	28. Chocolate
	29. Condensed Milk

TABLE V

DRINKS PERMITTED

Sweetened with Saccharin only

1. Natural and Carbonated Waters	8. Clabber
2. Lemonade	9. Cognac
3. Tea	10. Rum
4. Coffee	11. Whiskey
5. Van Houten's Cocoa	12. Moselle and Rhine Wines
6. Cracked Cocoa or Cocoa Nibs	13. Bordeaux, Burgundy, and other sugarless wines
7. Sweet and Sour Cream	

A spread from *Diabetic Cookery* by Rebecca W. Oppenheimer, first published in 1917

cardiovascular disease. Unfortunately, many physicians and dietitians around the nation are still recommending high carbohydrate intake for patients with diabetes, a recommendation that may harm the patients more than benefit them.[30]

I have since been informed that Landau has modified his views on the optimum diet for people with T2DM. Apparently he is no longer so certain that they should be eating high-carbohydrate diets. In addition, the CDE has initiated a trial of the effects of a very low-calorie diet in the management of T2DM, on the basis of evidence that this intervention may reverse T2DM in some patients.[31] For this, Dr Landau earns my deepest respect. There is perhaps nothing more difficult in clinical medicine than admitting an error.

In the same *Times* article, dietitians Tabitha Hume and Theresa Marais claimed that high-protein diets place 'undue stress on the kidneys which could lead to long-term damage'. Firstly, the LCHF diet is not a high-protein diet, and there is no published evidence showing that even the extremely high protein intakes of bodybuilders (2.8 grams protein per day) produce any evidence of kidney damage.[32]

A recent RCT found that a 'low-carbohydrate diet is as safe as Mediterranean or low-fat diets in preserving/improving renal function among moderately obese participants with or without type 2 diabetes (with mild renal impairment)'.[33] Similarly, a retrospective study of more than 11 000 US adults found that '[d]iets higher in plants and animal protein, independent of other dietary factors, are associated with cardiometabolic benefits, particularly improved central adiposity, with no apparent impairment of kidney function'.[34]

There is also evidence for the reversal of progressive renal failure with an LCHF diet in an obese diabetic patient, so that the authors question whether 'obesity caused by the combination of a high-carbohydrate diet and insulin may have contributed to the patient's failing kidney function'.[35] Secondly, there is clear evidence that the primary cause of kidney failure is T2DM.[36] And diabetes is caused by high-carbohydrate/high-sugar diets in people with IR. So the advice of these dietitians – to eat less protein and fat and more carbohydrates – can be directly linked to increasing rates of diabetic kidney failure.

Hume also suggested: 'If one avoids sugar completely the liver has to work overtime to produce glucose from fat and protein and this is unhealthy.' This is incorrect. My colleagues and I have subsequently shown that liver glucose production from protein and fat (gluconeogenesis) is the same in people eating either high-carbohydrate or high-fat diets.[37] Because the fat-adapted body is less reliant on glucose for metabolism, there is no need for the liver to 'work overtime' to produce glucose. In fact, the liver is working 'less hard'. In reality, it is high-carbohydrate diets that damage the liver by causing NAFLD in those with IR.[38] NAFLD causes the abnormal blood lipoprotein (lipid) profiles[39] that, together with insulin and inflammation, cause arterial damage in people with IR and T2DM.[40] Hume is therefore blaming the wrong macronutrient for causing bodily harm.

She also said that 'a lack of carbohydrates means the brain can struggle to produce serotonin. A lack of serotonin can lead to symptoms of depression such as anxiety, sleep disturbances and sadness.' Again, there is no published evidence to support this, because there is presently no method by which brain serotonin levels can be measured in living humans.

All the dietitians quoted in the *Times* article said that people who tried the LCHF diet 'all lost weight extremely fast but as soon as they start eating carbohydrates, they put on even more weight'. Hume went so far as to quote actress Jennifer Aniston, who famously said 'the carbs will find you'. Without realising it, these dietitians broke the omertà – the code of silence never to acknowledge that carbohydrates cause corpulence. In trying to argue that the LCHF eating plan causes weight gain, they inadvertently admitted that *carbohydrates cause obesity*.

By some convoluted (il)logic, their argument – that the moment you stop eating LCHF (which successfully produces weight loss) and reintroduce carbohydrates, you regain all the lost weight, and then some – is meant to cast the LCHF diet as the cause of weight gain, not the reintroduced carbohydrates. But what we should actually deduce is that, to avoid weight gain, humans should limit the amount of carbohydrates they eat (for life), exactly as the LCHF eating plan advocates.

On 9 October 2012, shortly after the publication of Dr Martinique Stilwell's article in the *Mail & Guardian* (see Chapter 3), the HPCSA issued a statement, quoting Professor Edelweiss Wentzel-Viljoen, then chairperson of the HPCSA Professional Board for Dietetics and Nutrition, who would later play a crucial supporting role in launching the HPCSA case against me (see Closure):

> 'Although low-carbohydrate diets containing less energy may have short-term beneficial effects on weight control and insulin resistance in some individuals, a healthy diet remains a balanced diet ... Exercise plays a very important role in reaching and maintaining a healthy weight. A healthy diet remains one that is balanced in terms of carbohydrates, protein and fats as well as vitamins and minerals. The best way to reach a healthy balanced way of eating is to follow the South African Food Based Dietary Guidelines,' Prof Wentzel-Viljoen explains.[41]

The statement also warned that high-protein, high-fat and low-carbohydrate diets 'have severe health consequences for those who follow them long term', and expressed concern about controversial and unhealthy diets 'being recommended by individuals who are not specialised in dietetics and nutrition'.

Of course, one of the dangers of talking about health and weight is that your own body shape reveals much about whether what you practise actually works. Chris Becker, an LCHF supporter, decided to investigate how well their own dietary advice was helping the senior HPCSA administrators control their weight. His conclusion, based on a comparison of photographs of me with those of senior HPCSA administrators, was that my dietary advice seemed to be working better for me than the HPCSA's advice was working for its employees. 'If these high-level government employees of the HPCSA are following their own, i.e. government dietary guidelines, well, then I don't need to say any more. Neither does Tim Noakes,' wrote Becker.[42]

The HPCSA statement introduced the concept of the 'healthy' 'balanced' diet without defining exactly what is meant by 'balanced'. I find it difficult to understand how a diet can be balanced if more than 50 per cent of its energy comes from a single nutrient – carbohydrate – for which the human body has no (i.e. zero) essential requirement. Surely a 'balanced' diet should contain, for example, one-third fat, one-third carbohydrate and one-third protein? And if not, why not?

The statement contained two other warnings that would become the rallying call for all those queuing up to attack me. The first, that the LCHF eating plan may have 'severe health consequences' in the long term is ironic coming from a former professor of dietetics and nutrition at Stellenbosch University, one of the three major universities in the Western Cape, under whose watch that province has become the T2DM capital of South Africa. Should Wentzel-Viljoen not be asking herself if there is even the tiniest possibility that the South African Food-based Dietary Guidelines, promoted by both the HPCSA and ADSA, could be the real cause of this problem?

The second is the board's implication that I am not qualified to give any dietary opinions, as I am 'not specialised in dietetics and nutrition'. Interestingly, when I had many fewer qualifications and was promoting the South African Food-based Dietary Guidelines throughout the country and to the rest of the world through my book, *Lore of Running*, not a single South African dietitian or professional board paid the slightest attention to what I was saying. It would appear that it is not my qualifications that are the problem; rather, it is what I am now saying publicly that has become the problem.

The timing of this statement is important, because it shows that already in October 2012 the HPCSA was taking an interest in my professional activities in nutrition, and that Wentzel-Viljoen was raising the initial 'concerns' from her position as chairperson of the most powerful and influential dietetics committee in the country.

Four months later, in February 2013, Dr Vash Mungal-Singh wrote an open letter to the press in her capacity as CEO of the HSFSA to express her opinion that my ideas were wrong and, indeed, dangerous. The letter began with the conventional statement that any diet, be it low fat or high fat, will cause weight loss provided it is calorie-restricted. 'Yet we know many people revert to their old eating habits,' Mungal-Singh wrote, 'and regain the lost weight, *plus more*.'[43] It was unclear what scientific point she was trying to make here, since the dietary advice I give is that unless one is prepared to continue with the LCHF eating plan for life, it is better not to start in the first place. This is something I have stated repeatedly.

The letter continued:

> The HSF does not say 'no' to fats! But the message is more nuanced. For good health we need some fat in our diet. The real issue is the quality of fats we eat, against the total kilojoules in the diet. While studies are unclear about the effect of saturated fats on health, there is solid proof that replacing saturated fats with unsaturated fats will improve cholesterol levels, reduce heart disease risk and prevent insulin resistance, a precursor of diabetes. Eating good fats in place of saturated fats lowers the risk of heart disease. *Replacement* is key.'

Mungal-Singh conveniently forgets to mention that the HSFSA has major conflicts of interest: it accepts funding from three companies that produce highly processed seed oils containing unhealthy omega-6 polyunsaturated fats and, until very recently, even more unhealthy trans fats (see Table 7.1). Among this group is Unilever, the world's largest producer of polyunsaturated 'vegetable' oils and, coincidentally, ice cream.

Table 7.1 HSFSA sponsors

Producers of polyunsaturated fats/margarine	Platinum sponsor	Willowton Group (Sunfoil Sunflower Oil, Sunshine D Margarine, Wooden Spoon Margarine)
	Gold sponsor	Unilever (Blue Brand Margarine, Flora, I Can't Believe It's Not Butter, Stork)
	Sponsors and partners	Unity Foods (Helios Sunflower Oil, Helios Margarine, Ruby Margarine, Golden Lite)
Producers of confectionery	Gold sponsor	Tiger Brands (Allsorts, Anytime, Beacon chocolates, Black Cat snacks, Fizzer, FizzPop, Jelly Tots, Jungle Oats Energy Bars, Maynards, Beacon mmmMallows, Smoothies, Sparkles, Toff-o-Luxe, Beacon Easter eggs)
Producers of breakfast cereals/grain products	Gold sponsor	Tiger Brands (Ace, Ace Instant Porridge, Albany, Aunt Caroline, Cresta Rice, Fattis and Monis, Golden Cloud, Jungle Oats, King Korn, Morvite, Simply Cereal) Unilever (Pot Noodle)
Producers of sugar-sweetened beverages	Gold sponsor	Tiger Brands (Energade Sports Drink, Oros, Halls, Roses)
Producers of ice cream	Gold sponsor	Unilever (Algida, Ben & Jerry's, Carte d'Or, Cornetto, Magnum, Ola, Viennetta, Wall's)
Academic/research institutions	Sponsors and partners	Cape Peninsula University of Technology Medical Research Council North West University Stellenbosch University Faculty of Health and Medical Sciences University of Cape Town Chronic Disease Initiative for Africa Communication and Marketing Department Division of Human Nutrition Hatter Institute of Cardiology Research Sports Science Institute of South Africa
Other government institutions	Sponsors and partners	Western Cape Department of Health

The list of HSFSA sponsors and the products they produce explains why the concept of eating real foods and avoiding cereal- and sugar-based products is so challenging to the HSFSA, as it is to all such organisations around the world. Nowhere is this conflict more apparent than in the HSFSA's Heart Mark programme. According to the current CEO of the HSFSA, Professor Pamela Naidoo: 'Reading food labels and lists of ingredients requires time and advanced knowledge in nutrition, which many consumers don't have. The Heart Mark offers the consumer a tool to make choosing healthier foods easier.'[44]

In other words, the public is not intelligent enough to understand that processed foods should not be eaten. So the HSFSA will 'health-wash' some of the very worst foods by calling them healthy and therefore save the ignorant consumer from ever realising just how unhealthy they are. In this way the HSFSA can health-wash a range of sugar-loaded, highly addictive products that are the direct cause of South Africa's obesity epidemic.

The effect of this industrial capture of health organisations is nowhere better demonstrated than in their slow reaction to research into the harmful effects of trans fats. Dr Mary Enig established in the 1970s already that trans fats produced by the chemical extraction of unstable polyunsaturated oils from seeds are unhealthy, yet only recently have heart foundations begun to acknowledge this fact.[45] And not one heart foundation anywhere has ever acknowledged their role in the promotion of this unhealthy foodstuff. Rather, it is as if their 40-year advocacy of so-called healthy polyunsaturated 'vegetable' oils containing trans fats simply never happened.

The reaction to Enig's discovery was predictable. As described in her book, no sooner had her first paper been published than representatives of the National Association of Margarine Manufacturers and the Institute for Shortening and Edible Oils came to visit her, warning her that unless she ceased her research, she would lose all her funding. Which is exactly what happened: 'The lipid group at the University of Maryland never got another penny for trans fat research, and as the professors retired, the group's effort was gradually abandoned.'[46] As a result, Enig's finding of a correlation between vegetable-fat consumption, trans-fat consumption and serious disease, including heart disease, was simply ignored and buried, as 'no one was doing [the research]'. Enig's career, like that of Professor John Yudkin, who tried to warn the world about sugar, was terminated as a result of industry's need to put profits before the health of people.

Getting back to Mungal-Singh, what is the evidence that unsaturated fats 'will improve cholesterol levels, reduce heart disease risk and prevent insulin resistance'? The first point is that even if polyunsaturated fats lower blood cholesterol concentrations, so what? We want to know whether or not replacing saturated fats with polyunsaturated fats allows us to live longer, healthier lives. Here, the balance of evidence from a series of RCTs is absolutely clear: there is no evidence that replacing saturated fats with polyunsaturated fats improves health outcomes. Let's consider two such studies.

Ancel Keys's diet-heart hypothesis predicts that saturated fats raise blood cholesterol concentrations, which then clog the coronary arteries, causing heart attacks. One way to test this hypothesis is to replace dietary saturated fats (from animal fats, common margarines and shortening) with omega-6 linoleic acid from either safflower oil and safflower-oil polyunsaturated margarine, or from corn oil and corn-oil polyunsaturated margarine. Two studies evaluated these two interventions: the Sydney Diet Heart Study (1966–1973) and the Minnesota Coronary Experiment (1968–1973), the latter directed by Keys himself.

For a variety of reasons, the data for both studies was not fully reported until Dr Christopher Ramsden and his colleagues from the NIH in Bethesda, USA, were able to recover the original data and subject it to an exhaustive, modern analysis. The findings of both studies were essentially identical. In their investigation into the Sydney Diet Heart Study, Ramsden *et al.* found that:

> In this cohort, substituting dietary linoleic acid in place of saturated fats increased the rates of death from all causes, coronary heart disease, and cardiovascular disease. An updated meta-analysis of linoleic acid intervention trials showed no evidence of cardiovascular benefit. These findings could have important implications for worldwide dietary advice to substitute omega 6 linoleic acid, or polyunsaturated fats in general, for saturated fats.[47]

In other words, there is no evidence that replacing saturated fats with polyunsaturated fats improves health.

Similarly, Ramsden's modern analysis of Keys's Minnesota Coronary Experiment found that: 'There was no evidence of benefit in the intervention group [those eating a diet where saturated fat was replaced with linoleic acid] for coronary atherosclerosis or myocardial infarcts.' In fact, they found 'a 22% higher risk of death for each 30 mg/dl (0.78 mmol/L) reduction in serum cholesterol'. This effect was especially apparent in those over 65 years old, so that after about 400 days on the diet, the cumulative number of deaths for those ingesting linoleic acid in place of saturated fat became progressively greater than for those who continued to eat saturated fats. 'In meta-analyses, these cholesterol lowering interventions showed no evidence of benefit on mortality from coronary heart disease ... or all cause mortality,' concluded Ramsden and his colleagues.[48]

There are other studies that support this interpretation. In fact, the very first study of vegetable-oil substitution for saturated fat was published in 1965. G.A. Rose and colleagues showed that whereas corn oil lowered the blood cholesterol concentrations of patients with heart disease, the proportion of heart patients who were still alive after two years was significantly less (52 per cent) in the group fed corn oil than in the group who continued to eat as they always had (75 per cent). The authors concluded that 'under the circumstances of this trial corn oil cannot be recommended in the treatment of ischaemic heart disease'.[49]

Another study conveniently hidden from view is the Helsinki Businessmen Study.[50] In that study, mortality was much higher in the intervention group, which was treated with medications to lower blood cholesterol concentrations and blood pressure, as well as 'intensive dietetic-hygienic measures' that would have included substituting saturated fats with vegetable oils. Predictably, the authors once more ignored the null hypothesis, concluding: 'These unexpected results may not question multifactorial prevention as such but do support the need for [more] research'. Interestingly, the blood glucose concentration taken one hour after glucose ingestion was the best predictor for mortality in the intervention group. This is compatible with the theory that IR is the real determinant of ill health. Could the findings also have been the result of the prescription of a higher-carbohydrate diet in the intervention group, as occurred in Rossouw's CORIS trial (see Chapter 4)?

In 2004, Dr Dariush Mozaffarian, a lifelong proponent of the health benefits of substituting polyunsaturated fats for dietary saturated fats,[51] who sits on the scientific advisory board of Unilever, the world's largest producer of polyunsaturated fats, completed a novel study of changes in coronary arterial narrowing due to atherosclerosis in 235 post-menopausal women in relation to what the women reported they ate. Inconveniently, the study found that 'a greater saturated fat intake is associated with less progression of coronary atherosclerosis, whereas carbohydrate intake is associated with greater progression'. Remarkably, in the text but not in the abstract, Mozaffarian and his colleagues were prepared to admit (as was clearly shown in the data) that both 'polyunsaturated fat and carbohydrate intakes were associated with greater progression'.[52]

As cardiovascular research scientist James DiNicolantonio and his colleagues assert, the totality of evidence shows that there is no definitive proof that replacing saturated fat in the diet with polyunsaturated fats will reduce the risk of heart attack or extend life.[53] Remarkably, a new meta-analysis concludes that: 'Due to null results and a small number of studies included **there is no strong evidence** that replacement of saturated fatty acids with unsaturated fatty acids may benefit lipid profiles in this population [my emphasis].'[54]

Interestingly, there are other scientific findings relating to the ingestion of polyunsaturated fats or 'vegetable oils' that are conveniently forgotten. Thus the ingestion of omega-6 rich linoleic acid in vegetable oil increased blood triglyceride concentrations in people with elevated blood triglyceride concentrations, whereas fish oils had the opposite effect.[55] Yet I have still to read the HSFSA warning those with hypertriglyceridaemia not to ingest vegetable oils, or to advise them that the LCHF diet reverses hypertriglyceridaemia.

Another study found that replacing saturated fat with an increased intake of polyunsaturated fat in vegetables increased blood concentrations of oxidised LDL-cholesterol and lipoprotein(a).[56] These are changes that would normally be considered as evidence for an increased risk for the future development of CHD, the opposite of what the HSFSA claims should happen when one replaces saturated fat with polyunsaturated fats in vegetable oils.

The HSFSA does not warn us that replacing saturated fat with refined carbohydrates, which is precisely what has happened in the US since the publication of the 1977 US Dietary Guidelines for Americans (Figure 17.9), adversely affects insulin secretion.[57] The HSFSA also never tells us of the potential benefits of exchanging carbohydrate in the diet for saturated fat. A recent study found that replacement of dietary saturated fat with monounsaturated fats or refined carbohydrates did not improve 'inflammatory and thrombogenic markers in abdominally overweight individuals'.[58] Instead, 'increased refined carbohydrates consumption adversely impacts fasting HDL subfractions'.

So the diet that the HSFSA promotes adversely affects what it labels 'good' cholesterol. Surely that cannot be 'good'? Or, as Steven Hamley concludes: 'Available evidence from adequately controlled randomised controlled trials suggest replacing SFA [saturated fatty acids] with mostly n-6 PUFA [polyunsaturated fatty acids] is unlikely to reduce CHD events, CHD mortality or total mortality. The suggestion of benefits reported in earlier meta-analyses is due to the inclusion of inadequately controlled trials. These findings have implications for current dietary recommendations.'[59] All this evidence should be the final nail in the coffin for the diet-heart hypothesis.[60] Anyone who claims otherwise is simply not telling the truth. In fact, there is clear evidence that cooking in 'vegetable' oils is likely to be very bad for our health.

Professor Martin Grootveld and colleagues from the De Montfort University Leicester conducted an experiment in which participants were given vegetable oil, sunflower oil, corn oil, olive oil, cold-pressed rapeseed oil, goose fat, lard and butter to use for their daily cooking. Participants collected the leftovers and returned them to the scientists, who then analysed the returned fats and oils for their content of aldehydes, chemicals that have been linked to heart disease, cancer and dementia. The researchers found that sunflower and corn oil produced aldehydes at levels 20 times higher than recommended by the World Health Organization (WHO), and that the longer these oils were heated, the greater the production of toxic aldehydes. Olive oil, rapeseed oil, butter and goose fat, however, produced far fewer aldehydes.

As a result of this analysis, Grootveld recommended that, to reduce aldehyde production, people should cook with 'an oil or fat that is high in monounsaturated or saturated fats (preferably greater than 60% for one or the other, and more than 80% for the two combined), and low in polyunsaturates (less than 20%)'. He further suggested that we use 'olive oil for frying and cooking – even butter and lard are better than vegetable oil when used at high temperatures'.[61]

Mungal-Singh does not acknowledge the science that disproves the stated position of the HSFSA. In fact, by encouraging the public to replace dietary saturated fats with polyunsaturated fats, the HSFSA has likely not prevented a single case of heart disease. Rather, it may have increased heart-attack rates in the elderly, and perhaps even cancer rates. The latter possibility is suggested by an original 1970s study and by what has become known as the Israeli paradox.

In a study published in 1971, M.L Pearce and S. Dayton described 'an eight-year controlled clinical trial of a diet high in polyunsaturated vegetable oils and low in saturated fat and cholesterol in preventing complications of atherosclerosis'. They found that while there were fewer deaths from heart attack in the vegetable-oil (experimental) group, overall mortality was the same in both groups. This was because of an almost twofold greater (31 versus 17) incidence of fatal cancers in the experimental group.[62]

Then there is the Israeli paradox, described by D. Yam, A. Eliraz and E.M. Berry in 1996 as follows:

> Israel has one of the highest dietary polyunsaturated/saturated fat ratios in the world; the consumption of omega-6 polyunsaturated fatty acids (PUFA) is about 8% higher than in the USA, and 10–12% higher than in most European countries. In fact, Israeli Jews may be regarded as a population-based dietary experiment of the effect of a high omega-6 PUFA diet, a diet that until recently was widely recommended. Despite such national habits, there is paradoxically a high prevalence of cardiovascular diseases, hypertension, non-insulin-dependent diabetes mellitus and obesity – all diseases that are associated with hyperinsulinemia (HI) and insulin resistance (IR), and grouped together as the insulin resistance syndrome or syndrome X. There is also an increased cancer incidence and mortality rate, especially in women, compared with western countries. Studies suggest that high omega-6 linoleic acid consumption might aggravate HI and IR, in addition to being a substrate for lipid peroxidation and free radical formation. Thus, rather than being beneficial, high omega-6 PUFA diets may have some long-term side effects, within the cluster of hyperinsulinemia, atherosclerosis and tumorigenesis.[63]

Perhaps the reason why the HSFSA does not ever address the dangers of polyunsaturated fats is because it receives life-sustaining funding from Unilever.

In the ultimate irony, Mungal-Singh writes in her open letter on behalf of the HSFSA: 'We trust that Prof Noakes is not recommending that people increase their trans fat intake (this is a fat too!). We know that trans fats significantly increase the risk for cardiovascular disease and so should be avoided.' Until very recently, every heart foundation in the world was guilty of ignoring the evidence about the dangers of trans fats, which were first flagged in 1978.

Under the heading 'Not all carbohydrates are bad', Mungal-Singh suggests that: 'There is no doubt that unrefined or wholegrain carbohydrates are healthy and protective against certain diseases including cancer.' Once again, there is absolutely no direct evidence from appropriate RCTs that wholegrain carbohydrates do anything for our health.

Mungal-Singh then makes this important admission:

In reality, when people cut back on fat, they fill up on foods full of refined carbohydrates (e.g. white bread, sugary drinks) or use fat-free products without the healthy fats and which contain hidden sugars. The result is an increased risk for obesity, CVD and diabetes, which is why we recommend replacing foods high in bad fats with foods high in good fats – not with refined carbohydrates.

Hang on, was it not the HSFSA that advised us to cut the fat, to eat 'fat-free products' and to replace the missing calories with carbohydrates, including even refined carbohydrates and sugar? Is the CEO of the HSFSA now admitting that this substitution is the cause of the diabetes/obesity epidemic? And what is her solution? To replace bad fats with good fats – which is precisely what we promote in *The Real Meal Revolution*. The only difference is that we suggest also replacing the bad carbohydrates **and wholegrain carbohydrates** (that are without proven health benefits and which may be harmful to the majority) with good fats.

Next, Mungal-Singh turns her attention to the 'matter of over-simplifying the causes of heart disease'. 'It is common knowledge,' she writes, 'that the causes of heart disease are multi-factorial, and are not exclusive to only blood cholesterol and a high fat diet as claimed. In fact, overweight and obesity are one of the risk factors. Maintaining a healthy weight requires much more than a diet. It means having to balance your energy intake with energy used through exercise.' She says that, as a result of my advocacy of the LCHF eating plan, 'the exercise message gets lost in the debate – which is a danger'.

Clearly, Mungal-Singh has not read my *Lore of Running*, which emphasises the crucial importance of exercise for all-round health, but not for weight control. Perhaps the lean Mungal-Singh has yet to learn that she is not lean because she exercises, any more than I and the likes of Bruce Fordyce and Oscar Chalupsky progressively gained weight in our middle years because we are lazy. It is difficult to accuse Bruce of laziness: in his athletic life he completed more than 200 standard marathons and perhaps another 50 ultra-marathons. Similarly, Oscar, who won the Molokai Challenge surf-ski race a remarkable 12 times, between the ages of 20 and 49.[64] Yet so much exercise could not prevent weight gain in these athletes' middle ages, as both became progressively more insulin resistant. (I address this issue further in Chapter 17, where I discuss the evidence that one cannot outrun a bad diet.)

The truth is that if you have to exercise to control your weight, then your diet is wrong. Those of us who have lost weight on the LCHF eating plan have learnt that you cannot outrun a bad diet, and that Mungal-Singh is absolutely correct: it is the carbohydrates in the diet that are driving the obesity epidemic, not the fats.

Mungal-Singh completes her letter with the following statement:

Perhaps the recent debate will feed your need to believe that you can indulge in butter, bacon, biltong and boerewors. Unfortunately, this cannot be without moderation, nor can it be in isolation of other factors ... To ignore other contributing factors, behaviours and living context that lead to heart disease would be erroneous and dangerous.

Again, nothing in *The Real Meal Revolution* disagrees with this statement.

The letter received 14 comments within the first 48 hours of its publication on *Health24*. The vast majority of commentators challenged the statements of the HSFSA and preferred my position. Perhaps if the HSFSA listened to public opinion it would be able to reduce the tsunami of arterial disease caused by T2DM and their advice to eat LFHC diets.

As the Banting movement continued to gain traction across the length and breadth of South Africa, perhaps predictably in 2016 the HSFSA felt it necessary to once again warn South Africans of the dangers and stupidity of adopting the LCHF eating plan. This time they put up an article on their website titled 'The highs and lows of a low-carb-high-fat (LCHF) diet'.[65]

The article[*] begins with a backhanded compliment: 'We have heard many accounts of people who lost weight using a LCHF approach by making radical changes to their eating habits.' However: 'To follow a LCHF-diet long-term is possible but requires extreme dedication, restriction of a wide range of foods, and may in fact be more expensive.' They go on to say that while some people may be able to adhere to this approach long term, many are unable to sustain it, as it is 'such an extreme intervention'. But, they say, the HSFSA does acknowledge that short-term weight-loss strategies are sometimes 'necessary', but in the long term, they recommend 'a more balanced approach'.

Clearly the HSFSA has not yet heard that South Africa is the third most obese nation in the world and that this could be the result of their and ADSA's promotion of the low-fat diet.

The article continues with a false statement: that the Banting diet is an LCHF diet that is based on 'predominantly saturated fat sources and animal protein sources', and that it is usually – and according to them, often inadvertently – 'moderate to high in protein'. It then goes on to list some of the possible consequences of an LCHF diet:

---

* The HSFSA declined permission for the authors to publish the article in full in this book. It can be found on the HSFSA website at http://www.heartfoundation.co.za/topical-articles/highs-and-lows-low-carb-high-fat-lchf-diet.

- People with genetically elevated LDL cholesterol or with existing heart disease may increase their risk of atherosclerosis substantially by increasing their saturated fat intake. (Genetic defects leading to raised cholesterol are more common in some South African communities than anywhere else in the world!) [*This is not true: Arterial disease is caused by high-carbohydrate diets in those with IR, causing NAFLD and the serious form of atherogenic dyslipidaemia, as fully described in Chapter 17. The diet promoted by the HSFSA is the one that causes arterial disease.*]

- Individuals with a genetically elevated iron level may incur liver damage when they increase their red meat intake significantly. [*Where is the evidence for this statement? The LCHF diet is not a diet high in meat. People with genetically elevated iron levels are aware of their condition and know what they should and should not be eating. They do not need a heart foundation to tell them.*]

- People with asymptomatic undiagnosed kidney disease (a common condition often present in people with diabetes), may accelerate their kidney disease by an even modest increase in protein intake. [*This statement has no basis in fact. People with undiagnosed kidney disease are most likely to have T2DM, as described earlier in this chapter. Eating a high-fat diet that better controls their diabetes will reduce the probability that they will develop kidney failure. In contrast, continuing to eat the high-carbohydrate diet promoted by the HSFSA will worsen their diabetes.*]

- Decreasing intake of dietary fibre may increase the risk of bowel conditions such as constipation, diverticular disease and bowel cancer. [*As Dr Caryn Zinn clearly showed during her expert testimony in the HPSCA hearing, the LCHF diet provides more dietary fibre than the diet the HSFSA promotes. The LCHF diet promotes the intake of fibre-rich, low-carbohydrate vegetables and fruits like avocados.*]

- Liver is often recommended as an affordable LCHF food choice but is also a very rich source of vitamin A. Consuming liver during early pregnancy may cause birth defects. As little as 20–100g liver exceeds the World Health Organization recommended maximum daily intake of vitamin A during pregnancy. [*Most South Africans eating the traditional maize-based diet are vitamin-A deficient and would benefit from vitamin-A supplementation. I am unaware of anyone in South Africa eating more than 20 grams liver daily. Who and where is that person?*]

- Very restrictive high fat diets may be low in various vitamins and minerals, depending on which foods are being eliminated. [*This is another bogus statement. The evidence is that high-fat diets provide more vitamins and minerals because they are more nutrient dense than the diet that the HSFSA promotes. In addition, as Weston Price argues (see Chapter 16), without sufficient fat in the diet it is not possible to absorb effectively the (lower) vitamin and mineral contents of the nutrient-poor, low-fat diet promoted by the HSFSA.*]

- Diets high in animal protein, sodium and/or low in calcium may increase the risk for osteoporosis. [*This is another bogus statement for which there is no scientific evidence.* [66] *Osteoporosis is a modern disease of nutrition that did not exist before humans began eating 'healthy' wholegrains at the start of the Agricultural Revolution 12 000 years ago. Indeed, the introduction of cereal and grains into the human diet was associated with a dramatic reduction in human height and the first appearance of bone diseases and dental caries. It is diets high in cereals and grains and low in fat-soluble vitamins, especially Vitamin D, which cause osteoporosis (See Chapter 16.*]

The HSFSA then says that, as even the best diets can be 'badly executed', they recommend that anyone who attempts to follow 'an extreme diet such as a[n] LCHF diet does so under medical supervision'. And anyone with diabetes, high cholesterol or high blood pressure is advised to monitor their kidney function, blood pressure and LDL cholesterol.

Indeed. And they will notice that their kidney function, blood pressure and LDL cholesterol all improve on the LCHF diet.[67] These improvements will soon convince them that following the Banting diet is far more healthy than following the diet the HSFSA recommends.

The anti-Banting propaganda continues with another backhanded compliment. They say that although a low-carb diet can assist type-2 diabetics with weight loss, and may aid in blood sugar control, this can also be achieved with a diet consisting of moderate, good-quality carbohydrates. The latter statement is again simply not true, as the evidence presented earlier in this chapter makes clear: adequate control of T2DM, including the potential to put the disease into remission, can only be achieved with diets that limit carbohydrate intake to about 25 grams per day.

The HSFSA goes on to say that they have no evidence that an LCHF diet prevents the development of heart disease, and that it may even accelerate this process in some individuals. They recommend a more moderate approach, which includes 'a reduction in energy intake from excess carbohydrates AND/OR fat, and choosing good quality carbohydrates and fats'. As I show in Chapter 17, there is no evidence that the diet currently promoted by the HSFSA 'prevents the development of heart disease'. Instead, all the evidence suggests that their diet promotes T2DM and, hence, heart disease. So one might legitimately ask on what scientific basis the HSFSA promotes its allegedly 'heart-healthy' diet.

The article concludes by saying that although the Banting diet has promoted awareness around nutrition and health in South Africa, the HSFSA does not agree with all the elements that make up this diet. They then list the foods they believe South Africans should eat, and recommend a reduced intake of sugar and processed foods. Their aim, they say, is to beat obesity, heart disease and diabetes in South Africans by recommending that they eat healthier foods like 'unrefined grains', healthy oils, fruit and vegetables, and limit the intake of salt, sugars and saturated fats. One wonders if the HSFSA has ever considered why their own message has failed to achieve the requisite results.

In a recent rant on the South African Heart Association (SAHA) website, 'the sole organization representing the professional interests of all cardiologists and cardio-thoracic surgeons in the country', the association repeated much of the same misinformation, while including the interesting statement that the Banting diet's 'rationale is based on a world-wide epidemic of obesity and type 2 diabetes, which is multi-factorial in its development, but to an extent is due to widespread consumption of sugar-sweetened beverages'.[68]

This is an interesting admission, given that the HSFSA, a non-governmental organisation linked to SAHA, allows its 'healthy' Heart Mark to be used on no fewer than 14 sugar-sweetened beverages,[69] as well as 23 breakfast cereals, the taste of the majority of which may be 'enhanced' with added sugar.

The article continues: 'There are two problems with the Banting diet: Firstly it is an untested hypothesis, and secondly it comes at considerable cost as it is accompanied by a deterioration in adherents' lipid profiles, which is certain to increase the likelihood of cardiovascular disease. The SA Heart Association cannot condone the Banting diet until conclusive proof of the long-term beneficial effects of increasing dietary saturated fat have been demonstrated.'

Which raises the question: If SAHA is really so concerned that its pronouncements be based on hard scientific evidence, why does it continue to promote a diet for which, despite 50 years of research, there is still no 'conclusive proof of the long-term beneficial effects' (Chapter 13)? And how can it claim that the Banting diet is an 'untested hypothesis'? Or that Banting exclusively promotes a diet high in saturated fat? Is SAHA not aware that any diet that promotes an increased fat intake must promote an increased consumption of all three types of fat: mono- and polyunsaturated fats, as well as saturated fats (see Table 8.2)? Is SAHA simply ignorant of all this information, or is it wilfully misleading the South African public?

And when will SAHA acknowledge that abnormal lipid profiles – the atherogenic dyslipidaemia that causes coronary heart disease – are driven by carbohydrates, not fats, in those who are insulin resistant (Chapter 17)? So that a diet high in fat improves the lipid profiles of those with metabolic syndrome[70] besides providing additional beneficial effects, including significantly reduced blood pressures,[71] lessened hyperinsulinaemia and reduced hyperglycaemia.

The problem for both the HSFSA and SAHA is that, in the not too distant future, both will be forced to face their moments of truth when the educated public finally grasps that it has been misled by these surrogates for Big Pharma and Big Food and that, in its naiveté, it trusted too certainly.

It will not be a benign moment for either organisation.

This book will only accelerate the arrival of that moment.

If the goal of the HSFSA and SAHA truly is 'to help South Africans beat obesity, heart disease and also diabetes', they could quite easily achieve this by listening to the evidence. Their inability to engage with the evidence proves that they have a different agenda.

The diet that the HSFSA, SAHA and ADSA have promoted for the past few decades has failed absolutely to stem the tsunami of obesity and T2DM that we now face. In fact, as I argue in Chapter 17, it has caused the very medical disaster that it claims to prevent. The basic text of Narcotics Anonymous, an organisation specialising in the treatment of drug addiction, includes the following: 'Insanity is repeating the same mistakes and expecting different results.' The HSFSA and ADSA need to address their shared addiction to providing marketing misinformation on behalf of their funders (Table 7.1). This misinformation is not evidence-based; it is known to be wrong; and it has caused, and continues to cause, great harm to the health of many South Africans, most especially those with IR.

Perhaps the single most important factor in the development of my academic career was the founding, with Morné du Plessis, of the Sports Science Institute of South Africa and its subsequent growth. This was made possible thanks to generous funding from Discovery Health, which allowed us to increase our research productivity exponentially. But perhaps predictably, when I discovered the LCHF diet in December 2010, my relationship with Discovery Health became strained.

The reason for this tension was Discovery Health's reliance on the 'evidence' for the health benefits of the LFHC diet, despite the fact that no such evidence exists. In addition, Discovery Health continues to focus on the role of cholesterol in the prediction of heart-attack risk, completely ignoring the key role of IR and NAFLD. I remain perplexed as to how a company that prides itself on innovation – on being at the cutting edge of human health promotion – can still be getting it so completely and utterly wrong.

With time, Discovery Health withdrew its funding from both me and the institute. And so I was surprised when I received an invitation from the head of Discovery Vitality to defend the Banting diet at the Discovery Vitality Summit in Johannesburg on 1 August 2014. The original list of speakers that I was told would be engaged in the debate when I accepted the invitation was rather different from the group I faced on the day. In particular, UCT professor of nutrition and dietetics Marjanne Senekal had been replaced by two key players in the publication of the Naudé review: Professor Celeste Naudé and her co-author, Professor Jimmy Volmink, dean of Stellenbosch University's Faculty of Medicine and Health Sciences.

First up was Mungal-Singh representing the HSFSA. She offered similar opinions to those expressed in her open letter the previous year, but in the end she seemed almost to embrace my proposal that we should all avoid eating processed foods. Remarkably, her talk focused on what the HSFSA found acceptable about the LCHF/Banting diet. 'We agree on the need to avoid sugar, processed foods and refined carbohydrates,' she stated. 'We need to have more whole foods.' As a result, we should all focus on the 'common enemy' of ultra-processed foods laden with sugar, salt and refined carbohydrates, because 'that's what's killing us'. (This was pretty much what we wrote in *The Real Meal Revolution*.)

Next up was Naudé. As she spoke, the thought occurred to me that her rejection of the LCHF diet is perhaps because it advocates the consumption of meat. She appears to favour vegetarianism, as, I have learnt, do many of the more publicly vocal South African dietitians. My conclusion was based on her reasoning of why humans should avoid eating red meat. Her 'evidence-base' was a raft of observational (associational) studies that can never prove causation – as she should know, being a specialist in this field.

Volmink's lecture was on the nature of scientific evidence, and the relative value of anecdotes, longitudinal observational (associational) studies and RCTs, somewhat along the lines of what he had said at the conclusion of the Centenary Debate (Chapter 4). Surprisingly, as director of the Centre for Evidence-based Health Care at the University of Stellenbosch, he failed to make the obvious point that almost all the evidence on which the current dietary guidelines are based comes from longitudinal observational studies that have little or no scientific validity. Association, he should by now know, does not prove causation.

Here is what Gary Taubes has to say in *Good Calories, Bad Calories*:

The only way to establish cause and effect with any reliability is to do 'controlled' experiments, or controlled *trials*, as they're called in medicine. Such trials [RCTs] attempt to avoid all the chaotic complexities of comparing populations, towns, and ethnic groups. Instead, they try to create two identical situations – two groups of subjects, in this case – and then change only one variable to see what happens. They 'control' for all the other possible variables that might affect the outcome being studied. Ideally, such trials will randomly assign subjects into an experimental group, which receives the treatment being tested – a drug for instance, or a special diet – and a group, which receives a placebo or eats their usual meals or some standard fare.[72]

In their lectures, Volmink and Naudé should have emphasised that longitudinal observational (associational) studies can only ever identify 'possibilities', i.e. possible causal relationships between different variables. These studies can never identify 'probabilities', i.e. real causal relationships between two variables (for example, between red meat intake and cancer, or between eating saturated fat and developing CHD).

Volmink should have explained that the evidence-base for the nutritional sciences is profoundly weak, almost non-existent, because almost all this evidence comes from longitudinal associational studies that cannot identify causation. He should have informed the audience of some of the conclusions that Dr John Ioannidis, professor of medicine at Stanford University and author of many of the definitive articles on the failings of evidence-based medicine,[73] has come to:

> In nutrition, there has been so much observational and mechanistic research that thousands of spuriously significant associations have already been produced and translated in heavily opinionated, debated recommendations. Getting another significant result in a field that is already saturated with so many significant results offers no information gain: we still (think we) know what (we thought) we knew. Conversely, 'negative' results offer high information gain, because they change our probably false beliefs about potentially effective interventions … we should hope to get more 'negative' results in the future.[74]

The legion of false positive findings explains why '[a]lmost every single nutrient imaginable has peer reviewed publications associating it with almost any outcome … Many findings are implausible. Relative risks that suggest we can halve the burden of cancer with just a couple of servings a day of a single nutrient still circulate widely in peer reviewed journals'.[75] As a result, these findings predict that 'if we increase or decrease (as appropriate) intake of any of several nutrients by 2 servings/day, cancer will almost disappear worldwide; manipulating the uptake of a single nutrient suffices'.[76] To rid nutrition science of this impossible conclusion, Ioannidis and his colleagues provide guidelines 'for improving the conduct, reporting and communication of nutrition-related research to ground discussion in evidence rather than solely on beliefs'.[77]

Why did neither Volmink nor Naudé highlight this fundamental problem in nutrition science, specifically that it is a discipline based on belief, not critically derived evidence? Perhaps because then they would have had to question the real value of much of the work produced in their research unit, including the Naudé review. As I discuss further in Chapter 17, it is Ioannidis's opinion that only about 3 per cent of meta-analyses are 'decent and clinically useful'. 'The production of systematic reviews and meta-analyses has reached epidemic proportions,' he writes. 'Possibly, the large majority of produced systematic reviews and meta-analyses are unnecessary, misleading, and/or conflicted.' The main driver of this epidemic is the irresistible attraction of 'easily produced publishable units or marketing tools'.[78] Or, in the case of the Naudé review, the persecution of an unwelcome opinion.

As James le Fanu writes in his book *The Rise and Fall of Modern Medicine*: 'epidemiological studies are easy to perform ... and thus rapidly filled the vacuum of ignorance ... This self-imposed insistence on rigorous methodology is missing from contemporary epidemiology; indeed the most striking feature is the insouciance with which epidemiologists announce their findings, as if they do not expect anyone to take them seriously. It would, after all, be a very serious matter if drinking alcohol *really* did cause breast cancer.'[79] In an earlier version of his book, Le Fanu even suggested: 'Meanwhile the simple expedient of closing down most university departments of epidemiology could both extinguish this endlessly fertile source of anxiety-mongering while simultaneously releasing funds for serious research.'

The final anti-Noakes speaker at the debate was Dr Anthony Dalby, a Johannesburg-based cardiologist in private practice, whom I have known since 1976, when we were both researchers in Professor Lionel Opie's unit at UCT. While the other speakers may have been somewhat measured in their criticisms of me and the Banting diet, Dalby came over as the original Big Pharma attack dog.

The first important point to make about his lecture is what was missing. Dalby failed to declare his conflicts of interest. He did not acknowledge that since 1994 he has served as national lead investigator for South Africa on the international steering committees of 39 phase III drug trials in a variety of cardiac conditions. He should have at least declared whether or not he has ever received remuneration for undertaking these studies and, if so, the magnitude of that remuneration. He also failed to declare that he serves on the advisory boards of leading health and pharmaceutical companies, including Aspen, AstraZeneca, Boehringer Ingelheim, Eli Lilly and Company, Novartis, Pfizer, Sanofi, Servier and Discovery Health. In addition, he represented the South African Heart Association in its discussion with Discovery Health in developing guidelines for the prescription of lipid-lowering drugs by South African doctors.

Dalby did not mention that it was he who first suggested that the pharmaceutical industry should be involved in the formulation of the South African guidelines for the management of high blood cholesterol concentrations.[80] How could anyone think that, in contributing to the guidelines, the industry would have any interest other than its own commercial welfare by ensuring that it 'captures' academics, those practising physicians who are key opinion leaders and regulatory bodies?

Dalby also did not acknowledge that there is little evidence for much of what cardiologists do in their daily practice. Acknowledging the remarkable ineffectiveness of statin drugs would have been a good start. Dalby publishes papers in local medical journals extolling their virtues, especially when combined with regular exercise and dietary change: 'Lifestyle changes combined with statin therapy provide potent protection against coronary heart disease,' he and Opie wrote in one such paper.[81] This statement has no factual basis, because, to my knowledge, no study has yet reported on the effects of lifestyle changes *combined* with statin therapy. Similarly, I wonder if Dalby ever warns the general public that neither coronary bypass surgery nor the stenting of coronary arteries prolongs life (see Chapter 3).

Dalby later fulminated about my 'criminal' behaviour, yet he did not mention that in 2009/10, five of the pharmaceutical companies for whom he works in an advisory capacity – Pfizer, Novartis, Sanofi, AstraZeneca and Eli Lilly – were fined a total of $4.7 billion for various fraudulent (i.e. criminal) activities.[82]

I also wonder if Dalby ever informs patients who participate in the pharmaceutical trials he oversees that their data belongs solely to the company funding the trial, and that the company has the right to do pretty much whatever it likes with that information. Danish physician and author Dr Peter Gøtzsche believes that these trials are so lacking in transparency that an honest patient consent form should read:

> I agree to participate in this trial, which I understand has no scientific value but will be helpful for the company in marketing their drug. I also understand that if the results do not please the company, they may be manipulated and distorted until they do, and that if this also fails, the results may be buried for no one to see outside the company. Finally I understand and accept that should there be too many serious harms of the drugs, these will either not be published, or they will be called something else in order not to raise concerns in patients or lower sales of the company's drugs.[83]

Interestingly, the one personal fact that Dalby did declare in his lecture was that he is, in his own words, 'obese'. Having admitted this, he should perhaps also have mentioned whether or not he has IR, NAFLD and metabolic syndrome, and, if so, precisely why he feels he developed these conditions and what, if anything, he is doing to correct them.

Dalby's lecture was the standard defence of the absolute infallibility of the diet-heart and lipid hypotheses. According to his argument, the key drivers of heart disease are fat in the diet and cholesterol in the blood. As a result, any increase in blood cholesterol concentrations caused by a high-fat diet must cause arterial disease and early death from a fatal heart attack. One of his patients, he reported, had more than doubled her blood cholesterol concentration, from 5 to

13 mmol/L, when she went on the Banting diet. This single case, he argued, proves that my advice to increase dietary fat intake is 'criminal'.[84]

As part of his tirade, Dalby read the disclaimer in *The Real Meal Revolution*:

> The information and material provided in this publication is representative of the authors' opinions and views. It is meant for educational and informational purposes only and is not meant to prevent, diagnose, treat or cure any disease. The content should not be construed as professional medical advice. As the authors are not offering prescriptive or professional medical advice they cannot be responsible or liable for the decisions and actions which readers undertake as a result of reading this content. Should the reader need professional assistance, a qualified physician or health care practitioner should be consulted.

To Dalby, this was evidence that my co-authors and I were the cynical purveyors of death and destruction. The fact that this disclaimer is the work of the publishers, to protect themselves, and is present in every similar book ever published, was lost on Dalby. The equivalent would be Dalby's own use of medical professional liability insurance. I would never assume that he takes out medical malpractice insurance so that he can act 'criminally' as a cardiologist.

As the talks continued, I began to wonder what had brought together this quartet – comprising the head of a non-governmental organisation, two academics and a private cardiologist who was South Africa's leading proponent of the use of statin drugs – to 'debate' the Banting/LCHF diet under the banner of Discovery Health. Four against one was hardly designed to be a balanced debate.

In my lecture, I argued that the single most important factor determining what we should be eating is our individual level of IR. This, I proposed, is the underlying condition causing obesity, T2DM, gout, hypertension and atherogenic dyslipidaemia in those eating high-carbohydrate diets. (Only later would I appreciate that cancer and dementia fall in the same category.)

Next I spoke about the work of Dr Gerald Reaven, considered the father of IR,[85] which shows that chronically elevated blood insulin concentrations explain how high-carbohydrate diets lead to this constellation of medical conditions in those with IR.[86] Thus, I proposed, the key feature of a 'balanced diet' is that it should minimise insulin secretion at all times.

I wound down with a brief review of the absence of evidence that saturated fats cause heart disease, before concluding with a short overview of the work of Harvard's Dr Alessio Fasano that shows how gluten and gliadin present in wheat, rye and barley causes the leaky gut syndrome that contributes to another array of medical conditions which remain poorly managed.[87]

At the conclusion of the debate, the head of Vitality Wellness, Dr Craig Nossel, was asked whether the Vitality HealthyFood benefit would be revised to fit with my recommendations. He answered: 'We have a responsibility to 3 million people in South Africa and millions globally so we can't afford to take any chances with their health. We stress that a healthy, balanced diet is important and this is reflected in the HealthyFood benefit offered through Vitality.'[88] Not documented was his throwaway line to the effect that I might be able to tear the pages about high-carbohydrate diets from *Lore of Running* when my opinion changed, but Discovery Health had to act more 'responsibly'.

There is a final interesting point to make about the debate and my relationship with Discovery.

Two years earlier, I had been invited by Discovery Health to speak at the annual Discovery Leadership Summit. I was a last-minute replacement for Archbishop Emeritus Desmond Tutu, who had withdrawn because British prime minister Tony Blair was on the speaker list. I spoke on the power of the mind in sport and had the great privilege of introducing and then interviewing the South African golden boy of swimming, Chad le Clos. Le Clos had recently returned from the 2012 London Olympics, where he had beaten the greatest Olympian, Michael Phelps, by 0.05 seconds to win gold in the 200-metre butterfly.

After the talk, the various celebrity speakers and I eagerly signed our books for members of the audience (mine was *Challenging Beliefs*). Just two years later, at the Discovery Vitality Summit, I was informed that there would be no place for me to sign copies of *The Real Meal Revolution*, and that it would be neither on sale nor on display at the event.

It was a clear measure of how far I had fallen in their eyes.

The 'debate' at the Discovery Vitality Summit provided the perfect excuse for University of Stellenbosch–embedded journalist Wilma Stassen to write a second article attacking the Banting/LCHF diet, and me. Published in *Health-E News* on 11 August 2014, and titled 'Noakes diet particularly dangerous for Afrikaans population', the piece clearly originated from the conference, as much prominence was given to Dalby's personal attack on me.

Stassen begins her article by implying that my advice is dangerous because 'some patients with high cholesterol have exchanged their cholesterol-lowering medication (called statins) for the LCHF diet, with detrimental results'.[89]

Nowhere in *The Real Meal Revolution* do I specifically state that people with high cholesterol should abandon their statins and follow the LCHF diet. I may believe that this is exactly what the evidence shows to be the best advice for people, especially women, who have 'high cholesterol' levels but no heart disease, but I do not prescribe behaviour. My job is simply to provide evidence.

Instead of asking me for my opinion, Stassen sets up a straw-man argument. 'Cardiologist Dr Anthony Dalby describes Noakes' advice to heart patients to exchange cholesterol-lowering drugs for his diet as "criminal", she writes. Yet, as I have said, I have never advised heart patients to replace their statins with the LCHF diet.

Stassen continues:

International obesity expert Professor Tessa van der Merwe says there are 'many health risks connected with the LHCF [*sic*] diet'. It could exacerbate heart disease, worsen diabetes and osteoporosis and cause gall and kidney stones, says Van der Merwe, honorary Professor of Endocrinology at the University of Pretoria. 'If you have got familial hypercholesterolemia (FH), the chances that you will develop a sinister cholesterol profile is a reality', she adds. FH is caused by a genetic disorder that causes high LDL ('bad') cholesterol. It is particularly common in the Afrikaans-speaking population, where there is a 1:70 occurrence in comparison to a 1:500 in the general population.

Van der Merwe conveniently fails to acknowledge her conflict of interest: that she works in a medical institution that promotes bariatric surgery over nutrition to manage obesity. She also does not ask how, if the incidences of diabetes, osteoporosis, and gall and kidney stones have all increased since 1977, when humans were told to remove fat from their diet, these epidemics can be attributed to an increased fat intake following the adoption by some people of the high-fat diet after the publication of *The Real Meal Revolution* in 2013. The cognitive dissonance of the professionals unable to acknowledge this conceptual paradox is addressed in a Credit Suisse report published in 2015, which suggests that: 'Health care officials and government bodies have been consistently behind developments on the [nutrition] research front.'[90]

Then there is this condition called familial hypercholesterolaemia. When a patient presents with an elevated total blood cholesterol concentration of 7.5 mmol/L or greater, cardiologists are quick to diagnose FH. We are taught that FH is a fatal condition that provides the absolute proof that cholesterol is the direct cause of arterial clogging and heart attacks.

But the truth is vastly different. In fact, it is the exact opposite.

Almost all conventionally trained cardiologists try to convince us that the best predictor of heart-attack risk is 'cholesterol load', which is an individual's lifetime average blood cholesterol concentration multiplied by their age. Thus, the higher the average lifetime blood cholesterol concentration and the older the individual, the greater the damage to his (mainly, but also her) coronary arteries. So, according to this logic, an elevated blood cholesterol concentration is like an internal time bomb, just waiting to explode.

This model therefore predicts that heart-attack risk in people with FH increases as they age and as their coronary arteries become progressively more clogged, until they eventually succumb to fatal heart disease by middle age.

To prove this hypothesis, all we need are studies of the life histories of a large number of people with FH. Fortunately, there are a handful of longitudinal scientific studies that have looked at this, and the results they provide are revolutionary. For my analysis, I have borrowed unashamedly from a blog by Dr Zoë Harcombe on this topic.[91]

Harcombe reports that in 1991 the Simon Broome Register Group found that people with FH were at a greater risk of dying between the ages of 20 and 39, but thereafter, this mortality difference lessened, so that mortality was no higher for people with FH aged 60 to 74 than it was for those of the same age without FH.[92] A second study derived from the Simon Broome Register Group found that death from CHD was 2.5 times higher for FH sufferers than the general population, but the all-cause death rate was no higher.[93] Thus, writes Harcombe, 'patients with Heterozygous FH were dying more of CHD, but less from cancer and thus the death rate was no higher overall'. Harcombe concludes:

> The combined findings from these two Simon Broome Register Group papers show that, if you genuinely have FH and you are aged 60 or over you should be pleased to know that you have a lower risk of cancer and no greater risk of heart disease. If you have FH and are aged 39 or higher, you are already past the highest risk period of your life for heart disease. Even in the 20–39 age group, there were 6 deaths in 774 person years studied – less than a 1 in 100 incident rate and that's in 1 in 500 people.

A Dutch study that traced two centuries of descendants of an ancestor with FH found that mortality in those with untreated FH varied dramatically between individuals and changed with time; mortality was no higher in FH carriers during the 19th and early 20th centuries, yet rose after 1915 to peak between 1935 and 1964, before falling again. The authors noted that: 'During the decades with excess mortality, survival in the branches of the pedigree differed significantly, ranging from normal life expectancy to severe excess mortality ... [so that] such large variation in mortality in two directions (over time and within generations) in a pedigree indicates that the disorder has strong interactions with environmental factors.'[94] The authors also suggested that in the 19th century, FH might have conferred a survival advantage against infectious diseases. Another study, published 15 years earlier, also reported normal life expectancy in some people living with FH before 1880.[95] And another, published 25 years earlier, found that people with FH did not have a reduced life expectancy.[96]

Even more perplexing for the cholesterol activists is the recent finding that in people with FH, blood cholesterol concentration has essentially no predictive value for heart attack or stroke in the next 5–10 years.[97] Instead, in order of significance, the following factors increased risk for a cardiovascular event: age (above 60 years), obesity, previous history of CVD, age (30–59 years), overweight, diabetes, use of the drug ezetimibe, high blood pressure, patient on maximum combined therapy, patient on maximum lipid-lowering therapy, male, premature family history of CVD, patient on maximum statin dose, and active smoking.

In other words, people with FH who are at risk of heart attack are those who have the conventional risk factors, most especially IR and perhaps blood-clotting abnormalities,[98] in which total blood cholesterol concentration plays no role. Recent genetic studies confirm that 'not all FH patients present the same CVD risk and accurate stratification of CVD risk in FH is imperative'. They further suggest that using genetic risk scores 'could lead to a more personalized approach to therapy'.[99]

The key point perhaps is that many people with FH will have a completely normal life expectancy despite living for seven or more decades with 'criminally elevated' blood cholesterol concentrations, whereas others with FH will die young from heart disease. This has important implications for our understanding of how to treat patients with FH, and how we interpret non-randomised studies of treatment outcomes in these patients. What you believe determines what you believe. And there is perhaps no better example of this than the current medical management of FH. Suppose the first patient with FH whom a doctor ever encounters dies at the age of 21 from extensive coronary artery disease and a fatal heart attack. How would that doctor not prescribe statin drugs to every other patient with FH in his practice, especially if everything he reads in the medical literature advertises the dangers of cholesterol in people with FH? For if high cholesterol can kill someone in their 20s, imagine what even moderately elevated cholesterol values are doing to the coronary arteries of all the doctor's other patients, whether or not they have FH.

What these studies show is that FH is not a uniformly fatal disease. Rather, there appears to be a 'protective effect of age', the opposite of what one would predict if it is solely exposure of the coronary arteries to years of high blood cholesterol concentrations that causes fatal heart attacks. Worse, in our current state of uncertainty, medical science is unable to distinguish between patients with FH who are likely to die at a young age and those who will have a normal life expectancy. All this becomes extremely important when we review the evidence that experts who work closely with the pharmaceutical industry use to convince us that statins are effective in mitigating FH.

The two trials usually quoted as proof of statins' effectiveness were neither randomised nor properly controlled.[100] As a result, we cannot be certain whether the apparently beneficial effects of statin prescription were simply because the populations studied consisted of older FH individuals (over age 39) with a normal life expectancy. But if you have been taught that (1) elevated blood cholesterol concentrations cause arterial disease; (2) the higher the blood cholesterol values, the sooner death from heart disease will occur; and (3) all people with FH must die young from heart disease, it follows that if a study finds that FH sufferers taking statins can have a normal life expectancy, then statins must be remarkably effective drugs. That an identical outcome could result even if the statins were ineffective will never be considered or conveyed to the medical profession, because it might just be another death blow for the lipid hypothesis (see Chapter 17).

If 'high cholesterol' is the exclusive cause of heart disease, how is it that elevated cholesterol levels suddenly become unimportant when people with FH pass the magical age of 39? The answer must be that it is not cholesterol that is causing arterial disease in those with FH, but something else. Because the blood cholesterol concentrations in people with FH who develop heart disease are no different from those who do not.[101] Imagine that: in the disease that we are told provides definitive proof that cholesterol causes heart disease, blood cholesterol concentration cannot distinguish between people who will develop coronary artery disease and those who will not. Then there is the question of why, in those with FH who develop coronary artery disease, it is only the arteries supplying the heart and not the brain that are affected.[102] Yet the brain arteries are exposed to the same high blood cholesterol concentrations.

Clearly something other than cholesterol is causing heart attacks in people with FH. The most probable explanation is that the genetic condition that causes FH is itself benign if it results solely in an increased blood cholesterol concentration. Rather, it is another genetic condition that sometimes, but not always, co-exists with FH and that increases the risk of heart disease. It seems probable that this factor has to do with an increased likelihood for developing blood clots[103] or perhaps plaque rupture, or even a co-existing insulin resistance.

Cardiologists should be telling older patients whose blood cholesterol levels rise on the Banting diet – perhaps exposing their FH genotype – that they are well past the age at which FH confers any increased risk of heart attack. And that they can take some comfort from the fact that, statistically, they are much less likely to develop cancer.

Returning to Stassen's article, she goes on to deliver what she clearly considers to be the Dalby knockout punch: the anecdote of the woman who 'dumped her statins for Noakes' diet' and whose blood cholesterol concentration increased from 5.1 to 12.9 mmol/L. 'But when the 39-year-old woman returned to a normal diet and resumed her medication,' observes Stassen, 'her cholesterol dropped substantially to 7.3.'

Stassen fails to ask Dalby for the evidence that prescribing statins to a woman without any sign of arterial disease will improve her life expectancy. Possibly because the answer is that there is very little evidence that statins improve life expectancy in women whose only abnormality is a raised blood cholesterol concentration.[104] The truth is that these drugs carry the risk of serious long-term side effects, including an increased risk for muscle breakdown,[105] peripheral neuropathy,[106] worsening blood glucose control shown as increasing HbA1c concentrations,[107] T2DM,[108] liver dysfunction, acute renal failure and cataract,[109] Parkinson's disease,[110] cancer,[111] and perhaps cognitive problems,[112] including transient global amnesia.[113] Others argue that statins worsen arterial disease and promote heart failure.[114] Hence their indiscriminate use might also be labelled 'criminal'.

My favourite author on this topic is cardiologist Barbara Roberts MD, who directs the Women's Cardiac Center at the Miriam Hospital in Rhode Island. In her book *The Truth About Statins*, she writes:

> I am seeing more and more healthy women in their thirties being put on this drug because their physicians don't read the fine print. A healthy woman in her thirties can expect to live another fifty years. It makes no sense at all to go on powerful medicines with the potential for serious, life-threatening side effects – for decades – when they have no proven benefit. Especially since you can get all the benefits of statins without taking them, simply by changing your lifestyle.[115]

Further support for the ineffectiveness of statins in treating postmenopausal women comes from a Women's Health Initiative study, ironically co-authored by Jacques Rossouw.[116] It found that postmenopausal women with T2DM had a 39 per cent greater risk of developing heart disease, even when treated with statins – the same risk as those who were not treated with statins. Rossouw did not refer to this in the Centenary Debate, because it further confirms that IR, and not cholesterol, leads to heart disease.

Which brings me to a point emphasised by Peter Gøtzsche in his book *Deadly Medicines and Organised Crime*:

> It's important to realise that drugs are never safe. Life jackets on boats are good to have, as they may save your life. They won't kill you. Drugs are not like that. Taking a statin may reduce your risk of dying from heart disease, but it will also increase your risk of dying from some other causes. Not much, but one of the statins, cerivastatin (Baycol), was taken off the market after patients had died because of muscle damage and renal failure.[117]

Importantly, Dalby fails to mention that at age 39, his patient is approaching the age at which the blood cholesterol concentration is without value in predicting risk of future heart attack.[118] Whereas low blood cholesterol concentrations consistently predict increased risk of cancer;[119] shorter life expectancy, especially in the elderly[120] and, most especially, in the very elderly[121] (see Figure 7.4); increased mortality in advanced heart failure;[122] increased risk for infection during life,[123] including a greater likelihood of contracting[124] and dying from HIV/AIDS;[125] in some but not all studies, an increased risk for developing dementia or Parkinsonism;[126] and increased risk for suicide[127] and violent behaviour.[128]

So the question becomes: Why would you want to treat an elevated blood cholesterol concentration in a female, especially one over 60 years of age, who has no clinical evidence for heart disease? Why not focus on treating the real causes of ill health, which are the complications caused by IR and persistent hyperinsulinaemia? What if these are of much greater importance than trying to treat a probably meaningless 'raised' blood cholesterol concentration?

Figure 7.4

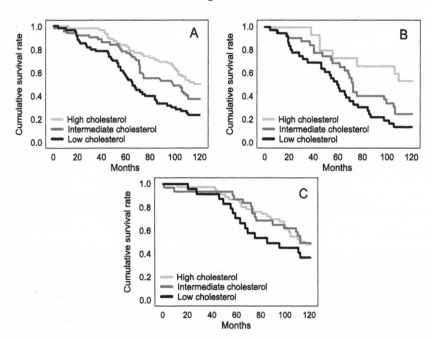

Cumulative survival curves in all 85-year-old participants (A), in men (B) and in women (C) based on the categories of blood cholesterol concentrations – high, intermediate or low. Note that there is a graded effect so that those with the highest blood cholesterol concentrations have the greatest survival. This effect is more marked in elderly men than in women. Reproduced from Takata *et al.*

Stassen next invites the opinion of another UCT professor, David Marais, who states: 'Statins make a tremendous difference in heart-disease risk in people with FH, as they will not be able to control their cholesterol through lifestyle.' He adds:

In persons with the common range of cholesterol, there is a definite association with risk but other factors such as age, smoking, hypertension, obesity and others, may *predominate* in their contribution to risk so that intervention with cholesterol lowering treatment will not have as large an impact as it has in the very high risk of FH [my emphasis].

What Marais does not add is that hypertension, obesity and diabetes (which he also failed to mention is the strongest risk factor for heart disease other than NAFLD and metabolic syndrome) are merely signs of an underlying insulin resistance in people eating high-carbohydrate diets. And that the most effective treatment of IR is the LCHF diet. If the LCHF diet can reverse obesity, hypertension and metabolic syndrome, as our Canadian study has shown,[129] and can effectively manage T2DM, then surely it should be any cardiologist's first choice in the management of heart disease?

Marais should acknowledge that the LCHF eating plan might have a special role in the management of heart disease, even if it can only reverse the 'other factors' that he admits contribute to its development. Recall that even in FH, environmental factors including diet are critically important in determining health outcomes.[130]

Stassen does present my IR theory of heart disease, but counters it by saying, 'Marais says there is more than enough scientific evidence to show that [*sic*] impact of blood cholesterol on coronary heart disease.' As I describe in detail in Chapter 17, there is no such evidence, and there is still no definitive evidence that an elevated blood cholesterol concentration is the direct cause of arterial disease.

The article ends with Van der Merwe saying:

> The whole concept of insulin resistance being the root of all evil comes from a poor understanding of metabolic and biochemical pathways ... An elevated insulin level purely means that your pancreas is stimulated by the capacity of your body to over secrete insulin. It doesn't mean to say that you have IR. IR only becomes a reality when you've developed glucose intolerance ... and the glucose is spilling over into the blood stream.

Van der Merwe falls into that group of endocrinologists who believe that T2DM is an inevitable consequence of being human in the 21st century. So the IR that causes the disease can simply be ignored. When the obese patient with IR finally develops T2DM and 'glucose is spilling over into the blood stream', he or she can always be treated with insulin. Or bariatric surgery. So what's the problem?

The problem is that T2DM patients treated with insulin do rather poorly in the long term, as we have seen. Our key responsibility should therefore be to ensure that people with IR do not develop T2DM. But it seems that some endocrinologists, like cardiologists, are not particularly partial to preventive medicine. I wonder why that is?

Is it because our profession has become programmed to produce customers for the pharmaceutical industry, instead of cures for sick patients?

8

The Banting for Babies Tweet

'A man's errors are his portals of discovery.'
— James Joyce, Irish novelist

On the suggestion of Lewis Pugh, whom I assisted in his ice-cold-water swims in the Arctic and Antarctic, I joined Twitter on 9 April 2012. Lewis suggested that this would be a great medium to expose my ideas about the low-carbohydrate diet to a global audience. Although acting on his advice would ultimately lead to the HPCSA's hearing against me, it was one of the best pieces of guidance I have ever received, because Twitter is perhaps the best educational tool I have yet encountered.

I began by 'following' those physicians and scientists who are at the forefront of the science and practise of LCHF diets. Immediately, my understanding of this topic began to increase dramatically. There is no other medium that, if properly used, can provide 24-hour coverage of exactly what is happening around the world in one's specific areas of academic interest.

But to enjoy all the advantages of Twitter, I first had to develop immunity to its evil offshoot: the personal attacks of the Twitter trolls, the porch dogs of the internet community, as well as those of the activists and the astroturfers.[1] Just as I was learning how to handle their annoying attentions, something much more threatening started to emerge.

Once *The Real Meal Revolution* had been released in November 2013, I began to receive invitations to talk about the book and the Banting revolution that it had sparked. Over the next 14 months, I would give more than 100 talks to as many as 30 000 South Africans across the length and breadth of the country. Without fail, the reception was the same. I would speak for about an hour, answer questions for another 45 minutes, and then autograph books and interact with the book buyers for perhaps another hour or two, depending on the size of the audience.

I doubt that any South African doctor or scientist in history has ever spent so much time interacting with the South African public on a single medical/scientific topic. This unique, in-your-face experience has taught me exactly what it is that the South African public wants to know about nutrition. An experience,

I might add, not shared by colleagues hiding in the academic ivory tower, express-ing their displeasure from on high.

One such talk, on 28 January 2014, formed part of the Extraordinary South Africans Series. It was no different from any of the other lectures that I would give over the next 12 months, except that it lasted a little longer, about 75 minutes, and included introductory material about my challenging of established dogmas. I ended the introduction with a summary of what I then considered to be the 'Four Absolutes for Healthy Nutrition':

- Healthy nutrition requires the best possible nutrition for the gut and the brain.
- What you eat determines what you eat.
- Absolutely no sugar or artificial sweeteners.
- Keep carbohydrates between 0 and 200 grams per day, depending on your level of insulin resistance.

I then discussed how we had been taught to fear fat (lipophobia); how there is no evidence that a high-fat diet causes heart disease; how obesity and T2DM rates rose dramatically after the introduction of the 1977 US dietary guidelines; and how the insulin model of obesity could easily explain why exposing populations with high rates of IR to high-carbohydrate diets produced the diabetes/obesity epidemic. I indicated that all the evidence supporting this interpretation was available in *The Real Meal Revolution*.

I began to wrap up with a review of my recently published paper in the *SAMJ*, describing the stories of the five 'miracle' responses to LCHF contained therein,[2] before ending, as I tend to do, with quotes from eminent persons. Thus, I quoted American historian Daniel Boorstin, whose statements would prove frighteningly predictive of what was about to happen to me:

> The greatest obstacle to discovery is not ignorance – it is the illusion of know-ledge ... I have observed that the world has suffered far less from ignorance than from pretensions to knowledge. It is not skeptics or explorers but fanat-ics and ideologues who menace decency and progress. No agnostic ever burned anyone at the stake ...

My concluding slides stated the following:
- Current dietary guidelines based on lipophobia are not evidence-based and are harmful.
- Adoption of the 1977 Dietary Guidelines for Americans caused the global epidemic of obesity and diabetes after 1980.
- This can be explained by exposing those with IR to inappropriately high carbohydrate intakes.

- Carbohydrate-rich diets are the cause of a wide range of modern chronic diseases of lifestyle.

So that:
- The hidden role of carbohydrates in our ill health needs to be acknowledged.
- Diabetes and obesity are carbohydrate-dependent diseases.
- All cancers are carbohydrate-dependent diseases.
- Dementia is a carbohydrate-dependent disease (type-III diabetes mellitus).
- Certain bowel disorders are carbohydrate-dependent diseases.

My final slide quoted the words of biologist Louis Agassiz: 'Every scientific truth goes through three states: first, people say it conflicts with the Bible; next, they say it has been discovered before; lastly, they say they always believed it.'

These were the themes that I would take with me as I travelled across South Africa speaking about the biology of the LCHF diet and why this eating plan should be the first choice for all those with IR and who have difficulty controlling either their hunger or their weight when eating the typically prescribed LFHC 'prudent' diet. In none of my talks did I ever detail what anyone should eat – in other words, not once did I prescribe a detailed diet for anyone, either in private or in public. That is not my job. I am a scientist interested in informing the public about science, something I have been doing for more than 45 years.

Importantly, in that talk, as in all my others (which ante-dated publication of our book on child nutrition, *Raising Superheroes*), I made no mention of breastfeeding or infant nutrition. And so I was perhaps a little surprised during the question time when I was asked to explain why, if breast milk contains carbohydrate, it does not prove that humans have an essential need for carbohydrates. Since the talk had focused solely on nutrition in adults, I considered the question unusual, but thought no more about it.

Over the next few days I became aware via Twitter and social media that a group of Johannesburg dietitians, who practise jointly as Nutritional Solutions Registered Dietitians (NSRDs), had been present at the talk. In a subsequent blog post on their website, published on 31 January 2014 and titled 'Prof Tim Noakes: Clarifying the Controversy', they proudly stated that each had recorded my talk.[3] This is the first time in 42 years of public speaking that anyone has admitted publicly to taping what I said without having the decency to first inform me. Why had they done this, I wondered, since essentially all the material is in *The Real Meal Revolution* or on YouTube?

It is important at this point to note that one of the NSRDs was Claire Julsing Strydom, the dietitian who would lodge the complaint about me with the HPCSA on 6 February 2014, less than a week after this first post appeared.

On their blog, the NSRDs wrote that they had decided to attend the lecture to discover what dietary 'advice is being dished out'. In which case they must have been disappointed, because, as I have said, I do not 'dish out' dietary advice in my talks. Among others, they made the following points:

[Noakes] constructs his argument cleverly by starting with disregarding the majority of nutrition studies – 'pharmaceutical industries support doctors and research', and '90% of nutrition research is associated evidence, association does not prove causation' ... most of the audience left feeling slightly overwhelmed and confused by the actual advice [to restrict carbohydrates by eating more fat, to eat only when hungry and only once a day] that was given – besides of course that bacon, liver and eggs should be staple foods from 6 months onwards ... We were also very interested in the way the Dietetics profession was described; somewhat dowdy, backward thinkers, close minded and heavily relying on the food pyramid from back in 1977.

They concluded by saying that they would be 'developing a series of blogs that will be posted over the next few days which will hopefully provide some evidence-based, objective guidance and a better understanding of healthy eating'.

A number of the comments at the end of the post were extremely supportive of what I had said. In response to one comment from a user defending me and alleging that I had been misquoted, the NSRDs observed: 'it is concerning how easily information that Prof Noakes is disseminating, can be misinterpreted. It is this issue that causes us, and a number of other health professionals, grave concern.' So it is not what I am saying that is wrong – it is how it 'can be misinterpreted'. But, I would argue, it can only be misinterpreted because it conflicts so absolutely with what the NSRDs advocate.

On 1 February, I responded with the following comment:

My talk was not primarily about what people should eat. It is about the absence of science behind the current dietary guidelines. I then state what I think nutrition should be about especially for those with insulin resistance. I wish you would represent what I said more honestly. Suggest you listen to all 13 hours of what I have said on the internet as has clearly Jan Nel (above). Why not focus on the absence of evidence for the 1977 Dietary Guidelines that was the main point I made in the lecture? The rest follows from that but is not my main message.

My point is that the internet has changed everything. The general public is now better informed on nutritional issues than ever before in our collective history. They are searching for what works. If they are given by me or anyone else information that does not work, they will no longer feel compelled to listen to that advice. They will simply go onto the internet to find what others have found to work for them. And they will follow that advice.

The success of *Real Meal Revolution* is because the book provides a simple explanation of what people who are struggling with their weight or health, because they are insulin-resistant, should be eating. They try this 'unhealthy' diet and suddenly find renewed vigour and health as did I. Then they wonder why they had been mislead to believe that what they had been eating and which caused their ill health continues to be promoted as healthy for all by a majority of dieticians globally. That is the question that you need to answer. Because if you fail to answer it, your profession will pass into history as an interesting anomaly. And it will happen very quickly. In this modern world with modern communication, bad ideas can become obsolete very quickly (think Nokia and Blackberry). My profession, especially the medical care of chronic illness, faces exactly the same problem.

I always say that your profession is the most important of all the caring professions. You need to embrace and act on these ideas and not see them as threatening.

I look forward to reading your blogs on insulin resistance and the use of HbA1c in monitoring health and preventing the diabetes epidemic.

We really should be friends.

It was at this point that Stellenbosch dietetics graduate Marlene Ellmer entered the debate. She would become an active participant in the HPCSA hearing, including offering to be an expert witness against me. But as the trial drew nearer, she had second thoughts and withdrew. She did, however, provide a summary of the evidence she wished to present (see Chapter 10).

In her first comment on the NSRD blog post, published on 2 February, Ellmer began:

I think the important issue here is that nutrition information is sent out to the general public in an assertive and effective way, which could be potentially dangerous and harmful to a nation's general health over the long-term. I can draw the comparison to a dermatologist who stands up and dishes out information about a heart condition and in the process discredits all the cardiologists.

Ellmer seemed unaware that I am an A1-rated scientist in nutrition who has published more than 150 publications dealing specifically with nutrition topics, and that for just those articles I have an H-index of 45, higher than that of any of the nutrition experts who would testify against me and whose publications deal solely with nutrition. As far as I can tell, besides her master's thesis,[4] Ellmer herself has co-authored a single publication in a peer-reviewed journal.[5] Neither deals with nutrition for health.

She continued by saying that 'Tim Noakes makes the argument that we all got sick from a low fat, high carbohydrate diet over the past 20 years', then adds the non-sequitur, 'so why should we take the risk of making the same mistake all over again'. Except, of course, for the fact that the diet I am proposing is the diet that humans ate for more than two million years before the introduction of the 1977 US dietary guidelines, and which was associated with low rates of obesity and diabetes in all populations around the globe (see Chapter 16). What new evidence do we need to prove that the diet we ate in the 1960s, which was much lower in carbohydrate, was unhealthy?

In another response, on 5 February, Ellmer stated that: 'There is not [sic] such thing as a low carb diet without high protein.' This erroneous statement suggested that perhaps her understanding of the LCHF diet was based on emotion, not fact. She continued: 'What worries me is if messages are sent to the public that are not well researched or important research are [sic] ignored to state a case and also when these diets are advocated for children who rely on their ignorant parents to feed them well. I will always stand up against that.'

She concluded by proposing that: 'A good person to follow for excellent but "less sexy" advice for how to be totally disease proof is Dr. David Katz ... My money would be on him if then not "trusting a dietitian with nutrition".'

I will deal with Katz and how money helps influence which nutritional 'science' he supports later.

It is interesting that Ellmer's concern about messages being 'sent to the public' does not extend to the current dietary guidelines, which are not evidence-based and which have clearly caused great harm. And neither Ellmer nor any of the NSRDs address the comments of people who found benefit in the LCHF diet. For example, on 3 February Etienne Marais wrote:

> Most of the top LCHF advocates openly say it's not for everyone, but it's certainly for me. Curious about why we have never heard about this from dietitians, I entered into an e-mail discussion with a few dietitians in South Africa. All I have got is negative scare tactics about health risks, which frankly I don't believe because LCHF is as old as the hills and if this was really known then people like Dr Eric Westman ... would have been sued a long time ago!! ... Gone are hunger pangs and the need to snack all the time.

The NSRDs produced a further three blogs, which continued the debate that ended with my final response six months later, on 4 July 2014. This is important, because it shows that I was actively involved in discussions with these dietitians at the same time that at least one of them was working with the HPCSA to ensure that I would be charged for expressing my opinions on social media (see Closure).

In the second blog, published on 6 February, the NSRDs responded to seven points I had made in my comment on their initial blog.[6] None of the responses was particularly enlightening or presented any hard science to disprove what I had said or written. Most were defensive.

In response to my question of why they had not highlighted my contention that the 1977 US dietary guidelines are not evidence-based, they wrote: 'Why focus on something that was used 37 years ago? Dietary guidelines have changes [*sic*], nutrition is an evolving science. Getting stuck on evidence for outdated guidelines will get us nowhere – for us to move forward in this debate we suggest that the focus is on current research.'

This is a disingenuous response. The dietary guidelines have not changed since 1977, and they are still not evidence-based, as Nina Teicholz[7] and Zoë Harcombe[8] have clearly shown. The guidelines continue to be based on the dogma that dietary fat causes heart disease; a falsehood that remains the basis for the nutritional advice provided by the NSRDs. It is not I who continues to promote 'outdated guidelines'.

In response to my suggestion that the public is now better informed than ever because of social media, the NSRDs responded: 'Better informed, or misinformed? … The problem is that there is information out there that is also harmful and misleading, with quick fixes and false promises, leaving people conflicted, unsure and more confused than ever.'

They miss the point that the internet exposes false information and quackery even more effectively than it promotes correct information. The public is only confused to the extent that people are now finally realising that those in whom they put their trust were wrong. Once the truth is known, the public will no longer be confused. The confusion now lies with the dietitians, who must adapt to a new reality; a reality in which most of what they have been taught has been proved to be wrong.

To my suggestion that *The Real Meal Revolution* is successful because it provides a simple explanation and solution for the problem of weight control and obesity, the NSRDs offered the standard answer: 'A simple explanation to a complex problem is a concern in any scientific field.' Their problem is that millions of formerly obese or overweight people have now discovered that there *is* a simple solution to their weight issues: eat fewer carbs and no sugar, stop eating addictively, lose the feeling of hunger and watch the weight fall off. There is nothing complex about it.

This blog attracted 46 responses, including a number from people who have benefited from the LCHF diet and who wished to share their experiences. Andrew hinted at the problem: 'From an outsider's perspective, it looks as if Prof. Noakes – in saying that dietitians the world over, are essentially giving their patients the wrong advice – has indeed hit a nerve … For me, what is becoming increasingly evident, is that people seem to have lost faith in the dietitian industry, and are very clearly turning to their own guidelines based on what they read on the internet.' While Charles Nankin noted: 'What is perhaps more intriguing is to understand how and why our trusted institutions and industries are leading us into this mess on a global scale.'

Johan van Niekerk described how his father had adopted the LCHF ketogenic diet in preference to chemotherapy and had successfully survived what had been diagnosed as a terminal cancer. He added:

I have no faith in registered dieticians. The fact that *The Real Meal Revolution* is the no. 1 selling book in South Africa is testament to the fact that the rest of South Africans don't trust dieticians. The prudent diet was advocated for many years and it makes us sick. I've seen results first hand, this shook our foundations and caused us to wake up. As a family we have never been healthier and never felt better and never performed better ... Registered dieticians don't make the grade. Professor Noakes and many other researchers such as prof Eric Westman do however and I trust their guidance, supported by proof, clinical studies and randomised trials. The fact that more and more medical doctors are following the diet is overwhelming.

Ellmer responded thus:

To hear that South Africans do not trust dietitians based on a book that is a recent best seller, really makes me wonder what the public understand about a role of a dietitian and what has happened to common sense and logic. To quote the person you love and trust with your life: 'Group think?'

We are but the messengers. We implement guidelines to the best of our knowledge and available science, we work very hard to keep up to date with medical and nutritional sciences. We do the best we can at any given point in time.

We first attempt to do no harm. We don't sell books to make our point, because that forms part of our daily job. That is what we get paid for. We do not publish millions of fan letters telling us how we have changed their lives, because its [sic] part of our daily job, what we get paid for. We do get acknowledged daily in our patient's [sic] lives. We do receive fan mail and gratitude and thank you's. You just don't hear about it because I do not announce it on 5FM.

Whether a dietitian is right or wrong, to be judged by the amount of fans, or the fact that a book sells so well, surely is a very one-sided view?

If you as a family to do [sic] better and healthier according to a diet book by Tim Noakes, then wonderful for you. But to blame the worlds [sic] problems and shoot the messenger, and nullifying a role of a dietitian is unnecessary.

This is the classic straw-man argument that would increasingly be employed by my critics. Van Niekerk's point is that the prudent low-fat diet has not worked for him and his family, and because this is the only diet that South African dietitians are allowed to prescribe, he has lost faith in the profession.

Instead of addressing his argument, Ellmer launches into an ad hominem attack, casting me as an egotist who writes books for financial gain (which is untrue – I donate all the royalties from all my books) and who craves media attention and praise. She does not understand that what I speak and write about in public is the result of 40 years of daily toil in the pursuit of science, or that, as we now have a diet that can reverse obesity and put T2DM into remission,[9] the new reality is that from now on dietitians will be judged on the results they produce in their patients and not on how effectively they can badmouth those who promote ideas with which they disagree.

Van Niekerk was not convinced by her response, explaining in another comment that the only way he could control his weight when eating the prudent diet was to train for the Ironman triathlon:

If you are not active enough you just have a constant battle with picking up weight, **controlling hunger and cravings** [my emphasis] and trying to eat low glycemic to avoid spikes and falling asleep at your desk.

The only alternative was to really get very active. The road to and taking part in an Iron Man event solved it all. I could eat as much as I needed and still lose weight. I just had to train vigorously twice a day. In a modern world with demands of a professional career you can only be that active up to a point. After scaling down on such vigorous activity you start picking up weight again and then the starving and cravings control the rest of your day.

I've been to at least three dieticians for advice, none of the diets are the same. **Although they make sense nutritionally I'm constantly hungry** [my emphasis].

For me it's about quality of life. After adopting the 'Banting' or 'Modified Paleo with dairy' or 'Noakes' or 'Westman' or what ever you want to call it diet, my quality of life has improved. In fact, I have not heard a single complaint from anyone who I talk to about this way of living. I don't get hungry, I never have cravings, I can do a olympic triathlon without eating breakfast and not eating anything in a better time than in the past. My total cholesterol is down [from] 6.8mmol/l to 4.9mmol/l. I have not been ill since starting this lifestyle and my allergic rhinitis subsided.

Another dietitian, Magda Uys Pieters, also accused *The Real Meal Revolution* of demonising dietitians. In fact, the word 'dietitian' does not appear in the index, and I was unable to trace any reference, good or bad, to the profession anywhere in the book. Instead, the book focuses its criticism of the current obesity/diabetes epidemic squarely on the development and promotion of the 1977 US dietary guidelines, which were not drawn up by dietitians, but by a government agency.

Regardless, Pieters wrote:

As a dietician(RD) I feel very frustrated because our profession IS being attacked/damaged by the whole Tim Noakes debacle! If you read all the comments, you would swear we as dieticians are responsible for all the Obesity, Diabetes etc. as if ALL overweight people followed recommendation set out by a dietician! NO! Most people don't care a tick about guidelines, they eat & drink merrily whatever taste good, and only seek advice AFTER their health deteriorates, so the cancer, diabetes, insulin resistance, obesity start LONG before they visit a registered dietician.

This is the classic defence of blaming the victim for any unfavourable outcomes. The truth is that, while carefully adapting their dietary patterns to those prescribed by the 1977 US dietary guidelines, Americans have become fatter and sicker. A report by the Credit Suisse Research Institute titled 'Fat: The New Health Paradigm'[10] includes the following table (Table 8.1) listing the changes in dietary intake patterns in the US from 1971 to 2009:

Table 8.1 Potential nutritional drivers of the obesity epidemic that began after 1977

		1971–1975	2009–2010	% change 1971–2009
Potential drivers				
Calorie intake (NHANES)		1 955	2 195	12%
Macronutrients (NHANES)				
Carbohydrates	Grams per day	215	280	+30
	% of daily energy intake	44	51	
Protein	Grams per day	82	88	+7
	% of daily energy intake	17	16	
Fat	Grams per day	79	80.5	+2
	% of daily energy intake	37	36	
Saturated fat	Grams per day	29	27	-7
	% of daily energy intake	14	11	
Food (FAOSTAT) (grams per day)				
Eggs		48	38	-21
Butter + lard		23	14	-39
Corn		17	34	+100
Wheat		180	218	+21
Vegetable oils		44	83	+89
Red meat		235	179	-24
Chicken		59	141	+139
Dairy		669	703	-5
Sugar		133	166	+25

Table 8.1 clearly shows that, compared to what they ate in 1971, by 2010 Americans were on average eating 12 per cent more calories, 30 per cent more carbohydrates, comprising 100 per cent more corn, 21 per cent more wheat and 25 per cent more

sugar. There had been a simultaneous 7 per cent reduction in saturated-fat intake as the result of an astonishing 89 per cent increase in vegetable-oil consumption, a 39 per cent reduction in butter and lard use, a 5 per cent reduction in dairy consumption, a 24 per cent reduction in red meat consumption and a 21 per cent reduction in eggs, all balanced with a 139 per cent increase in the consumption of (skinless, low-fat) chicken. With the exception of the rise in sugar intake, these changes align with what the 1977 dietary guidelines advocated. The unintended consequence of taking fat out of the diet was its replacement with sugar – this was not something that the people who drew up the guidelines ever considered.

I defended myself against the charges in the latest blog:

My goal is not to demonise dieticians (I focus almost exclusively on the distortion of science and the inability of my profession to see the reality especially as it relates to diet and heart disease) but to point out that current dietary advice is not working. There is no evidence that this is because the public is deviating greatly from these guidelines. They are eating low fat, high carbohydrate diets as they have been told to do. Interestingly the real deviation is in the carbohydrate intake. Those South African populations eating the most carbohydrate are amongst the illest – a paradox that no one seems too keen to address.

But the other evidence is that when people do the opposite to the guidelines and reduce their carbohydrate intakes, they suddenly start to do a whole lot better in all the health measurements that we have.

My privilege is to be insulin resistant and to have eaten both the prudent diet and the high fat diet and to have observed the quite opposite effects on myself and my health. I wish more dieticians could share my personal experiences because it would definitely influence how they see the 'science'. And whether they are prepared to dig deeply into the very large body of evidence showing the benefits of low carbohydrate diets in those with insulin resistance. A good place to start might be with the premier researchers in the field – Jeff Volek and colleagues – *The Art and Science of Low Carbohydrate Living* and *The Art and Science of Low Carbohydrate Performance.*

Again, I focused on the question of hunger control, which the NSRDs seemed completely to ignore:

Finally the influence of fat and protein on satiety is never mentioned. The body is a complex organism with a brain that directs what we eat and how much. The brainless calories in/calories out model of obesity ignores the fact that nutrient poor, high carbohydrate diets do not satiate hunger and lead to the overconsumption of calories in very many. One needs to understand the control of hunger fully to appreciate this effect.

So in my opinion, promoting a high carbohydrate diet has to promote obesity simply because, for many, it does not satiate. And there is a strong biological explanation for this. Then you add in sugar addiction and the results are the explosive rise in obesity since 1980.

When other commenters supported my idea that the obesity/diabetes epidemic had to be the result of adopting the 1977 Dietary Guidelines for Americans, Ellmer conceded: 'If Tim Noakes simply said, promotion of low fat, high carbohydrate diets lead [*sic*] to obesity epidemic we would certainly not have this debate. I think many dietitians including myself actually agree with this statement of his.'

This is pretty much all I say in my lectures, besides detailing why this happens biologically, why we need to understand IR if we want to reverse the obesity/diabetes epidemic, and why carbohydrate restriction is the key factor in managing IR, and therefore obesity and diabetes.

The third blog post, written by Ellmer on 4 March 2014, introduced the topic 'Is the LCHF diet suitable and safe for infants?'[11] By now I knew that Strydom had lodged a complaint with the HPCSA, and since I had not spoken about this topic during any of my talks, I could only assume that Ellmer had written this latest blog to support Strydom's complaint. The blog did not contain anything of value, and did not muster any evidence that the LCHF diet is indeed unsafe for infants. But it clearly represented a shift in the focus of the blogs, which the NSRDs had promised before Strydom decided to report me to the HPCSA.

Ultimately, Ellmer failed to address the real issue: What are the (epigenetic) effects of mothers eating high-carbohydrate diets during pregnancy and weaning their infants onto these diets? The answer is that their infants will be increasingly insulin resistant and at greater risk of developing obesity and diabetes.[12]

The NSRDs seemed very keen to introduce Ellmer as their new anti-Noakes attack dog. Her special assignment would be to continue addressing the dangers of the LCHF diet for breastfeeding mothers and infants, presumably in anticipation of any potential HPCSA action against me. To this end, Ellmer concluded the series of blog posts on 5 March with a fourth, titled 'LCHF diets continued: Are they safe for pregnant and/or breastfeeding mothers?'[13]

With this blog, Ellmer tried to build the case that the LCHF diet is detrimental for pregnant mothers. The sole lines of evidence she could muster were the following:

• 'No human studies have been done in this area to date, but animal studies show a strong association between ketosis [produced by a reduced carbohydrate intake] and reduced milk production.' *Presumably Ellmer wishes us to conclude that the same will apply to human mothers who choose to reduce their carbohydrate intake when breastfeeding.*

- 'One study carried out in 3601 pregnant mothers showed that high levels of urinary ketones led to a >2-fold occurrence of oligohydramnios (amniotic fluid insufficiency) and a significant increase in foetal heart rate decelerations.' *Ellmer fails to mention that the pregnant mothers in this study suffered from starvation and dehydration, and that any disorders detected in their infants were likely an effect of malnutrition and associated poor socio-economic circumstances, not ketosis.*
- 'It is widely acknowledged from nutrition studies that with LCHF diets, protein intake increases and high protein intakes are associated with bone mineral loss and calcium excretion. A pregnant and breastfeeding mother's calcium requirements are higher than most adults, putting her at a risk for poor bone health.' *But the LCHF diet is not a high-protein diet, it is a high-fat diet – a distinction I would expect a registered dietitian to understand.*
- 'Excluding fruit and whole-grain from your diet may lead to inadequate intake of anti-oxidants and other nutrients and evidence has shown an association linking inadequate antioxidant status in utero and early childhood to an increase in the risk of allergic disease, amongst other concerns.' *This makes one wonder how hominin infants survived for two to three million years before the development of agriculture. According to Ellmer's logic, they should have all died, taking the human race with them.*

I commented on this blog some months later, on 4 July 2014, perhaps because by that time I had received confirmation that the HPCSA was considering an action against me.

After birth, the greatest threat to the long term health of the babies of mothers reading this website, is the development of insulin resistance, obesity and diabetes at increasingly younger ages. We know that each generation of children born to such mothers is getting fatter and is at higher risk of all these conditions. Since genes have not changed, this raises the possibility that epigenetic effects acting before and after the child's birth may play a role. One factor that has changed in the last 50 years is the advice to mothers to increase their carbohydrate intakes during pregnancy and to wean the child onto cereal-based, high carbohydrate diets. But ingested carbohydrates have no essential role in human nutrition whereas fat and protein most certainly do. It is not possible to build healthy bones, brains and bodies on diets that are high in carbohydrate with obligatory reductions in fat and protein contents. Worse carbohydrates raise blood glucose and insulin concentrations needlessly – there is no biological advantage to having continuously elevated blood glucose and insulin concentrations. My point is that exposing the foetus to high glucose and insulin concentrations during pregnancy by having the mother ingest unnecessary carbohydrates makes no sense since it could produce epigenetic effects that may cause the child to be more likely to develop insulin resistance, obesity and diabetes mellitus. Unless you can be absolutely certain that this is not the case, and that your advice is not increasing the probability that children exposed to high glucose and insulin concentrations before and after birth are not being needlessly predisposed to the development of these conditions, you should perhaps be less certain (dogmatic) that your advice is the only correct option. Thank you.

In time, Ellmer re-published these blogs on the website of her Somerset West dietetics practice, Vergelegen Dietitians. One of the blogs included the advert: 'Book a consultation with us and find out what type of weight loss diet will work best for you.' With these blogs, Ellmer self-identified as the South African dietitian most willing to speak about infant nutrition and who, equally importantly, was zealously antagonistic to me and my advocacy of the LCHF diet. And so, when Strydom and the head of the HPCSA's legal team, Advocate Meshack Mapholisa, were looking for expert witnesses to testify against me, Ellmer was one of the first they approached.

In the midst of all this blogging, on 3 February 2014, Twitter user Pippa Leenstra tweeted the following to me and Sally-Ann Creed, my co-author on *The Real Meal Revolution*:

@ProfTimNoakes @SalCreed is LCHF eating ok for breastfeeding mums? Worried about all the dairy + cauliflower = wind for babies??

That the tweet was addressed to both Sally-Ann and me, and specifically referenced LCHF, indicated that Leenstra was aware of *The Real Meal Revolution* and was writing to us as its authors. Most importantly, she asked about breastfeeding **mums** and expressed concern for **babies** – not a specific mum or baby, or even her baby, but mums and babies in general. In doing so, she clearly defined the context of her question. She was **not** asking for medical advice in order to treat herself and her child. Rather, she was asking for general information that might be applied to all breastfeeding mothers. This is a crucial distinction that should have dictated how the HPCSA dealt with the complaint against me.

The HPCSA's rules regarding what information a dietitian – and by extension a medical doctor such as myself – may give are very clear. Schedule 2(b)(ii) of the Health Professions Act 56 of 1974: 'Regulations Defining the Scope of the Profession of Dietetics' differentiates between dietetics information given as part of a medical consultation and that which serves to promote 'community nutrition', defined as 'the professional communication of scientifically-based nutrition knowledge, according to need, to individuals and groups within the community in order to motivate them to maintain or change nutritional behaviour in order to improve quality of life and to prevent nutrition-related diseases'.[14]

Because Leenstra was asking a 'we' question, I was completely within my rights to give general information without examining the 'patient'. And, crucially, by answering the question, I was not entering a doctor–patient relationship with Leenstra.

Two days later, on 5 February, I tweeted my response:

@PippaLeenstra @SalCreed Baby doesn't eat the dairy and cauliflower. Just very healthy high fat breast milk. Key is to ween [*sic*] baby onto LCHF.

In this tweet, what I did not say is as important as what I did. I did not answer Leenstra's question directly, because I personally had no knowledge of a link between dairy and cauliflower in the mother's diet and wind in the breastfed infant. Thus, in keeping with the nature of Twitter, which is an open public forum for the sharing of information, I left the answering of that particular question to anyone else who might have the relevant knowledge that I lacked; Sally-Ann Creed, for example. I also did not instruct mothers to stop breast-feeding. Rather, my tweet endorsed breastfeeding. As fully expressed in *Raising Superheroes*, I believe that mothers should breastfeed for as long as possible, aiming for two to three years if feasible.[15]

I added the part about weaning babies onto LCHF because I strongly believe that infants should not be weaned onto the usual high-carbohydrate, high-cereal diet, which, in my opinion, predisposes them to the development of IR, obesity and T2DM. Alan Greene, professor of paediatrics at Stanford University, shares my view: 'In fact, I think [white rice cereal] is the tap root of the child obesity epidemic ... The problem is that it is basically like feeding kids a spoonful of sugar ... I'm saying you might as well be putting soda in the bottle as feeding the white rice cereal.'[16] In retrospect, had I written that the key is to wean baby onto real foods (instead of LCHF), the HPCSA trial may never have happened. But I had run out of characters, and it was clear that Leenstra was referring to *The Real Meal Revolution*, which meant she had to understand that, in my book, LCHF and real foods are synonymous.

Leenstra responded with the following:

@ProfTimNoakes @SalCreed ok, but what I eat comes through into my milk, is that not problematic for baby and their winds at newborn stage?

I chose not to respond to this question for two reasons. First, Leenstra had now asked a direct 'I' question, so that any answer I gave might be construed as medical advice. And second, she was asking for information on a topic about which I have no special expertise. Since the focus of my Twitter account is the dissemination of scientific information, not medical information about topics on which I am not an expert, I did not reply, hoping rather that someone more knowledgeable than I on the subject would offer Leenstra the appropriate advice.

Which is exactly what happened. Within a few minutes of posting my tweet, Leenstra received a response from Ellmer, who described herself as a 'paeds dietitian':

> @PippaLeenstra Pippa, as a paeds dietitian I strongly advise against LCHF for breastfeeding mothers. #notokay

To which Leenstra responded:

> @Mellmer80 thx, why do u say that?

Ellmer chose not to answer her question on Twitter. Rather she suggested they take the discussion offline:

> @PippaLeenstra Why dont you email me on marlene.ellmer@gmail.com and I will explain. Ps food flavours are definately [sic] passed through BM

This tweet is important for one critical reason. Central to the HPCSA's case against me was their belief that my original tweet constituted medical advice given to a patient from whom I had failed to take an adequate medical history and whom I had not properly examined. The key contention was that my tweet established a doctor–patient relationship with Leenstra, and once a doctor–patient relationship exists, my registration with the HPCSA as a medical practitioner obliges me to fulfil certain 'duties of care'. The HPCSA would contend that I had failed to perform these responsibilities.

If this were the case – in other words, had I established such a doctor–patient relationship – then Ellmer's latest tweet constituted supersession. By providing her contact details to Leenstra, Ellmer was seeking to make Leenstra her patient; in effect, she was stealing my patient. And stealing another medical professional's patient is a breach of the HPCSA's rules. If I were to be charged for breaching the rules, then the HPCSA would have had to act against Ellmer, too.

On 6 February, Claire Julsing Strydom entered the discussion with the following tweets:

> @ProfTimNoakes @PippaLeenstra @SalCreed I AM HORRIFIED!! HOW CAN YOU GIVE ADVICE LIKE THIS????

@ProfTimNoakes @PippaLeenstra @SalCreed YOU HAVE GONE TOO FAR, BE SURE THAT I WILL BE REPORTING THIS TO THE HEALTH PROFESSIONAL COUNCIL SA

@ProfTimNoakes @PippaLeenstra Pippa I am a breastfeeding mom of a 4 month old & a RD [registered dietitian] with a MSc in dietetics this info is shocking.

@ProfTimNoakes @PippaLeenstra Pippa please contact me on 011 023 8051 or Claire@nutritionalsolutions.co.za for evidence based advice

Strydom, it seemed, was also now actively trying to steal my 'patient'.

That they did indeed 'chat' was confirmed by Strydom's next tweet:

@ProfTimNoakes @PippaLeenstra Was great chatting to you Pippa – good luck with your little one.

And by Leenstra's response:

@DietitianClaire @ProfTimNoakes thx for the call and advice Claire.

Had Leenstra been my patient, here was proof that supersession had taken place.

The next person to get involved was Anne Till. Till was one of the senior dietitians advising Discovery Health when I was the Discovery Health Professor of Exercise and Sports Science at UCT. She and I had participated in a documentary TV series in which my main contribution was to nod sagely while Till gave the standard nutritional advice embraced by Discovery and based on the USDA's food pyramid, loaded with 'healthy' grains.

Since then, Till had immigrated to the US, intent, she told me, on 'making Americans healthy'. Her participation on 7 February allowed Strydom to repeat her statement about my 'dangerous advice':

@AnneTillRD @MicheChelle @ProfTimNoakes thanks Anne. I can't just ignore such dangerous advice especially when it comes to infant nutrition

Strydom next told Till that she had reported me to the HPCSA:

@AnneTillRD it is out of control! I have reported the infant nutrition recommendations made by TN to the HPCSA we will see the response

My interest all along has been the promotion of a questioning science, so in my response to Strydom and Till the following day I asked whether the consequences of weaning infants onto high-carbohydrate, cereal-based foods could be the early onset of obesity and T2DM. At the time, I did not yet understand that the reason why the South African dietary guidelines promote weaning onto cereals is not because they are healthy, but because they are regarded as affordable to the 'masses'. I tweeted:

> @DietitianClaire @AnneTillRD What if the childhood obesity epidemic is caused by the high carb diets to which we now expose our children?

In response to Strydom's statement that she had reported me to the HPCSA, I indicated that I was keen to read her evidence that a high-carbohydrate diet is essential for infant health:

> @DietitianClaire @AnneTillRD Can't wait. Look forward to your published evidence that high carb diet essential for health of infants/kids

To another Twitter user, Strydom suggested on 8 February that feeding infants real foods would increase infant mortality rates:

> @albie_cilliers Shocking -reported it to HPCSA. How can he give advice like that in SA where infant mortality rates are already high

She does not ask if it is possible that the high-carbohydrate, cereal-based diets onto which the majority of South African infants are weaned could be the cause of South Africa's high infant mortality rates. As they say, insanity is repeating the same mistakes and expecting different results. And never considering an alternative explanation.

That same day, Strydom tweeted:

> @drgail3 @MicheChelle Please forward me the literature that indicates that it is safe to wean an infant onto a LCHF diet!

A challenge that all proponents of the LCHF diet experience almost daily is having to deal with the sceptics' question: Yes, but where is the data? Surprisingly, these same sceptics never ask the question of those who defend the 1977 US dietary guidelines.

In time, I discovered that this feigned scepticism is simply a front, because when we presented 12 days of testimony at the HPCSA hearing showing why the LCHF diet is safe, and indeed essential, for infants, those who had been the most vociferous in assuring South Africans that the LCHF diet is dangerous were notably absent.

Five days after her original tweet to me and Sally-Ann Creed, Leenstra re-entered the discussion:

@2catsandababy @ProfTimNoakes @SalCreed thx but I'll go with the dieticians recommendation

As a result, I considered my job done, and I disengaged. Leenstra had received the information she had sought. She had made her choice. That is why Twitter exists: to share knowledge that allows the interested participants to make their own informed decisions.

In a subsequent interview with *Netwerk24* on 28 November 2015, Leentra stated that she could not care less about the HPCSA hearing that her Tweet had precipitated and which she described as a 'circus'.[17] She explained that, in 2014, her husband had come home with *The Real Meal Revolution* and she had started to prepare his evening meals according to the Banting guidelines. At the time she was breastfeeding their then six-month-old son, and she wondered if the LCHF diet might affect him adversely. This is what motivated her tweet.

When she read my Twitter response, Leenstra said she laughed, because she had no intention of weaning her son onto a Banting diet. When Strydom phoned her the next day and 'pleaded' with her not to follow my advice, she felt it was a moot point because she had never planned to follow the diet anyway.

The dietitians, however, would not let it go. They continued to post tweets that provided insights into not only their own feelings on the topic, but also their understanding of human biology, as well as how they viewed themselves and their professional responsibilities.

On 15 February, Ellmer hinted that she had fears about the dangers of ketone bodies for the suckling infant:

@drgail3 @PippaLeenstra @SalCreed And we havent even started on effect of ketones transferred in BM to BF baby?

Reading the summary of her testimony for the HPCSA hearing, my conclusion is that, at the time Ellmer wrote this tweet, she had little understanding of the critical role that ketone bodies play in the development of the neonatal brain. Which is a little disturbing for someone who considers herself a 'paeds dietitian'.

The truth is that ketones are absolutely essential for early brain development in newborn and suckling infants (see Chapter 17). If registered dietitians in South Africa do not understand this because it is not included in their curriculum, then this poses a significant academic challenge.

On the same day, Ellmer indicated that dietitians have a responsibility to educate their colleagues (presumably she was referring to ignorant doctors like me):

@drgail3 @PippaLeenstra I hear you. The onus are on us to also ensure our colleauges [sic] are properly educated and up-to-date with science

Yet Ellmer was absent when Nina Teicholz, Zoë Harcombe, Caryn Zinn and I presented our testimony supporting our position during the HPCSA hearing. How can you be an educator if you are not prepared to consider all the published evidence? Does Ellmer believe that a 'proper education' is one that only considers current dietary dogma? Her absence from the hearing is even more startling when one considers this tweet, from 15 March, in which she underscored the importance of lifetime learning:

Powerful Chinese Proverb. http://t.co/hkVlnoooup We are never beyond learning and almost never so wise

Two days earlier, she had complained that LCHF proponents had failed to send her information on the Banting diet:

@snooplambylamb Ross I have asked for 3 LCHF proponents to send me lists of scientific studies to support their view and no reply so far

Yet when the opportunity to listen to world authorities on LCHF arrived on her doorstep, at no cost to her, she failed to turn up. This is a classic case of confirmation bias: we accept the ideas that we like uncritically, and then demand mathematical certainty for all the concepts we dislike.

Finally, she dismissed the 'science' in *The Real Meal Revolution* without ever explaining why:

@ProfTimNoakes If anything like the 'science' provided in RMR I will be dissappointed and dissillusioned [sic]. For sake of arg I will read it

On 3 April, Strydom tweeted that she and her colleagues were collecting the names of the many people whose health was suffering as a result of adopting the LCHF diet:

@ianlane88 @nooralrefae_RD @ProfTimNoakes we are collecting these case studies to hand over to the HPCSA.

I asked her what her control group would be, but she did not respond. No list was forthcoming at the HPCSA hearing.

On the same day, Strydom indicated that everything she says is 'evidence based':

> @cclauson i have studied nutrition for many years and have been in private practice for over a decade. Everything I say is evidence based

The only problem is that most of the current nutritional 'evidence' is fictitious, based on meaningless observational, associational studies, the weaknesses of which I discussed in Chapter 7. While Strydom's training may indeed be 'evidence based', there is little hard evidence to support what she has been taught. The focus of the HPCSA trial would gradually swing from the consideration of my unprofessional conduct to a review of the absence of any evidence for the current dietary guidelines and, by extension, for much of what dietitians currently prescribe.

Strydom also retweeted material from others who believe that dietary fat is harmful to human health. Two such tweets drew attention to the ideas of American physician David Katz, who would soon become a new best friend of ADSA, flying to Cape Town to be the keynote speaker at their 2016 Nutrition Congress. Katz, who appears to be a vegetarian and leader of the plant-based food movement, has had a chequered medical career. In 2015, he was found to have written laudatory reviews for one of his own books under a pseudonym.[18] He is also one of the most highly paid consultants to the food industry, leading US investigative journalist Russ Greene to dub him 'Junk Food's Slyest Defender'.* It seems highly improbable that Katz would come to South Africa to speak on ADSA's behalf without expecting a sizeable fee from the congress funders, the South African Sugar Association.

In an exposé on Katz in 2016, Greene concluded:

> Katz has managed to live two lives, one as a paid junk-food apologist, the other as an independent source for public health information. But what makes his story more remarkable is that he successfully played both roles under a single name. And the media and government failed to adequately vet him for conflicts of interest, all the while promoting his work to the unknowing public. Thanks to the CDC [Centers for Disease Control and Prevention], US taxpayers provided the 'core funds' for Katz's research.

---

* Greene lists the known amounts of money paid to Katz by various food companies for his consultancy or research support: Chobani (yoghurt) paid him $3 500 an hour to serve as an expert witness in a sugar lawsuit; The Hershey's Company paid him $731 000 to study the health benefits of cocoa; PepsiCo (Quaker Oats) paid him $633 000 to study the health benefits of oats; and KIND paid him $154 000 to promote 'low-sugar' KIND Bars. In addition, Katz has served as president of the Coca-Cola-funded American College of Lifestyle Management and was hired by Big Sugar as an expert witness in the defence of Refinery 29 (Western Sugar Cooperative, *et al.* vs Archer-Daniels-Midland, Inc., *et al.*).

Logically and physically, only one Dr. David Katz can exist. His public health persona may be a facade, but the million-plus he has accepted from junk food companies remain matters of fact.[19]

Interestingly, on her website, Strydom acknowledges that she is one of 120 members of the council of directors for the GLiMMER (Global Lifestyle Medicine Mobilizing to Effect Reform) Initiative, the goal of which is to be 'a global voice devoted to disseminating and applying what we know for sure about health promotion and disease prevention'. GLiMMER's founder is Dr David Katz, who advocates a low-fat diet and maintains that saturated fat is not good for health.[20]

Katz would not be the first industry-sponsored nutritionist to be invited to speak in South Africa on the benefits of a 'plant-based' diet. In April 2014, Strydom invited Sylvia Escott-Stump from the East Carolina University Department of Nutrition Science to speak at the annual Nutritional Solutions Continuing Nutrition Education (CNE) Event. When interviewed by Strydom, Escott-Stump opined:

> The cause of obesity is multifactorial and it is truly impossible to pinpoint a single cause ... Ideally, it is recommended to consume a typical daily intake based on the general food based dietary guidelines which includes 45–60% of total energy per day from carbohydrates ... The high protein, low carbohydrate diet does not make physiological sense ... The brain and red blood cells require a constant supply of glucose ... In summary, eliminating a key macronutrient such as carbohydrate is quite detrimental as the body needs a steady supply for various purposes.[21]

The interview, which appeared in the *South African Journal of Clinical Nutrition* (*SAJCN*), ended with the following disclosure: 'Kellogg Company of South Africa was one of the executive sponsors at the 2014 Nutritional Solutions CNE. This sponsorship made it possible for Ms. Sylvia Escott-Stump to travel to South Africa to present at this event.'

In 2012, when Escott-Stump was its president, the US Academy of Nutrition and Dietetics issued a press release opposing New York City's plan to ban the sale of sodas and other sugary beverages larger than 16 ounces in restaurants and entertainment venues.[22] Their opposition is understandable when you know that AND was sponsored by Abbott Nutrition (makers of infant formulas), Coca-Cola, Kellogg's, Mars, PepsiCo and Unilever to the tune of $3 million in 2011. On one occasion, Escott-Stump famously appeared wearing Coca-Cola red to promote Coca-Cola at a 2012 Coca-Cola event in her role as AND president.[23]

Strydom's tweets also exposed her ignorance of the nature of dietary fats. On 19 February 2014, she wrote:

@MarikaSboros I will still not advocate a diet made up of 60–75% saturated fats. Show me the evidence that shows this extreme is good!!

Regardless of the fact that the Banting diet does not promote eating 60–75 per cent saturated fat, the reality is that all foods contain three types of fat in different proportions (Table 8.2), so that it is impossible to eat a diet that is 60–75 per cent saturated fat – unless you lived on coconut oil or ghee alone.

Table 8.2 Fatty acid profile of commonly eaten fatty foods

Fatty acid profile		Saturated	Monounsaturated	Polyunsaturated		
			omega-7, omega-9	Total	omega-6	omega-3
Saturated fats	Chicken fat	31%	49%	20%	Depends on feeding	
	Duck and goose fat	35%	52%	13%	Depends on feeding	
	Lard (pork)	40%	48%	12%	Depends on feeding	
	Palm oil	50%	41%	9%	9%	0%
	Tallow (beef or mutton)	55%	40%	5%	Depends on feeding	
	Ghee	65%	31%	4%	Depends on feeding	
	Coconut oil	92%	6%	2%	2%	0%
Monounsaturated fats	Avocado oil	12%	70%	13%	12%	1%
	Olive oil	13%	75%	12%	10%	2%
	High oleic sunflower oil	7%	78%	15%	15%	0%
	High oleic sunflower oil	9%	83%	8%	8%	0%
Polyunsaturated fats	Peanut oil	18%	48%	34%	34%	0%
	Canola oil	5%	57%	35%	23%	12%
	Sesame oil	15%	42%	43%	43%	0%
	Cottonseed oil	26%	18%	54%	54%	1%
	Sunflower oil	10%	35%	55%	65%	0%
	Soybean oil	17%	25%	58%	51%	7%
	Safflower oil	8%	17%	75%	75%	0%
	Flaxseed oil	9%	18%	73%	16%	57%

One final tweet from Ellmer is of interest. On 2 July, she tweeted:

> @miridavdm @ProfTimNoakes Mirida it is not safe to continue banting whilst pregnant. We don't have the studies http://t.co/c8Nsd4vLt4

She admits that 'we don't have the studies', so on what grounds does she draw the conclusion that Banting is unsafe during pregnancy? Recall that by the time the HPCSA hearing came around, Ellmer had become rather less certain of her conviction that the LCHF diet is dangerous to infants. In fact, she was then so uncertain that she decided not to testify.

True to her word, Strydom submitted a formal complaint to the HPCSA in the form of an email sent at 08h47 on Thursday 6 February 2014. It read:

> To whom it may concern.
>
> I would like to file a report against Prof. Tim Noakes. He is giving incorrect medical (medical nutrition therapy) on twitter that is not evidence based. I have attached the tweet where Prof. Noakes advices [sic] a breastfeeding mother to wean her baby onto a low carbohydrate high fat diet.
>
> I urge the HPCSA to please take urgent action against this type of misconduct as Prof Noakes is a 'celebrity' in South Africa and the public does not have the knowledge to understand that the information he is advocating is not evidence based – it is especially dangerous to give this advice for infants and can potentially be life threatening. I await your response.
>
> Kind regards,
> Claire Julsing Strydom

The HPCSA forwarded the complaint to me on 20 February 2014. It is absolutely clear that, in contrast to what Strydom said under oath during the hearing and subsequently on Twitter and in the media, this complaint did not come from ADSA, of which she was president at the time. It came directly and solely from Strydom. This was made clear in all the correspondence I received from the HPCSA, which always listed the complainant as 'Ms CJ Strydom'. Additionally, the email complaint was sent less than two and a half hours after Strydom tweeted asking Leenstra to contact her 'for evidence based advice' – both the tweet and the complaint therefore arising before 9 a.m. This allowed no time to consult with ADSA, let alone for them to approve a complaint that was to be made on their behalf.

My initial reaction to the complaint was that it was utterly ludicrous. How could a dietitian, who claims in her lectures and blogs that everything she does is 'evidence based', lodge a complaint without a single academic reference to support her contention?

I sent a four-page response on 2 May 2014. By this stage, because I considered the complaint so absurd, I had not consulted anyone about what I should write. I simply could not conceive that such a trivial, unscientific rant could ever be formulated into a charge against me.

Dear Ms Mngadi,

Thank you for the registered mail of the 20th February 2014. The letter includes the complaints of Ms Claire Justing [sic] Strydom relating to a Tweet I made on 05/02/2014. My tweet included the statement: 'Key is to wean baby onto LC HF'. I have sent a copy of this correspondence also by registered mail.

Ms Strydom claims that I am 'giving incorrect medical advice .... that is not evidence based'. She claims that I am guilty of 'misconduct' as this advice is potentially life-threatening. She asks that the HPCSA takes urgent action against me.

As I understand the legal process, it is not sufficient for the prosecution simply to make a claim as does Ms Strydom in this case, that what I have said is 'not evidence-based'. *Rather Ms Strydom must provide the evidence-base to prove that my comments are 'life-threatening'.* This is particularly import-ant as she has made this claim publically [sic] on Twitter so that I, as the aggrieved party, might have grounds to take legal action against her for unpro-fessional conduct with respect to public statements about the competence of another medical professional. In providing this response, I do not forego my options in that regard.

Unfortunately Ms Strydom does not provide that 'evidence-base' for her belief; thus she has no case. The basis for her complaint is null. *The reason she cannot provide that 'evidence-base' is simply because no such evidence exists.* There are no randomised controlled clinical trials (RCTs) comparing the long-term effects of weaning babies onto the high carbohydrate low fat diet that she prescribes or its converse which I believe is the only healthy option. There are certainly no clinical trials showing that my approach is 'life threatening'. In the absence of that evidence, Ms Strydom is in the invidious position that she has publicly attacked a professional colleague without being able to provide the scientific evidence to support her potentially defamatory and certainly unprofessional statement.

The reason why she believes that babies should be weaned onto a high carbohydrate diet is simply because that is the dogma she has been taught in her training as a South African dietician. But to elevate that dogma to established truth requires that the appropriate RCTs be performed. In their absence, neither she nor I can be certain of what is the best diet on to which one should wean a child. As a result we are allowed to come to our own conclusions, based on our professional experience and training, and it is perfectly in my right to conclude that her advice is wrong and that children should not be weaned in the manner she has been taught.

The logic for my position is an extension of my argument (with which the HPCSA has publicly expressed its disagreement) that a high carbohydrate diet is the single most important factor driving the obesity and diabetes epidemic in this country and indeed globally. I have partially developed that argument in our new book *The Real Meal Revolution*. It is too complex to argue fully here. However I do submit another document from colleagues (attached) that in my opinion is the single most clearly stated counter-argument to the current dietary guidelines that Ms Strydom and all South African dieticians are taught.

I frequently make the point, emphasized in our book, that the novel high carbohydrate low fat guidelines which Ms Strydom promotes were adopted in the United States in 1977 without an adequate evidence-base and purely to bring down the price of food and maximize the wealth of North American farmers. The evidence that these guidelines were driven by political/economic considerations alone without concern for their long-term health consequences is absolutely clear in the published record. It is most unfortunate that in her training, Ms Strydom appears not to have been exposed to this evidence. If she were, she might have a different opinion of the veracity of what she has been taught.

But with regard to the weaning of children, my arguments are the following:

1. In his book *Nutrition and Physical Degeneration*, Weston Price reports historic data showing the remarkable health of traditional societies eating traditional foods. In a European context he reports the astonishing health (and absence of common diseases like diabetes, obesity, tuberculosis and dental caries) in Swiss people living in the isolated Loetschental Valley (before the 1940s when the modern high carbohydrate diet first reached that population). The people in that valley lived on rye, dairy products and the meat of cattle. Thus the entire population ate a low carbohydrate diet. The same findings were reported for persons living in the outer Hebrides (Scotland) in which oats replaced rye and the main source of protein and fat was the abundance of fish. In both populations, the children were extremely healthy. In Africa the Masai live on a very low carbohydrate diet as do the Inuit in the Arctic. There are no reports that the limited carbohydrate intake of the

children in those populations is 'life threatening'. If it were, the populations would not have survived as all the children would have died.

It is notable that when these populations adopt the modern 'healthy' diet promoted by Ms Strydom and others, they become remarkably less healthy than when they ate their traditional high fat low carbohydrate diets.

2. Humans have absolutely no essential requirement for carbohydrate. There is no human disease caused by carbohydrate deficiency. Carbohydrate in the body serves only 2 functions – it is either used as a source of energy or it is stored as fat. There is no other option.

The human body has a great capacity to produce all its energy (at rest) from the oxidation of fat. There is no need for humans at any age to ingest carbohydrate in order to provide their bodies with 'energy'.

3. A deficient intake of either protein or fat is associated with disease and ill health. These conditions are well described and common in malnourished South Africans. *Malnourished South Africans and those with obesity and diabetes (including children) are NOT eating a low carbohydrate high fat diet.* They are eating a high carbohydrate low fat diet. Sooner or later this fact will have to be acknowledged and the dietary advice given to South Africans will have to change. Until that happens South Africans will continue to grow yet fatter with higher rates of diabetes and other related diseases.

4. There is growing evidence that the first 1000 days of the child's life are crucial determinants of his or her long-term health and intelligence. During this period of rapid brain development, the greatest need is for a high fat intake to maximize brain growth. Carbohydrates, because they provide only energy and substrates for fat accumulation, cannot provide the key nutrient (fat) necessary for optimal brain growth. Thus the probability is that providing the growing child with a high carbohydrate diet in the first 1000 days of his or her life could rob the child of vital nutrients necessary for maximizing brain growth. Thus the prescription of a high carbohydrate low fat diet in the first 1000 days of life might reasonably be described as 'life determining', if not actually 'life threatening'.

Indeed there is an urgent need to study the effects of the almost absence of fat in the diets of the poorest South Africans on their brain development and subsequent intellectual development. Or conversely the effects of low carbohydrate high fat eating on the brain development of those South Africans who are the most deprived.

5. Each generation of children (including South Africans) is becoming progressively fatter. Whilst the argument favoured by South African dieticians is that this is because children are simply becoming lazier and are eating too much fat, the evidence does not support this. Why is it that this effect is present already in children of 1–2 years? It cannot be because they are doing too

little exercise and eating too much fat since there is no population in South Africa, other than those individuals who have recently converted in the past year or so, eating a high fat diet (and children are not physically active until they start walking).

Rather the evidence points to this being a generational epigenetic effect in children. Epigenetics refers to the effects of environmental factors which alter the way in which our genes act. Thus the argument is that mothers advised to eat high carbohydrate diets produce an intra-uterine environment in which the fetus becomes accustomed to frequent elevations in blood glucose and insulin concentrations every few hours. This, it is argued, sets up the metabolic profile (and perhaps conditions the brain) that favours the development of obesity and perhaps diabetes. Next if the infant is not breast-fed, it will be exposed to more carbohydrates in formula milk. Then according to Ms Strydom's advice the infant will be weaned onto a high carbohydrate diet which must further continue the epigenetic programming caused by frequent oscillations in blood glucose and insulin concentrations, thereby increasing the probability for obesity and diabetes in adulthood (and with the further disadvantage of sub-optimum brain development).

Finally after reading all the literature and seeking the advice of dieticians who promote weaning onto a high fat diet, I advised my son and daughter to raise their children on low carbohydrate high fat diets. As a result both my grandchildren are lean, alert, infrequently ill and with seemingly endless energy. Indeed they mirror all the benefits that I have achieved from following this eating plan. There is no evidence that my grandchildren are suffering as a result of this advice. Instead it appears quite the opposite. I am very happy that the one key benefit of this eating approach will be that they will not become obese and diabetic which must be the single greatest threat to their future health.

I look forward to the day when the HPCSA will call for an investigation of the veracity of the 'evidence base' on which South African dieticians are currently being trained and its effect on the obesity and diabetes epidemic that is crippling the health of this nation.

I remain,
Yours Sincerely,
Professor T.D. Noakes OMS
MBChB, MD, DSc, FACSM, (hon) FFSEM (UK)

As supportive evidence, I included a recently completed criticism of the New Zealand dietary guidelines, written by colleagues at the Auckland University of Technology (AUT).[24] I believed that I had said enough in my reply for any rational committee to dismiss the complaint. In any case, I knew that the HPCSA rules mandated that, before I could be formally charged, I had to be given the opportunity to present more complete arguments to a preliminary inquiry committee, which would then decide whether or not the matter should be taken further.

I was certain that on the basis that I had answered a 'we' question – as is my constitutional right and fully compliant with the HPCSA's own rules – and had given accepted international advice for weaning infants onto animal products as the ideal complementary foods (see Chapter 12), the complaint would be thrown out within a few hours.

How wrong I was. Behind the scenes, unimagined by me, things were beginning to hot up. Very soon my life would undergo a radical change.

PART II

NUTRITION ON TRIAL

9

The Hearing: June 2015

'Objectivity does not exist. It cannot exist.
The word is a hypocrisy which is sustained by the lie that the truth
stays in the middle. No, sir. Sometimes truth stays on one side only.'
– Oriana Fallaci, Italian journalist and war correspondent

When the first attempt at a hearing against Professor Tim Noakes rolled round in Cape Town in June 2015, it was easy to spot his supporters. They were dressed in bright-red T-shirts, the colour of the cover of Noakes's book *The Real Meal Revolution*. It had sold more than 160 000 copies in its first six months, making it South Africa's bestselling book ever. It quickly became the 'bible' of Banting, as the low-carbohydrate, high-fat lifestyle has become known in the country.

The book's success had infuriated doctors, dietitians and academics alike. Among them was dietitian Claire Julsing Strydom, who had reported him to the HPCSA in February 2014 for what the public had dubbed the 'Banting for babies' tweet. As Noakes's legal team would later note in their closing argument, these health professionals were furious with him not only because they disagreed with him on the science for optimum nutrition, but also because the public appeared to be listening more to Noakes than they were to them. In other words, they were losing influence, and business, to Noakes. *The Real Meal Revolution* thus appeared to be one of the reasons why Noakes's critics were so keen for the HPCSA to silence him.

Ironically, Noakes is only one of the book's four co-authors. He wrote a single chapter on the science for LCHF. A common criticism doctors and academics throw at Noakes is that the evidence he presents in *The Real Meal Revolution* has no value because it has not appeared in a peer-reviewed journal. This is simply not true: the evidence for LCHF that Noakes presents in the book and elsewhere *has* appeared in respected medical journals, including those that are peer-reviewed.

And, of course, Noakes is not alone in writing or contributing to bestselling books on medical and nutritional science. Objectively, then, the attacks on Noakes for his contribution to *The Real Meal Revolution* have no scientific basis.

They reveal nothing more than his critics' determination to discredit him, by fair means or foul.

Before the June 2015 hearing, I wasn't convinced of an organised campaign to discredit Noakes. I thought it was more likely a symptom of the chronic incompetency that has infected the HPCSA in recent years. That day, after watching its legal team at work in the hearing, however, I came away convinced that something was rotten in the state of the HPCSA.

As a journalist, I'm always aware of my ethical responsibilities when reporting on any dispute or court case. When I was training to be a journalist, lecturers drummed into me the need for accuracy, fairness, balance and objectivity. Accuracy, fairness and balance are not that difficult to get right – if all sides are prepared to talk to you. When one side refuses to talk, or lies, or deliberately feeds you misinformation, accuracy, fairness and balance become difficult, though not impossible, to achieve. Objectivity is another matter altogether, and not just for journalists. I began to understand that more as I covered the Noakes hearing.

I was the only journalist to cover all the hearings sessions, from June 2015 to the dramatic day that the verdict was delivered in April 2017. That did not just give me unique insight and perspective; it also gave me headaches trying to be accurate, fair, balanced and objective. From the outset, the HPCSA wasn't talking – or at least, it never said anything material. The same applied to ADSA and its former president, Strydom.

Objectively, I saw big problems with Strydom's complaint about Noakes's tweet, in which he said that the key is to wean infants onto LCHF foods. In her complaint to the HPCSA, Strydom alleged that the tweet was life-threatening to infants. That was pure emotion, and emotions are ephemeral creatures. But the biggest problem I had with Strydom's 'horrified' response to Noakes's tweet was that she provided no science whatsoever to support it.

Scientists consider objectivity as central to research – or at least the good ones do. It's the reason for valuing scientific knowledge. After all, as Polish-American psychoanalyst Helene Deutsch once said: 'The ultimate goal of all research is not objectivity, but truth.' Scientists also see objectivity as the basis for the authority of science in society. Historians say that the idea of objectivity as an absolute arose during the 20th century, when people venerated science. Objectivity does not reign quite so supreme in other areas of endeavour – history among them.

An article in the 1996 edition of *Kleio: A Journal of Historical Studies from Africa* looked at whether historians can be truly objective. The author concluded that they could not be, since historians can't reproduce the past to test hypotheses. He went on to examine what history is, and thus what kind of objectivity is possible among historians. One answer lies in the article's title: 'Absolute objectivity the ideal; perspectivism the reality'.[1]

While historians may baulk at the comparison, the work of a journalist is not unlike that of a historian. Objectivity bedevils both.

Washington State University communications professor Richard Taflinger even went so far as to say that, for journalists, objectivity is an 'unrealisable dream'. In a commentary on 'The Myth of Objectivity in Journalism', Taflinger wrote:

> The oft-stated and highly desired goal of modern journalism is objectivity, the detached and unprejudiced gathering and dissemination of news and information. Such objectivity can allow people to arrive at decisions about the world and events occurring in it without the journalist's subjective views influencing the acceptance or rejection of information. Few whose aim is a populace making decisions based on facts rather than prejudice or super-stition would argue with such a goal.
>
> It's a pity that such a goal is impossible to achieve. As long as human beings gather and disseminate news and information, objectivity is an unrealizable dream.[2]

When I set off on my journalistic path, it couldn't have been more different from the one on which I now travel. I started off as a hard-news reporter on the now-defunct, anti-apartheid *Rand Daily Mail*. That was during the worst excesses of the apartheid era in the late 1970s and early 1980s. Because of my interest in politics, religion and the state, I often volunteered to cover the court beat. The political trials were the most interesting and demanding from a journalistic perspective. These cases were the grim legacy of oppressive racial and security legislation that was a hallmark of the ruling National Party regime, when capital punishment was a pillar of the country's judicial system.

As a journalist, I found it difficult to stay 'objective' when injustice stared me in the face, as was the case in most political trials. I managed to be balanced and accurate when reporting on cases involving the death penalty, and I mostly managed to be fair to both sides. Objective? Not so much, as the state trampled, literally and figuratively, on people and their basic human rights on an almost daily basis.

Among weapons that the regime invoked to suppress political opposition was the doctrine of common cause. As legal experts will tell you, the doctrine origi-nates in English law. The general idea is that when a group of people participates in an unlawful activity in which someone is hurt or killed, all those involved may be held 'jointly liable'. As an American law professor explained it, in South Africa, the Appellate Division had so 'vastly expanded the common purpose doctrine in political cases' that many accused were 'sentenced to death despite having only a trivial role in a crime'.[3] 'Guilt by association' became a deadly web in which the state caught and killed off many of its opponents.

Thus, I had an early baptism of fire in the full might of the state and the use of the law as a weapon – aided and abetted by compliant judges and attorneys – to prosecute and persecute those who got in its way. It was almost a relief when, in the mid-1980s, I changed professional direction. I moved from the unpredictability of hard-news reporting to feature writing. I gravitated naturally towards research and writing on health and lifestyle. But it didn't take long to realise that I had not left religion and politics behind. Both infect lifestyle, health and nutrition.

This became increasingly apparent as I covered the Noakes trial and uncovered those behind it. Politics infests the debate around the role of sugar and other carbohydrates in the diet – South African researchers said as much in a review of the evidence in the *Bulletin of the World Health Organization* in 2003:

> The development of a dietary guideline for 'sugar' has been fraught with conflict and political pressure, both locally and internationally. These conflicts seem to arise primarily from the twin imperatives: the formulation of appropriate public health policy and the protection of commercial sugar interests. Both have fundamentally influenced the content and process of this debate.[4]

Interestingly, the authors acknowledge the fundamental link between sugar and obesity; however, they also go on to make a strong case for the inclusion of sugar in the diet. Even more interesting is that one of the authors is Professor Nelia Steyn, head of the Division of Human Nutrition at UCT. Steyn's opposition to Noakes and LCHF is well documented. She has received funding from the sugar industry for her research, and actively supports the role of sugar in the diet.[5] She also has links to the International Life Sciences Institute, as US investigative reporter Russ Greene discovered. Greene has revealed links between the ILSI and many doctors and academics connected directly or indirectly with the HPCSA's case against Noakes.[6]

On 22 May 2014, the HPCSA's Fourth Preliminary Committee of Inquiry met to consider Strydom's complaint and Noakes's explanation. 'Fourth' in this case simply denotes the HPCSA's committee that deals with complaints about the conduct of medical professionals. When the HPCSA receives a complaint against a health professional, it first goes before the relevant board. If the board decides that it is serious enough to require an investigation, the complaint is forwarded to the relevant preliminary inquiry committee. In Noakes's case, as he is also a medical doctor, the complaint went first to the Medical and Dental Board and then to the Fourth Preliminary Committee of Inquiry. After two days, the committee felt it did not have enough before it to decide whether or not Noakes should be charged, and set a date for a second meeting on 10 September 2014. At that meeting, the preliminary committee decided that Noakes should be charged with unprofessional conduct for giving unconventional advice to a breastfeeding mother on Twitter. (How the committee came to its decision became a fascinating trial within the trial. It involved academics at both Noakes's alma mater, UCT, and the University of the Witwatersrand. See Chapter 11 for details.) The official charge sheet read as follows:

> That you are guilty of unprofessional conduct, or conduct which, which when regard is had to your profession is unprofessional, in that during February 2014, you acted in a manner that is not in accordance with the norms and standards of your profession in that you provided unconventional advice on breastfeeding babies on social networks (tweet).

The HPCSA only got around to giving Noakes notice of the charge four months later, in January 2015. A hearing was scheduled for June.

By the beginning of 2015, the HPCSA's decision to charge Noakes, and his decision to contest the charge, was common knowledge. It was also common knowledge to anyone with even a basic understanding of LCHF what Noakes was actually saying in his tweet. He was suggesting that foods such as meat, fish, chicken, eggs, dairy and vegetables are good for infants. It's the same advice that both Strydom and ADSA now routinely give for infant weaning.

From the outset, I found the HPCSA's decision to charge Noakes with unprofessional conduct peculiar. After all, the HPCSA usually reserves such a charge for practitioners who have committed really serious offences, such as sexual misconduct, theft, grievous harm or causing the premature death of patients. The HPCSA does not have any ethical rules governing doctors' conduct on social media. As such, the charge was unprecedented.

The HPCSA's most high-profile charge of unprofessional conduct to date had been against Dr Wouter Basson, nicknamed 'Dr Death' by the press. Basson was the apartheid-era cardiologist who ran the ruling National Party government's chemical and biological warfare programme. His 'duties' allegedly included concocting lethal cocktails of muscle relaxants and other drugs, which the government then used against its opponents.

Basson got off all murder and attempted murder charges in a criminal trial in 2002. In 2006, the HPCSA eventually charged him with unprofessional conduct. The case dragged on until 2013, when the HPCSA's Professional Conduct Committee found Basson guilty on four aspects of the charge against him. The HPCSA has yet to decide on a suitable sanction, and Basson continues to fight the ruling on the grounds of bias on the part of the committee that heard the charge against him.

In Noakes's case, it appeared to me that the HPCSA was using its full might to prosecute a world-renowned scientist for little more than his views on butter, eggs, bacon and broccoli. He had not advocated infanticide. His tweet was not a code for mass murder.

The HPCSA is a statutory body and the country's regulatory agency. Its brief is to protect the public and guide health practitioners. As such, its hearings are not meant to be adversarial. They are set up to be dispassionate, impartial inquiries aimed at getting to the truth of a matter. There was nothing dispassionate or impartial about the HPCSA's reaction to Noakes's tweet and the lengths to which its legal team went to load the panel that heard the charge against him.

An aggravating factor in the case against Noakes was incompetence within the HPCSA. Over the years, the trickle of complaints that practitioners, professional associations and academic training institutions had lodged against the HPCSA had become a tsunami. In February 2015, the minister of health, Dr Aaron Motsoaledi, set up a government task team to investigate the HPCSA. The report was damning in the extreme. The task team found the HPCSA to be in a state of 'multi-system organizational dysfunction' that had prejudiced both practitioners and the public. Three of its top executives – the chief executive officer, chief operations officer and head of legal services – were found to be unfit to hold office. They would not cooperate with the task team, and they refused to stand down. The CEO was eventually replaced.[7]

Ironically, the chair of the government task team was UCT cardiology professor Bongani Mayosi, then head of the Department of Medicine. Mayosi was an author of the UCT professors' letter, published in a Cape Town newspaper in 2014. In it, the academics made what many consider to be damaging, inflammatory and highly defamatory claims against Noakes. Inter alia, they accused him of 'aggressively promoting' LCHF as a 'revolution', making 'outrageous unproven claims about disease prevention', not conforming to 'the tenets of good and responsible science', and breaching the university's 'commitment to academic freedom' (see Chapter 5).

From the outset, all the authors of that letter also refused to talk to me. As a journalist, the walls of silence I kept hitting just piqued my interest even more. I had to find other sources of information and evidence behind the hearing. And when it finally commenced on 4 June 2015, it was a revelation, though not in the way that the HPCSA had likely intended.

Sitting on one side of the room was the HPCSA's legal team, the 'pro-forma complainant' in legal terms. Head of the team was Advocate Meshack Mapholisa. Alongside him were Strydom as the complainant and two of the expert witnesses he intended calling: North-West University professor Herculina Salome Kruger and professor and paediatrician Dr Muhammad Ali Dhansay. Also present were two Cape Town attorneys, Janusz Luterek and Michiel Grobler. Mapholisa told the hearing that Luterek and Grobler were on a 'watching brief on behalf of ADSA' and 'representing its interests'. I found it odd that Strydom and ADSA needed legal representation, as neither was on trial. The reason would only become apparent as the hearing progressed.

On the other side of the room sat Noakes, the 'respondent', with his legal team comprising Cape Town instruction attorney Adam Pike of Pike Law, advocates Michael van der Nest SC and Alfred Cockrell SC from the Johannesburg Bar, and Dr Ravin 'Rocky' Ramdass, a physician and practising counsel from the Pietermaritzburg Bar.

In the middle sat the HPCSA's Professional Conduct Committee, which effectively acts as judge and jury in HPCSA hearings. Given the legal complexities in what should have been an uncomplicated case, the HPCSA had chosen the committee's chair wisely: Advocate Joan Adams from Pretoria.

After Adams opened the hearing, Van der Nest immediately raised an objection related to the composition of the Professional Conduct Committee. The defence team had informed the HPCSA the day before in writing of their objection, but had received no reply. Therefore, Van der Nest told Adams, the committee as currently constituted was *ultra vires* (outside the law). He explained that legislation under the Health Professions Act and the Act itself set up the HPCSA and regulated its various committees and boards. In this case, because Noakes was a medical doctor as well as a sports scientist, the HPCSA's Medical and Dental Board was required to set up the Professional Conduct Committee according to the Act's regulations.

Those regulations are simple enough. According to Regulation 6.2, and Section 15(5) of the Act, the committee 'must' (Van der Nest emphasised the imperative language) comprise at least: two public representatives, one of whom must be the chairperson; one member of the board (i.e. the Medical and Dental Board); one legal assessor; and three persons in the 'relevant profession' or discipline in which the respondent (i.e. Noakes) is registered.

Adams ticked one of the two public representative boxes. A Mr Joel Vogel ticked the other. General practitioner Dr Janet Giddy ticked two boxes, as a medical doctor and Medical and Dental Board member. University of the Witwatersrand paediatrics professor Haroon Saloojee ticked the box for a member in the 'relevant profession', in this case medical doctors, registered with the Medical and Dental Board. The Professional Conduct Committee therefore lacked one member of the 'relevant profession', a medical doctor registered with the HPCSA.

However, the biggest stumbling block was the HPCSA's last-minute inclusion of Stellenbosch University dietetics professor Renée Blaauw. Van der Nest pointed out that Blaauw ticked none of the boxes required to constitute the committee correctly. Blaauw was also the HPCSA's second attempt at loading the committee with a dietitian, in contravention of its own regulations.

The HPCSA had notified Noakes's legal team a little over a week before the hearing (it has to do so at least seven days before) that Professor Edelweiss Wentzel-Viljoen would be on the committee. Wentzel-Viljoen is a dietetics professor at North-West University. She is also chair of the HPCSA's Dietetics and Nutrition Board and an ADSA member. Not surprisingly, Pike had immediately lodged an objection in writing, requesting Wentzel-Viljoen's recusal. He noted that Wentzel-Viljoen was on record expressing opinions in public opposed to Noakes and LCHF (see Chapter 7). This raised the question of bias. When the HPCSA refused to recuse Wentzel-Viljoen, Pike wrote to her directly, requesting that she recuse herself. Wentzel-Viljoen initially declined, but a few days later she agreed.

The HPCSA then informed Noakes's team that it had appointed Blaauw in Wentzel-Viljoen's place. Interestingly, the timeline showed that the HPCSA had passed and signed the resolution appointing Blaauw to the Professional Conduct Committee on the same date as it appointed Wentzel-Viljoen. Pike sensed something amiss, procedurally. He told me at the time: 'It seemed improbable that the [HPCSA] Medical and Dental Board would appoint a panel, one with Blaauw and the other with Wentzel-Viljoen, on the same day.'

In their written objection to the composition of the committee, Noakes's lawyers had made fundamental legal points. One was that medical practitioners facing a charge of unprofessional conduct had the right to be judged by their peers and a member of the public. Another was that members of the HPCSA's Professional Conduct Committee must be, and must be seen to be, independent and objective. And before any HPCSA committee can hear and judge a matter, it has to abide by its own rules and constitute itself properly.

From my perspective, Blaauw would have had as hard a time as Wentzel-Viljoen of persuading any reasonable person that she would be free of bias. It was only brought to the attention of Noakes's legal team on the day of the June hearing that Blaauw is also an ADSA member. The HPCSA appeared oblivious to the conflict of interest that represented. It was as if they believed that Noakes would, or should, have no problem with the fox guarding the henhouse.

Furthermore, like Wentzel-Viljoen, Blaauw's bias in favour of sugar in the diet and against Noakes's views on nutrition was well documented. She had openly supported the South African Food-based Dietary Guidelines on sugar consumption, and had participated in a South African Sugar Association 'roadshow' on nutrition to fight non-communicable diseases.[8]

On the first day of the hearing, Van der Nest pointed out the dilemma Adams now faced. The hearing could not proceed until she ruled on the make-up of the committee. And it was debatable whether Adams could rule, because her committee was not, in fact, a committee.

Unsurprisingly, Mapholisa had a different interpretation of the regulations governing the composition of the committee. In trying hard to load the committee with a dietitian, he may have signalled early on that there was some kind of turf war playing out. Dietitians believe that they are best qualified to give nutrition advice to the public. Indeed, ADSA believes that dietitians should have a monopoly on dishing out dietary advice. They don't want Noakes giving nutrition advice, especially if it conflicts with their own and the country's official dietary guidelines. Mapholisa was also indicating the lengths to which the HPCSA would be prepared to go in order to find Noakes guilty.

Mapholisa said that the HPCSA Fourth Preliminary Committee of Inquiry, which had decided to charge Noakes, had been made up solely of medical doctors. That committee, he said, had deemed it fit to 'request for an expert opinion of a dietician to give advice'. That was because the committee members felt that they did not have the 'knowledge, experience and qualification to comment on diet issues'. Mapholisa argued that 'logic would require' that the Professional Conduct Committee should also have the right to bring in a dietitian. If not, he said, the committee would consist of 'the blind leading the blind' when it came to discerning issues of danger and diet. Mapholisa stressed the need for committee members with 'qualifications and experience in relation to infant nutritional diet'. It would be unfair, he said, to expect that 'people who do not have experience in diet issues should be burdened with this particular task of making a judge call on a particular topic which they do not understand'.

Mapholisa's argument hinted at another strategy that the HPCSA and its witnesses would employ in prosecuting Noakes: trying to undermine his extensive expertise and knowledge of nutrition for all ages. The HPCSA eventually expanded the charge to say that Noakes was acting 'outside his scope' of professional medical expertise by advising patients on nutrition.

Van der Nest argued that Mapholisa, as the pro-forma complainant in the case, could not unilaterally decide the make-up of the committee. The law was clear, Van der Nest said. Noakes had the right to be tried 'by his peers, his peers only, and by members of the public'. Dietitians were neither his peers, nor were they from a 'relevant profession'. Van der Nest also stressed that it was not only dietitians who could understand nutrition and medical issues. 'A body of peers, a body of general practitioners and of relevant [i.e. of the same] profession, is perfectly able to consider expert evidence from dietitians and nutritionists and come to a decision,' he said. Therefore, there was no need for a dietitian or nutritionist to be on the panel.

After an adjournment, Adams ruled that the Professional Conduct Committee was indeed not properly constituted. She also ruled that the Health Professions Act, under which the HPCSA was constituted, defined the minimum, not maximum, number of committee members. The responsibility for appointing another 'relevant' member rested squarely on the shoulders of the chair of the Medical and Dental Board, not herself or her committee, Adams said. This would not preclude the committee from co-opting other members, which could include a dietitian such as Blaauw. On the topic of possible bias, Adams said, with a perfectly straight face, that Blaauw had indicated 'her absolute objectivity'. I found that hard to believe – as if all anyone had to do to prove lack of bias to this committee was simply to say: 'Trust me. I am absolutely unbiased.'

Van der Nest countered that Adams could not rule on how the committee could rectify itself because it was not properly constituted to begin with. It was also not possible for the HPCSA to rectify the errors timeously, according to its own rules, to allow the hearing to proceed.

Van der Nest noted 'a few other fundamental difficulties'. One was Adams's ruling that the committee could add a dietitian or nutritionist. 'The problem is that it is a finding that you make while you are not a constituted committee,' he argued. 'Properly speaking', the committee did not exist, and so the chair of a non-existent committee could not rule. In addition, the Medical and Dental Board had erroneously placed Blaauw on the Professional Conduct Committee, Van der Nest said. Therefore the board, and not Adams or her committee, would have to rectify any errors.

The issue of whether Blaauw should recuse herself was independent of the question of whether there should be a dietitian on the committee, Van der Nest said. In reply, Mapholisa argued that Adams's decision stood and that Blaauw could be on the committee. 'She is going nowhere,' he said.

They went back and forth until Adams eventually delayed the hearing until November 2015.

Afterwards, I asked Mapholisa for comment on criticisms that the HPCSA had had more than enough time to constitute the Professional Conduct Committee correctly. After all, the decision to charge Noakes had been made in September 2014, and he had only been informed in January 2015. The HPCSA had thus had a four-month head start in planning the prosecution. Mapholisa declined to comment, saying that I had to go through the HPCSA's official communication channels.

Pike was more forthcoming. 'It was a bitter-sweet day,' he said. 'We came prepared to hit the ground running if the committee went ahead despite our objections. These delays happen all the time in contentious proceedings. We're happy that our view prevailed. Now we look forward to fighting the good fight in November.'

10

The Second Session: November 2015

'A delusion is something that people believe in despite a total lack of evidence.'
– Richard Dawkins, English ethologist, evolutionary biologist and author

An air of anticipation hung over the room when the second session of the HPCSA hearing commenced on 23 November 2015 at the Belmont Square Conference Centre in Rondebosch, Cape Town. As before, on one side sat the HPCSA's legal team with dietitian Claire Julsing Strydom and other witnesses. On the other side was Noakes, his legal team and one of the expert witnesses he hoped to call once the HPCSA closed its case, New Zealand–based South African dietitian and academic Dr Caryn Zinn.

Between them sat the HPCSA's Professional Conduct Committee and chair, Advocate Joan Adams. This time, the HPCSA had constituted the committee correctly. There were the usual legal and other 'housekeeping' matters to clear. The defence made application to be allowed to call a witness, Canadian professor Stephen Cunnane, via video link. The HPCSA wasted most of that first day arguing against the application.

Prosecutor Meshack Mapholisa argued that the HPCSA was a 'rigid creature of statute' that had to abide by rules governing witnesses' evidence. Witnesses had always given evidence in person, he said, and HPCSA regulations did not expressly allow evidence via video link. The HPCSA had never before been asked for permission to present evidence in such a manner. Video link would make cross-examination difficult, he said. It wouldn't be easy to pick up nuances of body language and demeanour. Someone could coach the witnesses off-camera or 'tamper' with them during toilet breaks. Mapholisa even claimed that some-one could pretend to be Cunnane and 'no one would be any the wiser'. He also cited the 'connection factor': that the technology could break down at any moment, causing 'intolerable interruptions and delays'. Another obstacle was 'load-shedding', the peculiarly South African term for the regular power blackouts that plagued the country at the time. With a flourish, Mapholisa ended by saying that evidence via video link would be 'highly prejudicial' to the HPCSA's case.

Advocate Michael van der Nest SC was restrained in reply. HPCSA regulations did not specifically forbid evidence via video link, he said. He cited extensive local and international case law in which similar medical tribunals and courts routinely allowed evidence via video link. Evidence via video link was no longer controversial, and the benefits were now 'almost trite', he said. Videoconferencing 'is an efficient and an effective way of providing oral evidence both in-chief and in cross-examination'. It is 'simply another tool for securing effective access to justice'.

There were good reasons why Noakes could not find local specialists to testify for him, Van der Nest said. Thus, he was compelled to look abroad. Cunnane's schedule and financial considerations meant that a video link would be necessary. It was in the interests of justice for the committee to hear 'as full a debate and as balanced a debate as possible', Van der Nest said. 'If giving the evidence contributes to that, that is in the interests of justice. If excluding it leads to the opposite, that is not in the interests of justice.'

After an adjournment, Adams gave her committee's unanimous decision: Noakes could allow witnesses via video link. She ruled, inter alia, that the HPCSA was a national institution that was expected to 'keep up with the times and the trends and with technology'. It was 'far-fetched' to assume bad faith on the part of experts in this case. It was unlikely that Cunnane would require 'coaching' or submit to 'tampering'. There was also 'no reasonable prospect' of anyone getting away with pretending to be him. It was 'unfathomable' that anyone would attempt such a fraud on international television and media channels.

It was also reasonable to assume that Noakes would be forced to look abroad for experts, Adams said. Local experts would have 'a reasonable concern that they would not necessarily want to align themselves publicly with such a high-profile case for whatever personal or professional reasons'. That should not hamper Noakes in presenting his case properly.

Next, Mapholisa announced that the HPCSA had amended the charge against Noakes, backdating it from February 2014 to include January 2014. The charge now read: 'That you are guilty of unprofessional conduct or conduct which, when regard is had to your profession, in that during the period between January 2014 and February 2014, you acted in a manner that is not in accordance with the norms and standards of your profession in that you provided unconventional advice on breastfeeding babies on social networks (tweet/s).'

Van der Nest did not oppose the amendment, but said that he would address it at a later stage. He noted that the charge was now 'inconsistent with the parameters of the points of inquiry'. Those points were the 'four corners of the charge', there to stop either side from straying beyond the perimeters of the charge.

When Mapholisa opened the HPCSA's case, he may well have thought that a guilty verdict was a done deal. He had what he probably considered to be four strong witnesses. Apart from Strydom as a factual witness, he had lined up three expert witnesses: North-West University professors Hester 'Este' Vorster and Salome Kruger, and paediatrician Dr Muhammad Ali Dhansay.

These were relatively low-level expert witnesses. I wondered why none was from South Africa's top three universities: UCT, Wits and Stellenbosch. After all, academics at UCT and Stellenbosch had been the most vocal and active in their opposition to Noakes and LCHF. The HPCSA would not answer my questions on the topic. None of its experts could rival Noakes's rating by the NRF as an A1 scientist in sports science and nutrition. (The NRF has since renewed his rating for a third consecutive five-year period.) Vorster has an A2 rating, Kruger a C2, and Dhansay no rating at all. And none of them could match Noakes's large 'academic footprint' – an H-index of 71. Vorster's H-index at the time was 22 or 24 (she couldn't recall which); Kruger's was 17; and if Dhansay had one at all, he did not divulge it.

Interestingly, all the HPCSA's witnesses downplayed Noakes's extensive scientific expertise in and knowledge of nutrition. In emailed correspondence, Kruger seemed to take exception to the idea that Noakes is a world authority on nutrition. She would only acknowledge him as an expert in sports science.

The HPCSA had actually intended to call another expert witness, registered paediatric dietitian Marlene Ellmer, who had been the first dietitian to respond to Noakes's tweet (see Chapter 8). Before the hearing began in June 2015, Ellmer was on the HPCSA's list of experts and they had sent Noakes's legal team a summary of her testimony. The document had been finalised on 4 May, indicating that up to a month before the hearing began, Ellmer still considered herself competent to give expert testimony on infant feeding.

In the summary of her evidence, Ellmer made the following points, all of which Noakes has easily dismissed:

- *Infants and young children are in the most nutritionally vulnerable stages of the life cycle.* Noakes obviously agrees. It's why he wrote *Raising Superheroes*. In the book, he explains why a high-fat diet is crucial during the first 1000 days of an infant's life.
- *Noakes's advice to wean onto a LCHF diet is not 'evidence based' and is beyond his scope of practice and qualifications.* For many reasons, this is not true: the information is evidence-based, and Noakes is qualified to give it.
- *Noakes's information can also be potentially harmful to the infant because he does not define the exact composition of a LCHF diet. As a result, the advice is confusing and open to misinterpretation.* That applies to any information. Twitter is restricted to 140 characters. Leenstra understood this when she posed her question. Had she sought a detailed response, she would have consulted her doctor or a dietitian.

- *Carbohydrates provide 'readily available energy for growth and development as well as mental development'. It is not clear whether or not 'the infant body can efficiently and timeously provide energy from protein and fat alone if carbohydrate is significantly reduced in the diet'.* Carbohydrate is not an essential nutrient. The infant, like the adult, has no requirement for carbohydrate. Noakes points out that even the US National Academy of Medicine acknowledges this (see Chapter 7).

- *The weaning diet should include 'meat and meat alternatives', and 'milk and milk products'.* This is exactly what the LCHF diet provides.

- *Low-carbohydrate, ketogenic diets used in the treatment of drug-resistant epilepsy produce a wide range of complications.* Ellmer does not understand that since it is not ethical to perform controlled clinical trials of the ketogenic diet (as the control group would continue to have multiple seizures), it can never be known if these are the complications of the underlying disease or of the diet. Conveniently, she assumes that the diet must be the cause. This is known as confirmation bias.

- *Although the diet is said to be low in protein, in fact, it will be high in protein if insufficient fat is eaten. High-protein diets can allegedly cause multiple complications in infants and children.* Correct, which is why Noakes emphasises that LCHF is a high-fat, not high-protein, diet.

- *'We currently have no evidence on the effect on growth, development and obesity risk of a high-protein or a high-fat complementary diet.'* Presumably, Ellmer is saying that we must therefore assume that these diets will be harmful. This is more confirmation bias.

- *Child health in South Africa is deteriorating. 'Poor dietary intake, food insecurity and poor quality of basic services are important contributors to this problem.'* Noakes has often asked whether the current advice to wean South African children onto high-carbohydrate, cereal-based diets might be the cause.

Wisely, Ellmer chose not to put herself and her reputation through the mental anguish of going up against Van der Nest and Ramdass. They would have made short work of her 'expert' evidence.

It is significant that Ellmer referred to ketogenic diets in her summary. Ketosis and ketogenic diets would keep turning up like bad scientific pennies during the hearing. All of the HPCSA's witnesses referred to ketogenic diets as if they were synonymous with danger and premature death. They all displayed surprising ignorance on the topic, conflating ketosis with ketoacidosis. The former is a natural, benign bodily state. The latter is potentially fatal, fortunately rare, and seen mostly in patients with uncontrolled type-1 diabetes.

To top it all, the HPCSA had not even charged Noakes with advising a ketogenic diet, dangerous or otherwise. His tweet said nothing at all about ketosis.

Why the witnesses kept bringing up the subject would only be revealed towards the end of the hearing, when a series of emails came to light and was placed on record in February 2016.

Mapholisa opened his case by calling Strydom. As a factual witness, Strydom was required to restrict herself to the events leading up to her complaint against Noakes. Yet she frequently ventured expert opinion on the content of his tweet.

Van der Nest lodged the first of many objections on procedural grounds. Strydom could only be called as an expert witness if the HPCSA had notified the defence seven days before the hearing and had provided a summary of her evidence, he said. Mapholisa appeared oblivious of the requirements, arguing that Strydom could give both factual and expert testimony simply because she was a dietitian. 'She is not just a layperson who, like myself, just reads about nutrition in a book or elsewhere,' Mapholisa said. 'She went to varsity, studied nutrition and I will submit that she can express an opinion in that regard as an expert as she is, in fact, qualified to do that.'

Adams disagreed and sustained Van der Nest's objections.

In giving testimony, Strydom added significant weight to my theory that the trial was partly a turf war. Dietitians don't want Noakes taking business away from them. As ADSA president, Strydom had frequently made it clear that dietitians should have a virtual monopoly on giving dietary advice to the public. In her evidence, she said that Noakes erred in his tweet by not referring Pippa Leenstra to a 'qualified' professional. In addition, ADSA dietitians especially don't like the fact that Noakes's advice conflicts significantly with South Africa's lucrative official dietary guidelines, which promote low fat and high carb. Not surprisingly, the guidelines became a main focus of the hearing.

Strydom also tried hard to distance herself as the complainant in the case. She claimed that she had lodged the complaint as ADSA president and not in her personal capacity. Yet her letter of complaint to the HPCSA and all the HPCSA's correspondence with Noakes and his lawyers make it clear that she had complained personally. Back in 2015, I asked Strydom via email about her status. She replied that she would 'prefer' that I said she had complained from the outset as ADSA president. When I queried her use of the verb 'prefer', she went silent and stayed that way.

I also queried whether Strydom had a mandate from ADSA to lodge her complaint. In face-to-face discussions and emails, current ADSA president Maryke Gallagher was evasive. She and other ADSA executive members would only confirm that they had signed a letter more than a year *after* Strydom lodged the complaint. In it, they stated that, as president, Strydom had the authority to lodge complaints on ADSA's behalf. Legal experts say that the letter was an attempt to alter facts after the event.

There were many other self-incriminating elements in Strydom's testimony. One was a throwaway comment she made about the Naudé review, which would come back to haunt her, the HPCSA and ADSA. It was the first hint in evidence on the record of an organised campaign by prominent doctors and academics to nail Noakes. 'Everybody was waiting for this publication,' Strydom said, referring to the review, 'because we could not simply go ahead and make [a] statement about Prof. Noakes's hypothesis or diet without looking at the evidence. So, everybody, *all these big organisations* were waiting on the publication of this information before we could make any kind of media statement [emphasis mine].'

Under cross-examination, Van der Nest referred Strydom to statements issued by ADSA, the HPCSA and other organisations in July 2014, hailing the Naudé review as the death of Banting and proof that Noakes was on the wrong scientific track. Interestingly, the Naudé review does not mention Noakes, Banting or even LCHF.

'It is not like the way you are saying it,' Strydom protested. 'It is not like everybody joined together to now make a statement against Prof. Noakes. We were all waiting for the evidence to be published.' With those statements, Strydom teed up the Naudé review as the key piece of evidence against Noakes, a manoeuvre that she and the HPCSA would come to regret.

Van der Nest also raised the influence of ADSA's sponsors – among them food and soft-drink companies such as Kellogg's, Unilever, ProNutro, Huletts and Coca-Cola – on the case against Noakes. Mapholisa objected on the grounds of irrelevance, but Adams overruled him. Strydom, unsurprisingly, denied any outside influence.

Strydom ventured into expert territory again by claiming that Noakes had entered into a doctor–patient relationship with the breastfeeding Leenstra on Twitter. She also claimed that Noakes's tweet was medical 'advice', not information. By communicating on a social media platform as a medical doctor, 'who is trusted and regarded as a celebrity in South Africa', Noakes had given 'advice' that constituted a 'public health message'. At this, Van der Nest sighed and objected again: 'This is so over the line, it is just not true.' Adams sustained the objection.

Strydom appeared oblivious of the many deep legal and ethical holes she was digging for herself and Ellmer. If Noakes had established a professional relationship with Leenstra, then so had she and Ellmer. Both had tweeted far more extensively to Leenstra than Noakes. And if Noakes had given medical 'advice', then so had she and Ellmer. By Strydom's own logic, she and Ellmer would also have been guilty of supersession. That's the legal term for one health professional taking over the patient of another, without his or her knowledge or permission. Both Strydom and Ellmer told Leenstra to ignore Noakes and contact them instead. Strydom even tweeted her contact details to Leenstra. Under cross-examination, Strydom claimed not to know about supersession. Van der Nest said that as ADSA president she would have known about it. 'You knew [on 5 and 6 February 2014] and you know today that it is not ethical for one health practitioner to take over the patient of another health professional,' Van der Nest told her. Strydom had no choice but to concede, and Van der Nest pressed the point home: 'You did not consider [Leenstra] to be the patient of either Prof. Noakes nor Ms Ellmer, because otherwise you would have been taking her over as a patient, and that was not what you were wanting to do, correct?' Strydom agreed and eventually conceded that there was no doctor–patient relationship.

When Van der Nest raised Strydom's 'horrified' reaction to Noakes's tweet in front of 300 million Twitter users, she conceded that she may 'have overreacted a little'. Van der Nest then asked Strydom to read out from the same booklet outlining the HPCSA's ethical guidelines for health professionals to which she had referred in her testimony, specifically that 'a practitioner shall not cast reflections on the probity, professional reputation or skill of another person registered under the Act or any Health Act'. Strydom was forced to concede that she had cast adverse reflections on Noakes's reputation and skill in her own tweets to Leenstra.

To Strydom's claim that Noakes's tweet posed a danger to the infant because it was 'unconventional', Van der Nest posed the salient question: 'Do you really believe that it is correct that someone who has an honestly held view, which you considered to be unconventional, should be struck off the roll of practitioners?' (This was one of the possible consequences of a guilty verdict.) Strydom conceded that she did not believe that to be fair. She also conceded that no patient had alleged any harm from Noakes's tweet. Even ADSA was not alleging any harm.

Hovering over all of this was a question that would crop up repeatedly during the hearing, one that the HPCSA resolutely refused to answer: If the HPCSA genuinely believed that Noakes had breached its rules, why had it not also charged Strydom and Ellmer? Crucially, under cross-examination Strydom conceded that Noakes had been debating the science of nutrition with her and many other dietitians on her business website, Nutritional Solutions. Van der Nest then made a significant point to which he would return later: 'Because [Noakes] refuses to agree with you, you have him prosecuted?' Strydom became flustered at this, and said that she was only concerned about Noakes giving 'dangerous' advice to the breastfeeding mother.

Van der Nest pointed out that the HPCSA had not charged Noakes with giving dangerous advice. In effect, Van der Nest told Strydom, she believed that she had a monopoly on free speech. She also believed that if she disagreed with Noakes, then the HPCSA had to prosecute him.

Hester Vorster was up next, and fared no better. Her evidence was based on a 20-page secret report, which the HPCSA's Fourth Preliminary Committee of

Inquiry had commissioned her to write. It later transpired that the committee had used Vorster's report as the basis for its decision to charge Noakes, without showing it to him first. The defence team acquired the report by accident, shortly before the June 2015 hearing.

Vorster attempted to defend the contents of her report in her testimony. She also ventured into ethics territory by claiming that Noakes had established a doctor–patient relationship with Leenstra by giving 'uncalled-for advice' to wean a baby onto LCHF. This illustrated his 'promotion of the LCHF diet at each opportunity', she said. According to Vorster, health professionals are obliged to warn lactating mothers about the effects of LCHF, among them that the diet may not provide all the nutrients infants need and 'that ketosis should be avoided'.

Noakes's tweet was 'irresponsible', she said. It went against South Africa's 'up-to-date' food-based dietary guidelines (which she wrote and updated in 2013), which, she said, included paediatric guidelines for babies and infants up to five years. These guidelines, Vorster told the hearing, are supported by the best available evidence, and are in line with the WHO, and the Australian, New Zealand and US guidelines.

Vorster also alleged that Noakes had breached the HPCSA's code of conduct by criticising dietetic training in South Africa. 'Maintaining an opposite viewpoint in public could also be seen as unprofessional,' Vorster stated, before recommending that the HPCSA 'take the matter up' with Noakes.

Vorster supported Strydom's view of dietitians as best placed to give dietary advice. Despite his A1 rating, she said that Noakes was someone 'who has not been trained sufficiently in nutrition and would not qualify for registration as a dietician or nutritionist to provide dietary advice on an individual level'. He should not have given advice that differed from 'what the dietetic profession and registered dieticians accept as correct'. The 'correct conduct' would have been for Noakes to refer Leenstra to a dietitian.

Vorster also criticised Noakes for his 'inappropriate' use of Twitter as a communication medium, yet she admitted that she knew little about the popular social network. That was an understatement. Vorster said that she had 'just sort of looked in Wikipedia' to find out about it. Twitter's 'inherent nature' and 'short sound-byte messages' made it an 'unsuitable medium' for health professionals to give dietary advice to the public, she said.

Advocate Rocky Ramdass did a thorough demolition job on Vorster's evidence in cross-examination. Ramdass is also a medical doctor, with more than 23 years' experience as a family physician. He referred to Vorster's qualifications, which included an undergraduate degree in home economics and a doctorate in physiology. She confirmed that she had no qualifications or training in dietetics, had never practised as a dietitian or seen patients, had not done any research into LCHF diets and was not an expert in medical bioethics.

Ramdass noted Vorster's lack of knowledge of what constituted a low-carbohydrate diet. Vorster suggested it was one in which 45 per cent of energy was derived from carbohydrate foods. He also noted that she showed little understanding of the role of IR in chronic diseases other than diabetes. Ramdass asked Vorster why she would not acknowledge that a high-carb diet could be the cause of chronic disease, and why she insisted that dietary fat was the culprit. He pressed her for the evidence behind her recommendation in the South African Food-based Dietary Guidelines for adults and children 'to make starches the basis of most meals'.

'The point I am making,' Ramdass told Vorster, 'is that industry has a huge role to play in the provision of carbohydrates for an unsuspecting community.'

Vorster disagreed. She referred to research, including the Transition and Health during Urbanisation of South Africans (THUSA) study in which she was involved.[1] She conceded that the sugar industry was one of the study's sponsors, but denied that it had any influence. 'We are actually against sugar intake,' Vorster said. 'In addition to developing this guideline, we published against an increase in sugar intake, advising a low-sugar intake in South Africa very recently.' Taking a sideswipe at Noakes, she said, 'He also had money from the Sugar Association in his earlier days of research.' Noakes has always been open about this fact.

Ramdass questioned Vorster's support for wholegrains in the diet despite solid evidence implicating grains in dental disease, obesity, heart disease and more. He also questioned her wholehearted support for mieliepap – a cheap, staple food for South Africa's rural poor. Vorster said that nutrition guidelines had to consider what rural populations were eating and what they could afford. Her comment could be considered shocking. Mieliepap is dirt cheap, but it is also heavily fortified and very high-carb. Many nutrition experts, Noakes included, argue that nutrition guidelines should be based on a food's nutrient density, not on cost. They also say that 'real' food, by definition, needs no fortification to make it nutritious.

Ramdass pointed to another anomaly in Vorster's evidence: official guidelines for infant weaning don't stipulate that starch should be the basis of most meals. He read out the guidelines:

Continue breastfeeding to two years and beyond. Gradually increase the amount of food, number of feedings and variety as your child gets older. Give your child meat, chicken, fish or egg every day or as often as possible. Give your child dark green leafy vegetables and orange coloured vegetables and fruit every day. Avoid giving tea, coffee and sugary drinks, high-sugar, high-fat, salty snacks to your child.

He pointed out that these recommendations are no different from what Noakes said in his tweet. The implication was not lost on either side.

Vorster made brief reference to ketosis in her evidence, but declined to elaborate under cross-examination. Instead, she suggested that Ramdass reserve his questions on that subject to 'our expert in that field, which is Professor Dhansay'. Dhansay later told the hearing that he was not an expert in ketosis.

Salome Kruger testified next. She did not help her case by admitting under cross-examination that she had written her expert report 'in a rush' the night before. She also said that she had 'not used much detail' and had not checked her report before submitting it.

In her testimony, Kruger alleged that, in his tweet, Noakes had essentially advised Leenstra to stop breastfeeding. 'Only one type of advice should be given to a mother of a newborn infant and that is exclusive breastfeeding,' Kruger said. Noakes should also have warned Leenstra 'not to wean the baby too early on any diet'. Kruger claimed that her concern was that Noakes's tweet was 'not in line with the commitment to promote, protect and support exclusive breastfeeding up to six months'.

She also said that she had 'noticed a tweet' (not the one that prompted Strydom's complaint) in which Noakes had suggested that ketogenic diets are healthy for babies. This pointed to why the HPCSA had extended the time period of the charge to include tweets before February 2014. Kruger believed that Noakes's suggestion constituted unprofessional conduct because it was not evidence-based. She was concerned about the 'long-term effects of the ketogenic diet on brain development'. This despite Noakes saying nothing about a ketogenic diet in his tweet.

Kruger is a co-author of the 'Complementary feeding' support paper for the South African Food-based Dietary Guidelines. She said that while Noakes's views on nutrition 'could be in line with the South African Food-based Dietary Guideline on complementary feeding', he had been unprofessional in tweeting advice that was not evidence-based.

She launched an attack on doctors who write 'popular' books. It was obvious she was talking about Noakes, the author of bestsellers aimed at the lay reader. Chief among them is *The Real Meal Revolution*. The frequent references to this book during the hearing fuelled the theory that its success was one of Strydom's reasons for complaining about him. Kruger claimed that, by definition, such books are not evidence-based. She was especially critical of US neurologist Dr David Perlmutter, author of the bestselling *Grain Brain: The Surprising Truth About Wheat, Carbs, and Sugar – Your Brain's Silent Killers*. Kruger described Perlmutter as 'once a brilliant scientist', now a mere 'popular book writer'.

Van der Nest objected frequently on the grounds of irrelevance. Undeterred, Kruger said that she used Perlmutter as an example to demonstrate 'the evidence-based process' to her students. She was about to cite a critique of Perlmutter's book by US assistant professor of religion Dr Alan Levinovitz when an irritated Van der Nest interjected: 'This really has to stop, Chair.' Adams sustained the objection.

Although she is not a qualified ethicist, Kruger ventured expert testimony in that area anyway, laying herself wide open to attack by Ramdass during cross-examination. He honed in on inconsistencies in her claim that Noakes had breached two ethical principles in his alleged doctor–patient relationship with Leenstra: non-maleficence (do no harm) and beneficence (do good). When he asked Kruger to name all four pillars of ethics, she could only name three, including respect for autonomy of the patient. Ramdass reminded her of the fourth: distributive justice (to treat all people equally and equitably). He questioned Kruger's failure to comment on the ethics of Strydom's disparaging remarks about Noakes in her tweets, and reminded her of her ethical duty to be balanced and objective when giving expert testimony. Kruger had no answer, other than to say that she had done what the HPCSA had asked: to focus only on Noakes.

Kruger echoed Vorster's claim that Noakes had 'defamed' nutrition departments and lecturers in South African universities by describing their dietary advice as 'dogma'. This prompted a question from Professional Conduct Committee member Dr Janet Giddy, who said that she failed to see where defamation was mentioned in the charge against Noakes. 'I am not sure why you put this into your report,' she told Kruger. Again, Kruger had no answer.

Next up was Dr Muhammad Ali Dhansay. He sounded confident enough as Mapholisa led his evidence, starting with his CV. Dhansay is a paediatrician, an extraordinary associate professor and external lecturer at Stellenbosch University's Division of Human Nutrition and Department of Paediatrics and Child Health respectively, and a member of the SAMRC Burden of Disease Research Unit. In his testimony, he did not disclose his links to the food and drug industries, or that he is a former president of the South African branch of the US-based International Life Sciences Institute, a Coca-Cola front organisation. (Russ Greene revealed Dhansay's links with the ILSI in his comprehensive report on Noakes's trial in January 2017.[2])

In his evidence, Dhansay claimed that Noakes had provided 'wholly inappropriate and irresponsible' nutritional advice about infant weaning to a mother. He said that Noakes's recommendation went 'against all international and national precepts and guidance', and that South Africa's prevalence of stunted growth would be exacerbated if parents abided by it.

He also brought up the topic of ketones and ketogenic diets, and attempted to discredit the work of Canadian ketogenic specialist Professor Stephen Cunnane (presumably in anticipation of Cunnane's expert testimony for the defence). Yet Dhansay's knowledge of ketone metabolism proved minimal. He also did not seem clear on the difference between a low-carbohydrate diet and a ketogenic diet. Under cross-examination, Ramdass showed that Dhansay also did not know the difference between causation and association in quoting research on the deaths of two children on a ketogenic diet.

When questioned about his opinions on the dangers of these diets, Dhansay made a comment that highlighted the HPCSA's bias against Noakes. He said that the HPCSA had given him a 'directive or guidance' to provide opinion on certain aspects of Noakes's tweet, including his alleged recommendation of a ketogenic diet to a breastfeeding mother. By now it had become apparent that the HPCSA had given a similar directive to all its expert witnesses on nutrition.

Dhansay was either unwilling or genuinely unable to say who had given him the directive to focus on ketogenic diets. And when he admitted that he was not a ketosis expert, Ramdass asked why, when the approach was made, he had not immediately informed the HPCSA. Dhansay was defensive. 'Nobody knows every-thing,' he said. 'I want to state, for the record, that as far as the physiology of ketones and so forth, it is not within my experience and area of expertise. How-ever, I do say that one can research and do background checks and so forth. So I am au fait with the literature, but I am not an expert in ketone metabolism.'

Ramdass pointed out that although Dhansay claimed to have 'no interest' in *The Real Meal Revolution* and *Raising Superheroes*, he had quoted extensively from them in his evidence. He also queried the rationale behind Dhansay's stated tendency to 'zoom' in and out when scanning research for points to include in his testimony. Dhansay explained that he meant 'not starting with the know-ledge, but being aware of the knowledge'. He said that he had read only about 40 per cent of the 4 000 pages that Noakes had submitted as part of his evidence. (By the end of the trial, it had increased to 6 000 pages.)

Ramdass completed his cross-examination of Dhansay at the close of the fifth day, Friday 27 November. It was clear that the HPCSA's case was in serious trouble. The defence had effectively undermined the evidence of all of its wit-nesses. Adams prepared to adjourn the hearing until Monday morning, when Noakes's defence team would have their turn. It was then that Mapholisa unex-pectedly announced that he would apply to call another witness – HPCSA legal officer Nkagisang Madube – to give factual evidence. That meant no seven-day notice requirement, as was the case with expert witnesses.

When Van der Nest asked for confirmation that this would be the HPCSA's last witness, Mapholisa was evasive. Eventually he admitted that he would apply to call more experts, but refused to divulge their names or the topics on which they would testify. Van der Nest was having none of it. Neither was a clearly exasperated Adams. The hearing was not the set of *Ally McBeal* or *Petrocelli*, she said, referencing popular American TV courtroom dramas. There would be no surprise witnesses 'coming into court with drums rolling [to] save the day'. That only worked in the movies, not in the South African legal system. '[South Africa] is a democracy,' Adams said. 'We have a Constitution and the Promotion of Administrative Justice Act.' Justice, fairness and Noakes's constitutional rights demanded that Mapholisa reveal the names and status of the witnesses, she said.

Mapholisa gave in, but only after the defence gave an undertaking to keep the names confidential. Adams adjourned the session until Monday 30 November.

When the hearing resumed, both sides were in full fight mode. Mapholisa brought his application to call two new expert witnesses. He named only one, Stellenbosch University psychiatry professor Willie Pienaar, as the second had not yet agreed. Mapholisa said that it would be highly prejudicial to the HPCSA if the Professional Conduct Committee did not agree to his application, which, he added, he had spent the weekend preparing at an internet café after his home computer crashed. He described Ramdass's claim that Kruger was not an expert on ethics as 'bizarre'. (Kruger has no formal qualifications in medical bioethics.) However, equally bizarre was Mapholisa's contention that it was the defence team's fault that he had to call more witnesses. In effect, he was admitting that Noakes's lawyers had done too good a job at discrediting his experts.

In support of his application, Mapholisa cited the HPCSA's hearing against Dr Wouter Basson, the man dubbed 'Dr Death'. Van der Nest was unimpressed. The comparison with Basson was 'odious', he said, and simply 'didn't hold up'. In Basson's case, his lawyers had argued that their first witness had made concessions and, in the interests of justice, he required another witness. Mapholisa was claiming the opposite. He was saying: 'We stand by Professor Kruger. We will rely on Professor Kruger.' In standing so firmly by Kruger's testimony, Mapholisa had no need to call another witness, Van der Nest said.

Van der Nest also objected on the grounds of procedural unfairness. He placed on record the chronology of applications and related events. Noakes tweeted on 5 February 2014. Strydom lodged the complaint with the HPCSA on 6 February. The HPCSA's Fourth Preliminary Committee of Inquiry charged him seven months later, on 10 September 2014. It then took another four months to deliver the five-line charge to Noakes, who only received it on 28 January 2015. In the interim, the HPCSA had commissioned Vorster's report and kept it secret from Noakes. The report dealt specifically with whether or not Leenstra was Noakes's patient and the suitability of Twitter as a medium for providing dietary advice. In other words, the HPCSA had flagged the 'ethics' issue long before it charged Noakes. It was not 'by any stretch a new issue', stated Van der Nest.

The HPCSA then took nine months to constitute the Professional Conduct Committee to hear the charge against him, in breach of its own rules at the first hearing attempt on 4 June 2015. The net effect, said Van der Nest, was that the hearing date was wasted, because the matter could not proceed, and costs were mounting. In the meantime, the HPCSA had mustered three experts, all professors, to address all aspects of its case. It had correctly given the list to the defence at a prehearing conference on 28 May 2015. By doing so, the HPCSA had placed on record that it had all the experts it needed to proceed. More importantly, each expert had produced summaries and expert opinions in advance dealing with the alleged doctor–patient relationship between Leenstra and Noakes.

Van der Nest argued that the HPCSA's costly delaying tactics had made the case more adversarial than was necessary. He noted that the HPCSA had, in fact, adopted an adversarial attitude from the outset, as he could not think of a single request of any material consequence made by the defence to which the HPCSA had agreed. 'These are proceedings that are quasi-criminal in nature,' he said. 'This is a prosecution, not a civil proceeding. There are very serious consequences arising out of it.'

Van der Nest pointed to Section 35(3)(d) of South Africa's Constitution, which states: 'Every accused person has a right to a fair trial, which includes the right to have their trial begin and conclude without unreasonable delay.' Against this background, Van der Nest laid out significant prejudice to Noakes, who had had a cloud hanging over his head since February 2014. The fact that his own professional body was prosecuting him and that it had played out in the press had caused significant distress to Noakes and his family. The case was a drain on Noakes both emotionally and financially. It was not fair to let it drag on, much less for two years with no end in sight. 'It is well known that justice delayed is justice denied, particularly in matters concerning reputation,' Van der Nest said.

Van der Nest cited a seminal High Court judgment on the regulations governing expert witnesses. The judge ruled that the main purpose of Rule 36(9)(b) of the 'Rules Regulating the Conduct of the Proceedings of the Several Provincial and Local Divisions of the High Court of South Africa'* was to 'remove the element of surprise, which in earlier times (regarded as an element affording a tactical advantage) frequently caused delays in the conduct of trials'.[3] Acceding to Mapholisa's request would 'impermissibly sanction a breach of the regulations' and lead to more costs, said Van der Nest. Any opportunity to wrap up the hearing before the December holidays was rapidly 'disappearing into the mist'.

Van der Nest said that Noakes was one of South Africa's few respected A1-rated scientists. He had dealt with this ordeal 'with dignity and in a way that

---

* Rule 36(9)(b) states: 'No person shall, save with the leave of the court or the consent of all parties to the suit, be entitled to call as a witness any person to give evidence as an expert upon any matter upon which the evidence of expert witnesses may be received unless he shall not less than ten days before the trial, have delivered a summary of such expert's opinion and his reasons therefor.' Uniform Rules of the Court, available at http://www.justice.gov.za/legislation/rules/UniformRulesCourt[26jun 2009].pdf.

wishes to assist you to get this completed ... When you look at prejudice, his prejudice is manifest.' On prejudice to the HPCSA, Van der Nest submitted that there was 'absolutely none'.

Finally, Van der Nest said that the Constitution embraced the concept of substantive fairness: 'We say this is substantially unfair and that the pro-forma complainant [Mapholisa] should not be permitted to do this and to call on your sympathy for having worked over the weekend in an internet café. That is just not appropriate.'

Adams ruled in Mapholisa's favour, but she acknowledged the effects of the case on Noakes, saying that she had participated in many HPCSA hearings and that, in general, healthcare professionals regarded these proceedings, where they were tried by their peers, as 'more traumatic than any court case'. HPCSA hearings are *sui generis* (unique), Adams said. They are not criminal or civil, but 'a bit of both'. The onus of proof is, therefore, on a balance of probabilities, not beyond reasonable doubt as in a criminal case. It is not unusual in court cases and hearings of this nature for what transpires during cross-examination to oblige one party to feel the need for further evidence. Mapholisa was not introducing new scientific or nutritional information; he was introducing another expert on professional ethics.

Adams also made the point that the introduction of new witnesses at such a late stage could backfire. 'I have, myself, called a second witness only to find out that I was better off without one,' she said. Her committee had unanimously decided that 'the prejudice suffered to [Mapholisa's] case would probably, in this particular scenario and in these circumstances, be more severe than that for [Noakes], and not quite as prejudicial to the respondent at this stage, as may seem to the public or the untrained eye'.

With that, Mapholisa called Madube, who was clearly intended to address an ethical dilemma in the HPCSA's case: the fact that the Fourth Preliminary Committee of Inquiry had secured a report from Vorster as evidence against Noakes, but had failed to share it with him before charging him.

Madube testified that the use of 'secret' reports was routine for HPCSA committees. His reasoning: committee members may not always have the specialised knowledge required to determine whether a complaint warrants a charge, in which case they are entitled to request an opinion from an expert to assist them in 'arriving at an amicable or full conclusion'. Madube described such documents as 'for the committee's eyes only'. 'It is a confidential document,' he said. The practitioner 'cannot respond to the document' because it 'is not for him'. Therefore he should 'not have knowledge of the document'.

In cross-examination, Van der Nest asked Madube to point out where in the HPCSA's rules governing preliminary inquiry committees it allowed evidence to be kept secret from health professionals. When Madube continued to insist that the committee could gather evidence for 'its eyes only', Van der Nest dismissed his response as 'staggering'.

Van der Nest asked Madube whether he knew the Latin phrase *audi alteram partem* (let the other side be heard). It is a common law principle that encompasses the right to a fair hearing and the opportunity to respond. Madube said he knew the phrase, but that it did not apply to HPCSA preliminary inquiry committees.

With barely disguised impatience, Van der Nest again asked Madube: 'Which is the secrecy provision in this section that permits [the HPCSA] to do that – please tell me the words?' Madube became belligerent and insisted that there was no 'secrecy provision'. Van der Nest charged that the HPCSA had considered it 'impractical, inconvenient and costly' to give Noakes the opportunity to see and respond to evidence against him before charging him. In response, Madube ventured the opinion that if Noakes wasn't happy with the law as the HPCSA applied it in this case, he could contest it in the Constitutional Court.

Remarkably, neither Mapholisa nor Madube appeared to see anything unethical in a committee hiding evidence from Noakes before charging him. But the most remarkable part of Madube's evidence was yet to come. It would show that Adams's comment about the potential for a surprise witness to backfire was prescient.

Madube made passing reference to a file on the prosecution team's table. The file had not been entered as evidence. When Van der Nest asked to see it, Mapholisa agreed. The file was duly entered as evidence and the cross-examination continued. After a short while, Van der Nest broke off to say that he had noticed 'something happening on the other end of the table'. Dr Janet Giddy had also noticed that 'something' was up: former HPCSA ombudsman and member of the prosecution Dr Abdul Bharday was removing pages from the file.

Van der Nest objected, saying that it should be kept intact for the defence team. Adams agreed and instructed Bharday to stop. It was the first indication that there was something special about the file's contents.

What does not appear in the transcript of the day's proceedings is the unseemly skirmish that took place later, when Madube refused to hand over the file to Noakes's attorney, Adam Pike. Mapholisa claimed there were duplicates in the file that the HPCSA simply wanted to remove to save the defence some time. Van der Nest did not believe him and insisted that Madube hand over the complete file to Pike. Madube's obvious reluctance and Mapholisa's obvious discomfort were further signs that there was something in the file that they did not want the defence to see. I started calling it the 'dodgy dossier', and so it turned out to be, as the next hearing session showed.

11

The Start of the Third Session: February 2016

'When truth is replaced by silence, the silence is a lie.'
– Yevgeny Yevtushenko, Soviet and Russian poet

Cape Town is the home of Banting in South Africa. It is where Professor Tim Noakes lives, and from where he singlehandedly set off the Banting revolution in 2011. The revolution spread quickly across a sick, fat and hungry nation, gathering millions of followers along the way. Reports began to pour in of people with obesity, T2DM and heart disease reversing their symptoms and, in many cases, coming off all medication simply by changing to low-carb, high-fat foods.

By the time the February 2016 hearing session rolled around, the flood of reports was drowning out the orthodox medical and dietetic opposition to LCHF. The power of the anointed was giving way to the wisdom of the crowds. You wouldn't have known it from the many doctors, dietitians and academics who still clung to their belief that diet can never effectively replace drugs in the treatment of life-threatening, chronic diseases. Many had chosen to involve themselves in the HPCSA's case against Noakes, and the February session would reveal just how murky their involvement had become.

Noakes's lawyers had gone through the file that the HPCSA had reluctantly handed over at the end of November 2015. Among other documents, it contained a compromising chain of email correspondence between members of the HPCSA's Fourth Preliminary Committee of Inquiry. It made the HPCSA look less like a 'rigid creature of statute', as Mapholisa had described it when trying to block the application to call a witness via video link, than a spiteful, Gollum-like creature hiding in a misty mountain cave, plotting to silence Noakes once and for all. Anyone reading it might more readily agree that the conspiracy theory of an organised campaign against Noakes was rapidly becoming fact.

The Fourth Preliminary Committee of Inquiry had a simple enough task: investigate the complaint that Strydom had lodged with the HPCSA against Noakes, and decide whether the complaint warranted a charge. To this end, they held two meetings. The first was in May 2014. At the second, in September 2014, the committee decided to charge Noakes. The significance of the delay between the first and second meetings becomes clear in the chain of email correspondence in the file, and points to what Noakes's lawyers diplomatically called potentially 'highly irregular' conduct on the part of the committee's members. That's a euphemism for unethical, and possibly illegal, actions in breach of the HPCSA's own rules and Noakes's constitutional rights.

In particular, the emails showed that committee members had involved themselves in the case against Noakes despite being *functus officio*. That's the legal term for 'having performed their office'. The committee had discharged its duty by deciding that the HPCSA should charge Noakes, and that should have been that. All members should have returned to their day jobs as academics. Instead, as the emails revealed, some went to great lengths to boost the chances for a guilty verdict. In other words, certain committee members appeared to have acted *ultra vires* – 'beyond their legal powers or authority'.

Unsurprisingly, given the large number of UCT academics involved in the ongoing and public attacks on Noakes, two of his former UCT colleagues had been on the committee: emeritus professor of surgery and former executive of the South African Medical Association John Terblanche; and UCT psychiatry professor and then SAMA president Denise White, who has since passed away. Interestingly, White was also a member of the HPCSA's Medical and Dental Board that first considered Strydom's complaint and decided to pass it on to the Fourth Preliminary Committee of Inquiry. I would have thought that was a clear conflict of interest.

The committee chair had been Professor Amaboo 'Ames' Dhai, director of the Steve Biko Centre for Bioethics at the University of the Witwatersrand. She is a medical doctor and a member of the Fellowship of Colleges of Obstetricians and Gynaecologists of South Africa, and has a master's degree in law and ethics. Wits describes her as 'an ethicist of international standing who can be credited with entrenching bioethics as an integral aspect of health sciences in SA'.[1]

Dhai's emails appeared to show her lack of understanding of basic legal principles, particularly the *audi alteram partem* principle (that all accused persons have the right to see all available evidence before being charged). After the Fourth Preliminary Committee of Inquiry's first meeting in May, Dhai had commissioned the Vorster report on the background to Strydom's complaint. As we know, Dhai did not let Noakes see and respond to the report before her committee used it as evidence in its decision to charge him in September 2014. Most alarming, however, was that Dhai appeared to see nothing wrong or unethical in keeping the Vorster report secret from Noakes.

The emails also showed how she exceeded her brief as committee chair. In one email, for example, she tried to tell Mapholisa how to conduct his case, even whom he should enlist to assist him, and bluntly told him to employ external lawyers. In another, Dhai refused to provide Mapholisa with the reasons for the committee's decision to charge Noakes, because, she said, Mapholisa had disregarded her 'instruction' to instruct external legal counsel. In yet another email, she suggested that the June 2015 hearing should not go ahead because the HPCSA was not ready to proceed. Clearly, Dhai believed that she had wide-ranging power and influence over the HPCSA's case.

Mapholisa appeared not to appreciate Dhai's inference that he was not up to the job. He ignored her instructions, 'to his credit', as Van der Nest later commented. Evidence on the record showed that Mapholisa had even threatened Dhai with a subpoena if she did not give the reasons for the committee's decision. Joan Adams described that action as 'brave' for someone in Mapholisa's position.

I emailed Dhai for comment. She did not reply. I then emailed Wits University's vice chancellor, Professor Adam Habib, cc'ing Dhai. Habib replied, but only to say that Dhai had assured him of 'no wrongdoing'. I emailed back to say that, in my opinion, that wasn't how universities should respond to serious accusations of misconduct by their academics. I suggested that it required a proper investigation. Habib did not reply to any further emails.

Terblanche's emails were just as illuminating. They revealed his enthusiastic attempts to mobilise UCT colleagues to give evidence against Noakes. Terblanche, too, was acting beyond his brief as a member of the preliminary inquiry committee. In one email, Terblanche offered to ask Professor Wim de Villiers, dean of UCT's Faculty of Health Sciences at the time, to give expert testimony against Noakes. In another, he suggested Noakes's friend and mentor Lionel Opie. Both De Villiers and Opie were signatories of the infamous UCT professors' letter, published in the *Cape Times* in August 2014. As it turned out, neither De Villiers nor Opie obliged. That was probably a smart move, given the ethical questions that the letter raised, as well as claims that it was a form of academic bullying. In another email, Terblanche helpfully included a copy of the professors' letter and suggested that the committee use it as evidence against Noakes. Interestingly, the email chain shows that none of Terblanche's fellow committee members objected to him exceeding his authority in this manner.

Terblanche also suggested using the contents of 'The Big Fat Debate', a section on UCT's Division of Human Nutrition website.[2] It's difficult to see much debate, robust or otherwise, on the site. What is easier to spot is bias in favour of the typically prescribed LFHC 'prudent' diet. It includes research by departmental head Nelia Steyn and Marjanne Senekal. Both have links to the sugar industry and the Coca-Cola front organisation International Life Sciences Institute.[3]

Senekal was a signatory of the UCT professors' letter, a co-author on the Naudé review, and later agreed to become a consultant for the HPCSA after its case started falling apart at the end of November 2015. The second section on

'The Big Fat Debate' is titled 'Further evidence for healthy balanced diets', and the first link is to the Naudé review published in *PLoS ONE* in July 2014.[4] The site does not include a link to the re-analysis of the Naudé review by Noakes and Dr Zoë Harcombe, published in the *SAMJ* in December 2016.[5] They found the Naudé review to be riddled with so many errors as to be fatally flawed.

'The Big Fat Debate' was quick to link to the UCT professors' letter, but failed to even mention Noakes's vehement and robust reply. Interestingly, the link to the letter has subsequently vanished, but all the remaining links relate exclusively to research favouring LFHC, and mirror much of the evidence that the HPCSA's expert witnesses presented against Noakes and Banting. For example, the very first section on the site's home page, dedicated to 'Evidence for a healthy and balanced diet', contains links to all 13 articles in the 'Food-Based Dietary Guidelines for South Africa 2013 No. 3 (Suppl)', published in the *South African Journal of Clinical Nutrition (SAJCN)*.[6] The introduction, by North-West University nutrition professor Hester Vorster, the first expert witness called by the HPCSA, extols the virtues of South Africa's official dietary guidelines, of which she was an author.[7] 'The Big Fat Debate' ignores ongoing controversy in scientific circles around the lack of science to support these low-fat, high-carb guidelines.

The *SAJCN* is a joint publication and mouthpiece of ADSA and the Nutrition Society of South Africa (NSSA). Vorster is a lifetime ADSA member and a member of the NSSA, as are the HPCSA's second expert witness, Salome Kruger, and many others involved in active opposition to Noakes.

Nelia Steyn is responsible for the second article on the site, in which she gives uncritical support for the dietary guidelines.[8] Vorster again writes the fourth article, this time on one of the most hotly contested aspects of dietary advice, especially for the country's poor: 'Make starchy foods part of most meals'.[9] The tenth article, by Cornelius Smuts and P.W. Wolmarans, addresses dietary fats. Titled 'The importance of the quality or type of fat in the diet', it does say that saturated fats 'will remain an integral part of the human diet'; however, it then pursues the conventional fat-phobic line against saturated fats, favouring foods high in polyunsaturated and monounsaturated fats, and vegetable oils.[10] All the articles support the premise of the diet-heart hypothesis that saturated fat causes heart disease. This hypothesis was a major pillar of the HPCSA's case against Noakes.

The second section on 'The Big Fat Debate' also includes a link to a 2013 *JAMA* article titled 'A call for an end to the diet debates'.[11] That probably says more than the academics intended about the real motivation behind their website. 'The Big Fat Debate' is not a debate at all, and perhaps was never intended to be one. It seems to be nothing more than an institutional attempt to suppress scientific debate by presenting one side of an argument.

At the end of the day, the email chain discovered in the file suggests that the Fourth Preliminary Committee of Inquiry intentionally deferred their decision to charge Noakes while they waited for certain documents – the Naudé review in particular – to be published. The emails all but confirm Strydom's own admission at the hearing in November 2015, when she said, 'everybody, all these big organisations were waiting on the publication of this information before we could make any kind of media statement'.

What legal and scientific experts have found most astonishing about the actions of various academics and affiliated universities involved in the case against Noakes is their deafening silence. I personally have emailed and placed phone calls to people up and down the universities' hierarchies, and it appears that those in positions of power and influence have closed ranks. They all seemed willing to defend the indefensible – in effect, to collude in the suppression of evidence and the attempted silencing of one scientist.

When the hearing resumed on Monday 8 February 2016, the HPCSA had recruited new soldiers in its ongoing battle against Noakes and Banting. It had an expensive new team of external lawyers in place, with Katlego Mmuoe of KK Mmuoe Attorneys as instructing attorney, and doctor-turned-advocate Ajay Bhoopchand as counsel. Mmuoe and Bhoopchand would have been aware of the gaping holes in the HPCSA's case after their witnesses' cross-examination by Ramdass and Van der Nest, and they would have been briefed on the file's potential to inflict further damage. But first they had to announce the unexpected loss of a major witness.

Recall how, at the last session in November 2015, HPCSA chief prosecutor Meshack Mapholisa had sprung a last-minute application for two new expert witnesses. At the time, he would only reveal the identity of one: Stellenbosch University psychiatry professor Willie Pienaar. Now it seemed that the other, Professor Jacques Rossouw, would not be appearing. Rossouw had recently retired from the US National Institutes of Health Women's Health Initiative, but was still employed by the NIH. He is one of Noakes's most vociferous and vicious critics. Noakes was therefore looking forward to a scientific debate with his arch-enemy on a very public platform. When Bhoopchand announced that Rossouw would not be appearing after all, it was a big disappointment on both sides.

Rossouw should have made enough time to secure a yes-or-no answer from the NIH to attend. The HPCSA had asked him in late January. All the NIH would tell me was that it did not give him permission in 'a timely manner'. It also said that Rossouw was currently 'unavailable' for an interview with me. My freedom-of-information request to the NIH revealed the rest in an email chain.[*]

---

[*] In an email to his superiors at the NIH, Rossouw refers to Noakes as 'a South African physician promoting the low carb high fat diet for all that ails mankind'. In refusing an interview with me, he calls me 'a shill for the physician'. Thus an interview will be 'mishandled', he claims.

Yet seven days before the February hearing, Rossouw was clearly ready and willing to be a witness. He had timeously submitted to the HPCSA a summary of the evidence he intended presenting, and the HPCSA had passed it on to Noakes's lawyers. So why did he really bale? Rossouw was in Cape Town in late January 2016. In preparation for his testimony, he would have read the transcripts of the November hearing. Like Marlene Ellmer, he would have known that the risk of exposing himself, and his reputation, to cross-examination by Van der Nest and Ramdass was high. Thus, in the end, Rossouw and the HPCSA chose the line of least resistance.

With the Rossouw matter out of the way, Van der Nest began to place on record the contents of the file obtained in November. He told the hearing that after viewing the file, Adam Pike had written to the HPCSA registrar, Dr Buyiswa Mjamba-Matshoba, as well as to Mapholisa and the chair of the Medical and Dental Board, Professor Letticia Mmaseloadi Moja, asking for information, including the reasons for the Fourth Preliminary Committee of Inquiry's decision to charge Noakes and all documentation on which that decision had been based.

Mjamba-Matshoba's response had been surprisingly blunt and obstructionist. Refusing the request, she said that Noakes would have to seek a ruling from the Professional Conduct Committee to order the HPCSA to release the information. Since the HPCSA is the parent body and appoints members to all its committees, it was like a parent passing on responsibility to one child and ignoring the delinquent behaviour of another. Mjamba-Matshoba was blithely ignoring the fact that the HPCSA's Fourth Preliminary Committee of Inquiry had a duty to provide Noakes with the reasons for charging him.

Van der Nest was forthright in his criticism. He said that the HPCSA was playing a 'game of cat and mouse' with Noakes. He applied to Adams for a ruling to compel Mjamba-Matshoba to provide information on three issues: the conduct of the Fourth Preliminary Committee of Inquiry; Dhai's refusal to provide reasons for her committee's decision to charge Noakes; and her failure to reveal all the evidence the committee had considered before making its decision. He included subsidiary questions about the influence of outside organisations on the decision to prosecute Noakes. Among them was the South African Medical Association.

This last seemed a reasonable enough request, given the well-documented antagonism towards Noakes and LCHF displayed by many SAMA doctors. The SAMA had also acceded to the demand from a group of ADSA dietitians to withdraw the CPD points it had initially granted for the Cape Town low-carb summit that Noakes co-hosted in February 2015 (see Chapter 1). The SAMA only reinstated the points when the conference organiser, Karen Thomson, threatened legal action.

If there was ever any hope that the HPCSA's new lawyers would take their client down a less adversarial path, Bhoopchand instantly dispelled it. He objected to Van der Nest's application, contending that the Professional Conduct Committee did not have the power to instruct Mjamba-Matshoba to comply with its statutory obligations. He claimed that Noakes's only redress was the High Court. He also contended that Noakes could have applied for any information he wanted using the Promotion of Access to Information Act (PAIA). The purpose of PAIA is to give effect to Section 32 of the Constitution, which provides for the right of access to information. It states that 'Everyone has the right of access to (a) any information held by the state; and (b) any information that is held by another person and that is required for the exercise or protection of any rights'. The motivation here is to entrench a culture of transparency and accountability in both public and private bodies. It also enables members of the public to exercise and protect all their rights more fully.

Bhoopchand denied any irregular conduct by Dhai and her fellow committee members. In effect, he argued that the committee could do as it pleased. By his reasoning, the committee was exempt from the principle of *audi alteram partem*. He also tried to have the file's incriminating evidence struck from the record altogether, claiming that the HPCSA had 'inadvertently' handed the file over to the defence and that Noakes was therefore not entitled to its contents. Terblanche's emails were 'personal and private', Bhoopchand said, before suggesting that the defence team had infringed Terblanche's rights under the Protection of Personal Information Act (commonly known as PoPI) by releasing the contents 'into the public sphere without his permission'.

In response, Van der Nest was a legal juggernaut, thundering through Bhoopchand's arguments. The HPCSA was 'playing quick and loose' with Noakes's rights by sending him 'from pillar to post', he said. The suggestion that his only redress was a High Court action was 'not only grossly unfair, but surprising'. There was nothing in law to suggest that Noakes should have made an application under PAIA in order to defend himself properly and fully.

South Africa was a democracy with a Constitution that included the Promotion of Administrative Justice Act (PAJA), Van der Nest said.

Legal experts say that PAJA seeks to make the executive (administration) of any statutory body effective and accountable to the public. When read with the Constitution, PAJA encompasses and embraces the Batho Pele ('People First') principles, which require public servants to deliver good service to the public. Lawmakers enacted PAJA specifically to promote and protect the rights of all South Africans to administrative action that is just and fair.[12]

In legal terms, administrative action is defined as a decision, taken or not taken, 'that is of an administrative nature made in terms of an empowering provision that is not specifically excluded from the PAJA'.[13] The decision can be made by an organ of state or a private person exercising a public power or performing a public function that adversely affects rights and that has a direct external legal effect.

Section 33 of the Constitution guarantees that 'everyone has the right to administrative action that is lawful, reasonable and procedurally fair'; and that 'everyone whose rights have been adversely affected by administrative action has the right to be given written reasons'.

In summary, PAJA ensures that administrative procedures are fair; gives people the right to ask for reasons from officials; and gives citizens the right to have the courts review any administrative action that impacts unfairly on them. As per PAJA, all administrators must follow fair procedure when making a decision and clearly provide the rationale. In other words, they have to explain any decisions taken. They also have to allow relevant parties to have their say before making any decision that might affect their rights – the *audi alteram partem* principle.

Van der Nest thus used the most powerful weapon at hand – South Africa's Constitution – to undermine Bhoopchand's arguments that the HPCSA's Fourth Preliminary Committee of Inquiry's actions were lawful. In this case, the committee's most important administrative action was its decision to charge Noakes. There was no argument that the committee's decision amounted to administrative action. There was also little argument that the HPCSA's action was procedurally unfair. The HPCSA had breached the principles of PAJA and, by extension, Noakes's constitutional rights. The HPCSA knew its obligations, Van der Nest said. It had agreed in writing to give Noakes written reasons in May 2015 for the decision to charge him, yet he was still waiting.

In effect, Bhoopchand had made a surprisingly narrow reading of the regulations. He also appeared to have glossed over the basic requirement that any law that contradicted the Constitution must be 'read down'. 'Reading down' is a legal mandate to courts to interpret an unconstitutional statute so as to bring it into line with the Constitution's liberal demands. Therefore, any rule or regulation that contradicts PAJA and the Constitution must be 'read down'.[14] The reasoning: PAJA is a constitutional statute, which the legislature promulgated as a constitutional right. That constitutional right still exists outside of PAJA. Since the Constitution is supreme, and PAJA is a constitutional statute, PAJA prevails over regulations or statutes, unless specifically excluded. The Health Professions Act, under which the HPCSA was set up, is not specifically excluded.

Van der Nest also showed that there is nothing in law to suggest that official correspondence by officials exercising a public function could be considered private or personal. PoPI was not designed to be a cover for the abuse of power by officials, he said. Terblanche's emails were not personal or confidential, as they all related to the HPCSA's prosecution. There was also nothing 'inadvertent' about how the defence had acquired the file. When Van der Nest had asked to view the contents of the file, Mapholisa had readily agreed. The HPCSA had therefore waived whatever privilege there might have been in not handing it over.

Van der Nest said that the HPCSA's response so far had raised serious questions of legality, justice and fairness. Chief among them: 'Where do the chair [Dhai] and members of a preliminary inquiry committee get the power to try and find expert witnesses to prosecute a case after the decision has been made and after that function has been exercised? Where does the chair get the power to try and tell the pro-forma complainant [Mapholisa] how to run his case, to postpone, to get someone else?' Van der Nest answered his own questions. They did not have those powers. It was also disconcerting, he said, that the HPCSA's registrar did not take as serious a view of the committee's behaviour as Noakes and his lawyers were taking.

When Adams ruled, she came down squarely on the side of the defence. It was 'astounding, to say the least', Adams said, that the HPCSA's Fourth Preliminary Committee of Inquiry had refused to provide written reasons for its decision to charge Noakes. It was in 'blatant defiance of the Constitution', PAJA and PAIA, she said, citing the *audi alteram partem* principle. Noakes's lawyers had made such requests repeatedly, as had Mapholisa and the HPCSA's own legal department. Mapholisa had displayed the 'utmost integrity under circumstances that were trying and traumatic' in attempting to extract the reasons from Dhai, noted Adams.

Once the HPCSA had placed Strydom's complaint before its Fourth Preliminary Committee of Inquiry, 'why would anyone on earth think ... that suddenly it is game over, all fair play out of the window?' Adams asked rhetorically. 'That simply does not make sense.' It was also 'unfathomable' that the committee could have made an informed decision without 'cogent reasons', she said.

Adams dismissed Bhoopchand's suggestion that Noakes's only recourse was an application to the High Court. It 'defies all logic', she said, to expect Noakes to incur exorbitant costs and extensive delays, and suffer severe prejudice, due to the failure of its own committee to comply with its mandate and the Constitution. She agreed that her committee did not have the power to order the registrar to extract the reasons from Dhai; however, they could request her to comply, and it would be 'a travesty of justice' if she did not.

In her ruling, Adams requested that Mjamba-Matshoba provide Noakes with written reasons for the Fourth Preliminary Committee of Inquiry's decision to charge him, along with all the documentation on which that decision was based, by 4 p.m. on Friday 12 February 2016. (The HPCSA met the deadline in form but not substance. All that Adam Pike would say was that Dhai gave 'sparse' reasons.)

The following day, Bhoopchand called Stellenbosch University psychiatry professor Willie Pienaar to give expert evidence on ethics. Once again, Pienaar's presence was best explained by the contents of the file. Besides compromising emails, it also contained notes made by Meshack Mapholisa. Two of them are particularly pertinent to explaining Pienaar's late inclusion as an expert witness for the HPCSA:

> We need to focus on the ethical complaint and the charge sheet and the crux of the matter; the case is not about whether Prof Tim Noakes current theory on diet is correct or not, it's about giving medical advice over social media on nutritional matters to a patient you have never met, never spoken to and know nothing about the medical history – in respect to the infant.
> […]
> This is not a hearing about Low Carbohydrate High Fat diets as opposed to the South African Dietary Guidelines which are evidence-based. The outcome of the hearing should not be a conclusion on whether Prof T Noakes theory of LCHF is right or wrong, it should be a conclusion on whether it is unprofessional or not to provide advice over social media to a patient, in this case a baby, about whom you have no history or other information e.g. medical conditions, deficiencies or other risk factor. We do not need a lecture on advantages or disadvantages of a Low Carbohydrate, High Fat diet and the fact of the matter is that professional medical nutritional advice was given over a social network and that is the crux of the complaint.

Mapholisa went on to list the expert witnesses that, at the time, he proposed to call: Pippa Leenstra, Marlene Ellmer, Salome Kruger and Muhammad Ali Dhansay. Ellmer, Kruger and Dhansay all have expertise in nutrition, not ethics. This indicated a surprising disconnect in Mapholisa's argument. When the hearing got underway, Ellmer had been replaced, not by an ethicist, but by another nutrition expert, Hester Vorster. There was still no ethicist in sight. With witnesses such as these, the focus of the trial was clearly always going to be on nutrition, not ethics.

As the hearing progressed in November 2015, Mapholisa must have seen that he was failing to deliver on the 'crux of the matter' and decided to secure a real ethicist. Seeing as Dhai, the 'doyenne' of South African ethics, had been chairperson of the Fourth Preliminary Committee of Inquiry, and was already party to the decision to charge Noakes, he had to cast a wider net. Still, his choice of Pienaar was surprising.

Pienaar is a big, chubby man with a mop of silvery hair and a genial, grandfatherly demeanour. His expertise is in psychiatry, although he does have a master's degree in philosophy and a special interest in medical ethics. He said that fully qualified medical bioethicists are 'thin on the ground'. That much is certainly true. Despite not having a doctorate in the subject, Pienaar is one of three bioethicists in Stellenbosch University's Faculty of Medicine and Health Sciences, and lectures part-time on bioethics.

Pienaar began his testimony confidently enough. He stated his belief that Noakes had a doctor–patient relationship with Leenstra on Twitter. He also claimed that Noakes had ended the doctor–patient relationship 'without a mutual understanding and consensus'. Pienaar called that 'another virtue that [doctors] treasure'. He argued that Leenstra's tweet to Noakes was an 'I' rather than a 'we' question, despite being in the third person: 'is LCHF eating ok for breastfeeding mums?' His reasoning: Leenstra was one person speaking to one doctor on Twitter. He also claimed that Noakes's tweet constituted medical advice, not information.

Pienaar readily admitted that he was not an expert on dietary requirements for newborns or infants, but commented on the subject anyway. As a clinician, he said, he knew that such diets were 'something special'. He suggested that the 'advice' that Noakes had given in his tweet was 'dangerous'. He expressed fear at the possible harm that could have come to the many millions across the globe who might have seen and acted on the tweet. As previous witnesses had done, Pienaar claimed that anyone reading Noakes's tweet was likely to interpret it as telling Leenstra to stop breastfeeding.

Pienaar also admitted that he was not active on Twitter. Under cross-examination, he said that he had 'wilfully' decided not to be on the popular social network. He clearly knew very little about the dynamics and etiquette of the 'Twitterverse'.

Pienaar said that if doctors gave out any medical advice on Twitter, patients would lose trust in them; the doctor–patient relationship would suffer; patients and the community would suffer; and ultimately the entire medical profession would suffer. He appeared blissfully unaware that doctors have been tweeting information regularly for years without any of these dire consequences. Pienaar also predicted that open social media would become a 'huge thing' (as if it were not already), and that doctors would have to look at issues of security, informal consent, the 'whole tooty'. He compared social media to 'morphine', which he called 'fantastic stuff'. He added that we 'cannot live without morphine, but it is very, very dangerous'. It was 'very, very wrong' for doctors to give advice on social media, he said.

Van der Nest listened with growing impatience to Pienaar's litany of fears about Twitter. He interrupted him at one stage, saying: 'I mean no disrespect, Professor, but you are a social media dinosaur.'

It was ultimately Pienaar's insistence that Noakes and Leenstra had a doctor–patient relationship that tripped him up under cross-examination and brought into question his credibility as an ethicist. The HPCSA attempted to use Pienaar to exploit a classic circular argument. According to this argument, Twitter does not allow a doctor to interact properly with a patient, as it does not allow for a proper medical consultation. The doctor is unable to take an adequate medical history and examine the patient, and therefore can't accurately diagnose and decide on a treatment strategy. The medium of Twitter therefore precludes any possibility of a traditional doctor–patient relationship.

The HPCSA would argue, through Pienaar, that, as a result, no professional should ever provide any form of medical information on Twitter. A more reasonable interpretation might simply be that all parties involved in any Twitter communication understand that the absence of any possibility to take a medical history, to perform an examination and to submit a medical bill means that whatever a doctor tweets, whether offering medical advice or sharing medical information, cannot ever constitute a doctor–patient relationship.

Yet in his testimony, Pienaar repeatedly stated that those doctors who do give medical opinions on Twitter are guilty of unprofessional conduct. His reasoning: engaging with someone on Twitter immediately sets up a doctor–patient relationship, and once a doctor–patient relationship exists, a doctor is obliged to fulfil certain 'duties of care'; and because the medium of Twitter does not allow for a proper medical consultation, the doctor in question cannot fulfil these responsibilities. But if, as the argument began, Twitter precludes any possibility of a doctor–patient relationship, how can any doctor on Twitter be accused of violating something that, by the HPCSA's own reasoning, cannot exist in the first place?

Pienaar got himself into further trouble with his assumption that simply telling someone to follow the LCHF diet constituted medical advice. It took him a long while to accept that, logically, the reverse must also then be true: telling someone *not* to follow the LCHF diet is, equally, medical advice. Van der Nest reminded Pienaar that two dietitians, Ellmer and Strydom, had responded to Leenstra on Twitter, and that both had told her not to follow Noakes's diet. Were they not then equally guilty? Pienaar tried to wriggle out of making any concessions by saying that Strydom and Ellmer had responded to what they considered to be wrong advice, and that the HPCSA had briefed him to consider only Noakes's conduct on Twitter.

But Van der Nest persisted. 'I'm not going to let you off that lightly,' he told the increasingly frazzled witness. By Pienaar's own admission, Leenstra now had two choices: Noakes saying that LCHF was good, and Strydom and Ellmer saying that it was bad. In the meantime, Ellmer told Leenstra to email her for further information. With this action, Leenstra was 'rapidly disappearing' as Noakes's patient – if she ever was one, Van der Nest said. And then Strydom stepped in again, tweeting Leenstra to contact her directly and providing her phone number. If Leenstra was indeed Noakes's patient, as Pienaar said, then surely this action, like Ellmer's, constituted supersession?

Pienaar hesitantly conceded that, by his own argument, Leenstra would have to be considered a patient of all three: Noakes, Strydom and Ellmer. As the legal and ethical implications of this dawned on him, he admitted that, in all likelihood, none of them had in fact had a professional relationship with Leenstra.

Crucially, Pienaar also conceded that no harm had come to Leenstra or her baby from Noakes's tweet. He tried to suggest that because Twitter was an open platform, things 'could have been different' for anyone else reading the tweet. In other words, there was potential for harm for anyone who read the tweet. Van der Nest focused on the glaring bias in this statement. Pienaar could just as easily have suggested that there was potential for good, he said. Pienaar could only stutter in reply: 'Absolutely. Absolutely. Again, I am not a scientist.'

Van der Nest was on a roll. He went for the jugular with Pienaar's observation that Leenstra had 'wisely decided' not to follow Noakes's advice. 'You began the exercise by saying you are completely neutral about the [LCHF] diet,' Van der Nest told Pienaar. 'It could be good or it could be bad. Yet you described the action of Pippa Leenstra in not following it as a wise decision. Now, if you were truly neutral you would never have described the decision not followed as a wise one.' Realising that he had overstepped the bounds of his expertise, Pienaar tried to back-pedal: 'I am not the scientific expert, but just as a clinician, and I do not want to put my foot into this, but I am still of the opinion ... that the dietary needs of ... neonate or infant or baby are specialised information.'

Unimpressed, Van der Nest remarked to Pienaar: 'Your petticoat of bias is showing.'

Pienaar eventually conceded that he should not have used the word 'wise'.

Pienaar's poor performance under cross-examination was not entirely his fault. It was glaringly obvious that the HPCSA had not briefed him properly. He was unfamiliar with the full context of the tweeted exchange between Leenstra, Noakes, Strydom and Ellmer. Van der Nest described it as a 'mystery' and 'inexplicable' that the HPCSA had withheld crucial information from its own witness.

After cross-examination, members of the Professional Conduct Committee were invited to ask questions. Dr Janet Giddy asked Pienaar whether, as a bio-ethical expert, he would recommend that the HPCSA charge Ellmer and Strydom as well – or did he have 'different rules for different people'? Clearly floundering, Pienaar said there were 'many, many perpetrators', but given Noakes's high profile, he should be singled out.

Giddy found that sentiment disturbing and repeated her question: 'I am asking you, as an ethicist, what is the ethical, right thing to do? ... We know in this particular case there were other, what you called perpetrators, which is quite a loaded word, if I might say. But what I am hearing you are saying, it is good to make an example of one perpetrator, but you are not worried about the other perpetrators?'

Pienaar confirmed his opinion that the HPCSA had to make an example of someone, and that it should be Noakes.

Thus, the HPCSA's case ended in even deeper trouble than it had been in November 2015. Pienaar, like all the other expert witnesses before him, had failed to sustain the claim of a doctor–patient relationship. He had also failed to uphold the argument that Noakes's tweet constituted medical advice, and not just information. And, just as crucially, he had conceded that there was no evidence of any harm.

12

Finally, Noakes Speaks

'The greatest enemy of knowledge is not ignorance,
it is the illusion of knowledge.'
– Daniel J. Boorstin, American historian

On the afternoon of Wednesday 10 February 2016, two years and six days after the tweet that started it all, Professor Tim Noakes began his defence in what the public had by now dubbed 'the Nutrition Trial of the 21st Century'.

Local and international interest in the hearing was high. At stake were Noakes's reputation, distinguished career and right to freedom of speech as a scientist. Costs for both sides were already in the stratosphere, perhaps more so for the HPCSA, which had recently acquired an expensive team of external lawyers. The HPCSA also appeared to have pockets as deep as its desire to find Noakes guilty. According to a reliable source, Advocate Ajay Bhoopchand would submit a bill of close to R1 million (the equivalent of around $62 500 at the time) for the eight-day hearing alone.

By the time Noakes began testifying, Bhoopchand and instructing attorney Katlego Mmuoe would have known that their client's case was possibly in terminal decline. None of their expert witnesses had held up well under cross-examination. Their only hope was for Bhoopchand to undermine the defence's evidence. It was a tall order: Noakes's evidence alone consisted of 6 000 pages, 1 200 slides, and more than 350 publications and articles. It would take him almost 40 hours to present, over two sessions, concluding on 17 October 2016.

An expectant silence settled over the room in the Cape Town conference centre as Advocate Rocky Ramdass led Noakes through his CV. At over 100 pages, it was the longest and most fecund CV, scientifically speaking, of the trial so far. Noakes sped through it, punctuating his words with an ironic smile – Ramdass would call it his 'habitual smile'. To the uninitiated, it could have seemed that Noakes was blowing his own trumpet – critics, and even supporters, sometimes accuse him of arrogance – but in this case, he was sending a signal to the HPCSA and the world that he was here to deliver a loud and clear message. It was one that his qualifications and knowledge gave him every right to dispense.

His credentials, research experience and A1 rating by the NRF dwarfed the prosecution witnesses', including the dietitian who had started it all, Claire Julsing Strydom. Next to Noakes's ruddy scientific pedigree, Strydom's looked positively anaemic. She was also conspicuous by her absence. Noakes later described her failure to attend as both 'disappointing and a lost opportunity'. Strydom might have learnt something. (Bhoopchand later said that he had advised Strydom not to attend, but would not say why.)

In going through his CV, Noakes said that he had 'to some extent started sports science and sports medicine' in South Africa. That was an understatement. Noakes is well known for his generosity of spirit in readily acknowledging the work of others. Among those is former South African rugby captain Morné du Plessis. In the early 1990s, Noakes and Du Plessis teamed up to found the Sports Science Institute of South Africa to fund research into sports performance and to house the laboratories of the UCT/MRC Research Unit for Exercise Science and Sports Medicine (ESSM), which Noakes had helped found and which he directed for 25 years. The application of this research would provide sportspeople of all disciplines with the evidence-based means to improve performance. Noakes and Du Plessis also wanted to use it as a platform to build public interest in the country's top sportspeople and build state pride. They achieved those aims and more.

Noakes listed key aspects of his work and experience spanning decades. This included supervision of the research of PhD and master's students, and his own extensive research in fields ranging from insulin and carbohydrate metabolism (not just glucose, but fructose as well), and cholesterol and triglyceride (blood fats) responses, to the modification of risk factors for heart disease through diet and peripheral artery disease as it relates to T2DM. As far back as 1978, Noakes's areas of scientific exploration at SSISA/ESSM have covered glucose metabolism (glycaemic control), lipid profiles and fat metabolism, and diabetes. All this was decades before his spectacular about-turn on the role of carbohydrates and fats at the end of 2010. His ESSM unit was also one of the first to investigate low-carb diets, including ketosis, for sports performance. In one fell swoop, Noakes decapitated the HPCSA's contention that his scientific knowledge and experience of nutrition was narrow and restricted to adults and athletes.

Noakes spoke eloquently about the effects the HPCSA hearing was having on him and his family. 'I would have done anything in my power to stop [this trial] happening because of the cost to me personally, and to my family,' he said. He choked up when he spoke of his family's support, in particular that of his wife, Marilyn. He also paid tribute to his legal team. (From the outset, Van der Nest and Ramdass had offered their services for free.) 'I wouldn't have got through it without them,' he said. 'It has been a tough time, financially very, very taxing. People just do not understand what the costs of an action like this are.' Noakes's critics gleefully took to social media to claim that he had 'broken down' while giving evidence, and the press picked up and ran with it. That was not true. As Noakes later explained, it was nothing more than cathartic relief that brought him close to tears – the relief of finally being able to speak up for himself and the enduring passion that drives him professionally: the search for scientific truth.

Noakes then outlined the framework within which he would present his evidence. He said that it would include describing his own data, which was 'relatively important to this whole case'. In Chapters 16 and 17, he gives an overview of the rigorous science that he presented in his own defence. Thus, it would be needless repetition here. Instead, I have identified key themes in his evidence and highlighted how he used the science to rebut the HPCSA's case against him.

The public had compared the HPCSA hearing to a modern-day Spanish Inquisition, and Noakes to Galileo. He took up the comparison with dramatic effect, quoting at length from *Galileo's Middle Finger* by American bioethicist Alice Dreger:

> Science and social justice require each other to be healthy, and both are critically important to human freedom. Without a just system, you cannot be free to do science, including science designed to better understand human identity; without science, and especially scientific understandings of human behaviors, you cannot know how to create a sustainably just system ... I have come to understand that the pursuit of evidence is probably the most pressing moral imperative of our time. All of our work as scholars, activists, and citizens of democracy depends on it. Yet it seems that ... we've built up a system in which scientists and social justice advocates are fighting in ways that poison the soil on which both depend. It's high time we think about this mess we've created, about what we're doing to each other and to democracy itself.[1]

Using Dreger, Noakes placed scientific evidence at the heart of the hearing: 'Evidence really is an ethical issue, the most important ethical issue in a modern democracy. If you want justice, you must work for truth. And if you want to work for truth, you must do a little more than wish for justice.'[2]

'You have to look at the totality of the evidence,' Noakes said. 'That's what I am doing. I am a totalist. I have obsessive compulsive disorder with facts. That's why I write like I do. If anyone tells me there's no evidence to support low-carbohydrate diets, I tell them they haven't read the literature.'

Reciting one of his favourite quotes, Noakes said: 'Everyone is entitled to their own opinion, but not to their own set of facts.'

'I tell my students that when a single strand of evidence conflicts with their beliefs, they better start questioning their views,' he said. Only those who refuse to look at the totality of evidence could conclude that his views on LCHF are 'unconventional'.

It was clear from the evidence Noakes presented that he had a dual purpose. He wanted to educate those who had charged him and to demolish the pillars of the charge. Using his natural teaching instincts and chatty style – which held the attention of his 'audience' throughout – he began to reveal why there are so many endocrinologists and cardiologists among his most vociferous critics: he had dared to challenge medical orthodoxy and the industries that had grown up around conventional treatment protocols for obesity, diabetes and heart disease.

In particular, he contradicted the pessimistic outlook of orthodox doctors and dietitians towards T2DM. They see diabetes as a chronic, degenerative condition that increases the risk of heart disease, kidney problems, blindness and amputation. Noakes challenged this thinking, as well as the orthodox medical model that has diabetics taking drugs for the rest of their lives. Optimism in the face of a T2DM diagnosis was a key theme of his evidence. Noakes has never called LCHF a 'cure' for diabetes. He has, however, said that it is a safe, effective and cheap method that can reverse all the symptoms of the condition. It's a matter of semantics, really, and many people around the world who use LCHF to manage their T2DM say that it is as close to a 'cure' for the condition as modern medicine has come thus far.

Noakes's evidence was a powerful mix of the personal and the professional. One of the first slides he presented was a photograph of him and his parents at his graduation in 1981. He had just received his Doctor of Medicine (MD) degree – a PhD equivalent that allowed him to teach and set up a sports-science course at UCT. His father, Reginald 'Bindy' Austin Noakes, had been diagnosed with T2DM a few months earlier. At the time, Reginald also had high blood pressure and other features of IR and the metabolic syndrome. He was the same age then (68) as Noakes is today. Within six years, he would lose his foot from the consequences of diabetic PAD. Within eight years, he would lose both legs and surrender his mind to the disease.

That faded photograph spoke volumes about what drives Noakes as a scientist, a medical doctor and an ordinary mortal: the search for truth and the desire to help people improve their health. It spoke particularly of Noakes's mission to save diabetics from the grim fate that had befallen his father after following orthodox dietary advice. At the time of his father's illness, dietitians and doctors (Noakes included) believed that diabetics needed regular carbohydrates to ensure there was enough glucose for the brain. Noakes did not blame the dietitian, Joan Huskisson, who advised his father. She gave advice that she thought was right at the time. She based her advice on a hypothesis that many doctors and dietitians still hold dear today: when prescribing diets for patients with T2DM, the sole consideration is that the brain requires glucose to function (see Chapter 7). 'This hypothesis is wrong,' said Noakes. The information that Huskisson gave his father was therefore 'utterly and completely false, a wrong assumption that has to lead to the wrong advice'.

Noakes had helped Huskisson to develop teaching in dietetics at UCT. Her advice was the same that experts continue to give diabetics today: eat a low-fat, high-carb diet. Huskisson wrote a book in 1990, funded by SASA, titled *Food: What's In It For You?* She gave Noakes a copy, in which she had inscribed: 'Tim – Thank you very much indeed for the ongoing support! It really is appreciated tremendously ... and No! I don't get royalties for copies sold.' (That highlighted another theme running through the hearing: the sugar industry and its toxic influence on dietary advice.)

In his evidence, Noakes quoted from a more recent book, by South African registered dietitian Hilda Lategan: 'Carbohydrates are an important source of energy in the body and glucose, which is the product of the digestion of carbohydrates ... is the only energy source for the brain ... It is, therefore, crucial for diabetics to include carbohydrate-rich foods at each meal.'[3]

Since his Damascene moment, dietitians have frequently accused Noakes of being antagonistic towards them and dietetics in general, and ADSA in particular. Neither is true. If anything, the HPCSA's witnesses showed that it is ADSA that has a 'beef' with Noakes, not the other way round.

Noakes related how devastated he was when he realised that his father had died not because he was not getting enough glucose to his brain, but because he had disseminated (widespread) arterial disease, which is now recognised as the cornerstone of diabetes. Reginald Noakes would also have had NAFLD, commonly known as 'fatty liver', although no one knew it at the time. Noakes presented robust research showing that high-carbohydrate diets cause NAFLD in people who are insulin resistant/diabetic. He also showed that NAFLD causes blood-fat abnormalities, and that it is these blood-fat abnormalities that, together with high blood insulin levels and inflammation, lead to disseminated arterial disease. Thus, he showed that T2DM is ultimately a condition of progressive, disseminated arterial disease. It progresses over decades, he told the hearing. It leads ultimately to complete obstruction of blood flow to the eyes, kidneys and lower limbs. The consequences couldn't be more severe: blindness, kidney failure and gangrene (and eventually amputation) of the limbs. This same arterial disease can lead to heart attacks and strokes, although these represent a 'fundamentally different process'.

Ultimately, Noakes said, the high-carbohydrate diet killed his father. He spoke with profound sadness about the consequences of not knowing what really ailed his father. If he had known then about NAFLD and its crucial role in T2DM and heart disease, he could have examined his father. 'We would have seen that my father had fatty liver with certain cholesterol abnormalities,' he said. 'These are called lipoprotein abnormalities, which are specific to NAFLD. We could have treated him, because what he needed to do was the opposite of the advice that was given.' Noakes said that hepatologists (liver specialists), and not cardiologists, would probably be the ones to treat heart disease in the future. It was the first of many gauntlets he'd throw to cardiologists in his evidence.

Another theme in Noakes's evidence was the diet-heart hypothesis that saturated fat causes heart disease. The hypothesis, which became a pillar of the HPCSA's case against him, is the platform on which drug companies built the multibillion-dollar statin industry. Statins are cholesterol-lowering drugs. They are also the world's most prescribed drugs. It's an understatement to say that Noakes is no fan of statins. While evidence shows that statins may have some use in secondary prevention (i.e. after a first heart attack or stroke), they don't work well for primary prevention. They also come with a long list of side effects, many severe enough to offset any benefits.

Noakes gave evidence in the hearing to show that the diet-heart hypothesis is currently unproven and therefore, by definition, should be considered unconventional and unscientific. He outlined how the hypothesis had spawned the lipophobia (fear of fat), demonisation of fat (especially saturated fat) and glorification of carbohydrates that began in the late 1970s. He described saturated fat as the victim of possibly the 'biggest scam in the history of modern medicine'.

'Carbs and insulin are driving obesity,' Noakes stated, 'not saturated fat.' When food-makers took saturated fat out of the diet, he said, they had to replace it with something to make food more palatable. That something was sugar and carbohydrates, two highly addictive substances. The consequences for global health have been nothing short of catastrophic: a pandemic of lifestyle diseases.

It is true that heart-attack rates have been falling in some countries since the late 1960s. Some scientists claim that this is proof that the low-fat diet prevents arterial disease. But Noakes offered an alternative explanation in his evidence: a reduction in smoking in these countries has reduced the number of patients experiencing the sudden plaque ruptures that cause heart attacks and strokes, he said. But while fewer people are dying of heart attacks, many more are developing T2DM as a consequence of LFHC diets. The disease burden of arterial disease has therefore simply shifted to the obstructive form found in T2DM. If the low-fat diet really prevented arterial disease, it should also have prevented the now much more prevalent obstructive form found in type-2 diabetics.

'I find it baffling why so many have difficulty understanding this obvious truth,' said Noakes. 'Perhaps it is inconvenient?'

Ironically, when Noakes himself first showed evidence of IR in the 1980s, he was helping drive the establishment of dietetics at UCT. It was only after his Damascene moment that he realised he had missed the signs that he was developing T2DM and that he had always been profoundly insulin resistant. He began to wonder what lay ahead. Would he lose his foot in six years and both legs in eight, as his father had? Would his cognitive functions deteriorate rapidly? His concern was not just personal. 'Diabetes is the biggest challenge we face in the world in medicine,' he told the hearing. 'Insulin resistance, which I have, is the most prevalent medical condition in the world and we do not teach it in our medical schools. That is wrong and that is partly why I am here today.'

In his evidence, Noakes addressed a myth that his critics frequently use to try to discredit him and LCHF. They claim that he only developed T2DM after going on an LCHF diet for three months in 2010, and that therefore the diet caused his condition. For proof, they cite the fact that Noakes still takes medication (metformin) to control his blood sugar. He easily dispatched the argument. It makes no sense, he said, to say that the diet he ate for 33 years did not cause his diabetes, but the one he ate for three months did. Anyone with even a basic knowledge of glucose metabolism knows that it takes years for T2DM to develop. Noakes explained that the reason why he still takes medication despite improving all his symptoms by eating LCHF foods is because he wants perfect blood sugar control. In this way, he hopes to further increase his chances of avoiding the grim fate that befell his father. He therefore chooses to add an appropriate dose of metformin.

Unsurprisingly, the role of dietary carbohydrate was another key theme in Noakes's evidence. He spoke ruefully of the consequences of buying into the prevailing dogma that 'carbohydrates are good for you and the more carbohydrates you have, the better'. He had himself bought into the conventional 'wisdom' that diabetics should eat low-fat diets because they were especially prone to arterial disease. But with his father's death, he had begun to question everything he had learnt in medical school. As a responsible and ethical scientist, Noakes said that he had always looked at what he thought was the totality of evidence; however, he had no idea at the time just how effectively experts in positions of power and influence, with vested interests in food and drug companies, were conspiring to suppress or hide evidence.

Good science was another theme. During his testimony, Noakes readily acknowledged where he had made errors in his research and described how he typically responded. One example was a large methodological error in a study he had co-authored. Titled 'High rates of exogenous carbohydrate oxidation from starch ingested during prolonged exercise', it was published in the *Journal of Applied Physiology* in 1991.[4] Noakes and his co-researchers had used a tracer to measure oxidation that did not track the starch. They therefore came to the wrong conclusions. They wrote a letter to the journal retracting their findings the moment they realised their error. 'The point,' Noakes told the hearing, 'is that if you make an error, you acknowledge it.' At least, that's what ethical scientists do.

Contrast that with the behaviour of the authors of the Naudé review, published in *PLoS ONE* in August 2014.[5] When Noakes and Dr Zoë Harcombe did their own analysis of the Naudé review, they found it to be riddled with so many errors and bias as to undermine its conclusions. After they published their findings in the *SAMJ* in December 2016,[6] the authors of the Naudé review immediately went on the defensive, attacking Noakes and Harcombe in a public statement in the *Cape Times*.[7] When they eventually published an official response in the *SAMJ* in March 2017, they declined to address the errors that Noakes and Harcombe had identified.[8]

The Naudé review was puzzling from the start. There was already a solid Brazilian meta-analysis and review from 2013 to show that very low carb/ketogenic diets were superior to low-fat diets for long-term weight loss.[9] Why had the Naudé review authors felt the need to add another meta-analysis supposedly addressing the same question? And why had the HPCSA and its witnesses used it as evidence against Noakes when it was on adult nutrition, not infant feeding? It lent credence to Noakes's theory that the purpose of the Naudé review was to target him and the growing support for LCHF in South Africa specifically. If true, the research remains suspect from a scientific perspective.

Not one to shy away from his own faults, Noakes told the hearing how, in his earlier research, he had committed a cardinal intellectual error of bias similar to the one that the Naudé-review authors had committed. Just as they had seemingly ignored evidence that did not confirm their beliefs, so, too, had Noakes and his co-authors in a study published in the *Journal of Applied Physiology* in 2006.[10] In a world-first, they compared a group of patients who had carbo-loaded before exercise with a placebo group. They expected the carbo-loaded group to show superior performance, and were surprised when the group showed no benefit when compared with the placebo. The scientifically correct thing to do would have been to acknowledge the null hypothesis and move on. Instead, when he came to write up the study, Noakes tried to explain why their data should have shown the effect they expected. Scientists call that 'hiding or avoiding the null hypothesis', he said, 'but it's just not on. You cannot get around a hypothesis by trying to explain why it did not work, and then saying it should have worked but didn't.'

Looking back on his behaviour, Noakes is embarrassed. 'We were biased,' he said in his evidence. 'We were so convinced that carbohydrates would help those people. We could not get our minds around the idea that actually, maybe, there was something else involved.' It was a measure of the abiding power of conventional 'wisdom' on the role of carbohydrate in the diet that prevailed for more than four decades. 'I wasn't ready [to admit that] in 2006. I only became ready in 2010. At this Damascene moment, I realised that I have been wrong on carbohydrates for 33 years.'

Noakes also illustrated a key point about the scientific method: that scientists don't have to be experts in a research area to come up with new ideas and evidence that impact on it. To that end, he traced how he had reached some of his most influential research conclusions, including how the brain regulates exercise performance. In 1996, he was the first to come up with the idea that the brain protects a person during exercise. Although he did not know too much about how the brain functions, Noakes came up with a model, now accepted in exercise sciences, that during exercise the brain determines performance. His research showed him, eventually, that 'the brain is in control, and the same applies in obesity'. It is the brain that drives obesity, and carbohydrates that drive the addictive behaviours that prevent the brain from controlling appetite and weight.

The key, Noakes said, is to look at the totality of evidence: 'If you look at the totality … if you put it all together, you can come up with the truth.' People miss the truth when they are 'too expert in small areas'. One of his strengths as a scientist, he said, is that he 'understands how the whole body functions, not just the heart, not just the lungs, not just the muscles'. That made him more able to 'put it all together'.

Ketosis and ketogenic diets formed another intriguing theme. The HPCSA's lawyers had only themselves to blame for opening the door for Noakes to introduce compelling evidence on the safety and efficacy of ketogenic diets. They had allowed their witnesses to claim over and over again that Noakes had advised a 'dangerous' ketogenic diet for infants, despite the fact that his tweet made no mention of such diets. And despite the fact that the HPCSA had not charged him with advising a ketogenic diet, dangerous or otherwise. None of the witnesses was an expert on the subject, so why keep bringing it up? As it turned out, there was method in the madness.

In her initial letter of complaint to the HPCSA, Strydom claimed that Noakes had advised 'medical (medical nutrition therapy)' in his tweet. The words made little sense, and so Noakes thought she had left out the word 'advice'. In his letter of response to the HPCSA, he thus wrote: 'Ms Strydom claims that I am "giving incorrect medical advice….that is not evidence based"'. Bhoopchand would later allege that Noakes's addition of the word 'advice' was a tacit acknowledgement that he had given advice, not information; knew that he had acted as a medical doctor, and therefore had a doctor–patient relationship with Leenstra. Noakes and his legal team had no problem undermining all these allegations.

The problem for Strydom was that accusing Noakes of giving 'medical nutrition therapy' in his tweet required significant graft after the fact in order for it to stand up to even the most basic scrutiny. The only relevant treatment remotely resembling medical nutrition therapy at the time was the successful and relatively routine medical use of extreme ketogenic diets to treat epilepsy in cases where drugs had failed. Strydom and the other witnesses therefore had to introduce ketosis and ketogenic diets into evidence if they wanted to connect Noakes's tweet to any sort of 'therapy'.

Noakes has never claimed to be an expert on ketosis and ketogenic diets; however, he has done extensive reading on and research into these diets. He can reasonably claim to be the most knowledgeable person in South Africa on the topic of LCHF in general and ketogenic diets in particular. In his evidence, he presented research to show that ketosis is a natural, benign state. He called it possibly 'the healthiest state there is'. He showed that ketone bodies are an effective fuel source and may also be important for long-term health. He pointed especially to the work of Professor Stephen Cunnane on the importance of ketones for infants' developing brains.[11] Noakes said that infants are born naturally in a state of ketosis. He showed that there is something about breast milk that makes it a 'ketogenic food', despite its relatively high carbohydrate content – along with its high fat content, of course. Researchers are not yet clear why, he said. Furthermore, as much as 25 per cent of the newborn's basic energy requirements in the first several days of life come from the use of ketones. Just as convincing is the finding that the foetus has a capacity to produce its own ketones independent of what its mother provides.

'When you read that, you cannot conclude that ketones are dangerous, toxic or damaging to the infants,' said Noakes. 'The only way you could conclude that ketones were dangerous for infants would be because you did not know the literature. You did not take the effort to go and read the literature as I have, and as we have reported in [*Raising Superheroes*].'

Bhoopchand was likely seeing more yawning chasms opening up in the HPCSA's case. He repeatedly objected to Noakes's evidence, arguing that, 'while interesting', much of it was irrelevant. He also claimed that Noakes was using the hearing as a 'platform' to gain media attention and support for LCHF. 'We have indicated that, we repeat that,' he said to Adams. He 'pleaded' with her and her 'honourable committee' to stop Noakes.

Van der Nest was barely civil in response. 'With all respect to our learned friend, that is outrageous,' he said, before pointing out that Noakes had not asked to be prosecuted. He had not asked to spend two years under a professional cloud, living with significant stress and having to spend a fortune on his own defence. 'Dietitians brought the case against Noakes because he disagreed with them,' Van der Nest said. 'Because he had the temerity to hold a different view to them, they thought he must be prosecuted.'

Looking directly at Bhoopchand, a steely Van der Nest said: 'Do not get upset when you prosecute someone and he puts up a fight. That is the consequence of prosecuting someone for a tweet that was ignored by the so-called patient, Ms Pippa Leenstra. That is why we are here. [Noakes] is the defendant. He is entitled to defend himself to the fullest, and he will.'

After an adjournment, Adams ruled that while the charge against Noakes might seem simple on the surface, it was complex. It made no sense, she said, for the HPCSA to charge Noakes with giving 'unconventional advice' only to deny him the opportunity to give evidence showing that his advice was not unconventional. The committee unanimously agreed, she said, that there was no reason to limit Noakes's constitutional right to defend himself fully.

Noakes went on to address the claim that he had breached official paediatrics guidelines by telling Leenstra to stop breastfeeding. Again, his tweet said nothing about stopping breastfeeding, and the HPCSA had not charged him with giving such advice. Noakes is also well known for endorsing breastfeeding exclusively for the first six months of an infant's life and for as long as possible thereafter. If anything, his tweeted comment about breast milk being 'high fat' and 'very healthy' was a ringing endorsement of breastfeeding. I would have thought even the HPCSA's lawyers and experts could see that.

Noakes spent a large portion of his evidence on another key theme of the case: South Africa's official dietary guidelines, or rather 'misguidelines', as he calls them. As we know, they closely follow the influential Dietary Guidelines for Americans that the US government launched on an unsuspecting public in 1977, with no solid evidence.

Noakes referenced the work of US investigative journalist Nina Teicholz, author of *The Big Fat Surprise*. (She would be another expert witness for Noakes, in October 2016.) The point Teicholz made about the guidelines, he said, is that they simply 'do not make sense ... They do not match up with the science that we have. They are causing so many [health] problems.' So where is the disconnect, he asked, and why is it so enduring?

Noakes also waded into the inappropriate influence of industry on nutrition advice. He added to compelling research from around the globe showing the insidious influence of food companies – especially the sugar and soft-drink industries – on top scientists and academics. Noakes referred to food-industry sponsorship of dietitians' associations worldwide, including ADSA. He described the extensive web of interconnections between vested interests, academia and the HPCSA's expert witnesses. For example, SASA and the SAMRC were funding the upcoming 2016 ADSA annual conference. Dr Muhammad Ali Dhansay works for the SAMRC.

Noakes has never let himself off lightly on the subject of conflicted research. He has openly admitted to receiving funding from SASA, Leppin and Bromor Foods in the past for his research, but that was only until he and his fellow researchers proved that their products did not work and were 'potentially not a good idea'. Unsurprisingly, at that stage he lost funding from the sugar industry as well as from Bromor Foods.

In retrospect, Noakes's evidence in his own defence benefited handsomely from what UK-based author Ian Leslie called the 'prevailing wind' of scientific evidence on sugar. 'We read almost every week of new research into the deleterious effects of sugar on our bodies,' Leslie wrote in *The Guardian* in 2016. 'Sugar has become dietary enemy number one.' [12]

Noakes showed how dietitians' associations and their members globally help food and drug companies to 'health-wash' products. Health-washing is a particularly iniquitous activity in which companies use dietitians to give a veneer of respectability to their products by suggesting their health benefits. An offshoot is what is known as astroturfing, which is just as sinister in intent. In an allusion to fake grass (AstroTurf), astroturfing has a specifically political connotation. In a Content Technologies study guide, Doris A. Graber defines it in terms of political campaigns: 'The goal of such a campaign is to disguise the efforts of a political or commercial entity as an independent public reaction to some political entity – a politician, political group, product, service or event.' [13] In nutrition science, astroturfing denotes campaigns or organisations that claim to act in the consumer's interest when their real aim is to benefit food, soft-drink or drug companies.

Research shows that companies such as Unilever, Nestlé and Coca-Cola have embraced astroturfing to create the impression of genuine, grassroots movements to peddle their corporate agendas. Coca-Cola is a particularly egregious example. Research in 2016 showed that the company spent $118.6 million on health research and partnerships in the US between 2011 and 2015. That included funding for a group criticised for downplaying the role of sugary drinks in obesity. [14]

While it is tempting to finger companies such as Coca-Cola as the sole guilty party, the issue is more complex. As Leslie noted: 'If, as seems increasingly likely, the nutritional advice on which we have relied for 40 years was profoundly flawed, this is not a mistake that can be laid at the door of corporate ogres. Nor can it be passed off as innocuous scientific error ... It suggests instead that this is something the scientists did to themselves – and, consequently, to us.' [15]

Noakes and his expert witnesses picked up on this theme: the active role that scientists themselves have played in dishing up bad dietary advice to the public. In their research, Harcombe, Teicholz and Noakes's third expert witness, New Zealand–based dietitian and academic Dr Caryn Zinn, have highlighted the many interests keen to protect the current guidelines.

Coincidentally (or not), Vorster wrote the 'secret' report that the HPCSA's Fourth Preliminary Committee of Inquiry commissioned and used as evidence to charge Noakes. In his evidence, Noakes easily rebutted all the claims in Vorster's report and said it was a pity that the committee members had not shown it to him before embarking on the prosecution. If they had, the hearing may never have taken place.

It became clear from all the evidence that it was not so much what Noakes had said in his tweet as what he did *not* say that led to his prosecution. In her testimony, Strydom conceded that she 'may have overreacted a little' to the tweet. Vorster and Kruger acknowledged that LCHF aligns closely with paediatric dietary guidelines that promote meat and vegetables as good first foods. However, the South African Food-based Dietary Guidelines also heavily promote cereals and grains – starchy foods – as the basis of most meals for adults and babies older than one year. And while all dietitians profess to support a reduced intake of sugar and other processed carbohydrates, few are prepared to say that sugar has no role in a supposedly healthy, 'balanced' diet.

Therein lies one of the keys to why so many dietitians are so keen to silence Noakes: he and other LCHF experts do not advise cereals and grains, even in their unrefined state.

Most entertaining in Noakes's evidence was his list of all 'the dogs that did not bark' in the case against him. That was a reference to Sir Arthur Conan Doyle's Sherlock Holmes story, *The Adventure of Silver Blaze*. Silver Blaze was a famous racehorse who went missing from his stable the night before a big race. The next day, the body of Silver Blaze's trainer was found in the countryside not far from the stables, the apparent victim of a murder. Holmes solved the case on the basis of a negative fact: that a dog at the stables had not barked on the night that Silver Blaze disappeared. 'That was the curious incident,' said Holmes.

Attorney Mike Skotnicki explains:

> The fact that the dog did not bark when you would expect it to do so while a horse was stolen led Holmes to the conclusion that the evildoer was not a stranger to the dog, but someone the dog recognized and thus would not cause him to bark. Holmes drew a conclusion from a fact (barking) that did not occur, which can be referred to as a 'negative fact', or for the purpose of this discussion, an expected fact absent from the record.[16]

Noakes made the point that the HPCSA hearing included a number of such negative facts.

The first negative fact was the absence of Pippa Leenstra. The person who had asked for the information on Twitter and who had the potential to suffer harm had not involved herself in any way with the prosecution. If Noakes's Tweet had caused harm to either her or her infant, then she should have laid the complaint. But Leenstra had indicated on Twitter and in subsequent media interviews that she had not even followed Noakes's advice.[17] In his evidence, Noakes dismissed outright the charge of having had a doctor–patient relationship with Leenstra. He said that she was a stranger to him. When he tweeted his reply to her question, there was no point at which he considered her to be his patient. Crucially, Noakes said that he interpreted her question to mean that she was simply asking for nutrition information, not medical advice. He pointed out that he had been providing nutrition information on Twitter regularly for years, including on LCHF.

Instead, Strydom had laid the complaint, allegedly on behalf of ADSA. Yet the Tweet could not have caused Strydom any direct harm. From this Noakes deduced that the complaint and subsequent hearing were clearly never about a single tweet. Had the hearing really been about the tweet, Leenstra would have been the key witness, barking very loudly. Instead, her silence was an obvious negative fact. The dogs that don't bark are 'the hardest to hear', Noakes said.

Reading the NSRD blogs on Strydom's business website, Nutritional Solutions, and especially the sentiments expressed by Marlene Ellmer (see Chapter 8), it seemed to Noakes that the real reason for the complaint was the effect of the publication of *The Real Meal Revolution* just three months before the Twitter debacle. *The Real Meal Revolution* was causing huge swathes of the South African public to question the current dietary advice they were receiving and, ultimately, to lose faith in their dietitians. The latter were clearly disgruntled, he said. Strydom's complaint to the HPCSA was therefore driven by a clear conflict of interest – a fact that should have been obvious to the members of the Fourth Preliminary Committee of Inquiry, who were responsible for deciding whether there were grounds to charge Noakes.

The second negative fact was that he was charged with giving unconventional advice on breastfeeding on social media. As mentioned previously, he did not give any information about breastfeeding in his tweet. Rather, he provided an opinion on weaning.

The third negative fact arose from the existence of *Raising Superheroes*, the follow-up book on infant and child nutrition written by Jonno Proudfoot, Bridget Surtees and Noakes. It had been published before the trial commenced in earnest in November 2015, and had even been reviewed by a committee of six ADSA dietitians, including Ellmer and current ADSA president Maryke Gallagher. In *Raising Superheroes*, Noakes wrote extensively on the science behind appropriate approaches to breastfeeding and infant weaning. If the hearing was really about his views on infant weaning, Noakes said, Strydom and the HPCSA should have presented evidence from the book that his advice was dangerous. But they did not, for the simple reason that there is no such evidence. The ADSA dietitians were unable to find fault with the weaning advice he provided in *Raising Superheroes*. The sole criticism they could muster in their book review was revealing:

> The authors clearly criticise the use of baby cereals or grains for children when complementary foods are introduced. It needs to be acknowledged that South Africa is a country with high levels of household food insecurity. Often, families cannot afford or access animal protein and vegetables or fruit daily. In such situations, grains such as oats and millet, appropriately fortified staples, such as maize and brown bread, and commercially produced enriched complementary foods, such as infant cereals, may provide cost-effective food options.[18]

It seemed that Noakes was on trial for refusing to promote an inferior weaning diet to vulnerable South Africans, in particular those who believed they could not afford the 'luxury' of the best possible diet for the future health of their children.

The fourth negative fact was that the most important body of scientific evidence used by Strydom and her team to bring their action against Noakes was not about breastfeeding, or weaning, or children, or even infants. It was the flawed Naudé review that deals exclusively with adult nutrition. That raised the question of what adult nutrition had to do with the initial charge laid against Noakes.

The fifth and final negative fact was that Strydom laid the complaint in February 2014 on the grounds that the LCHF diet was dangerous, especially for infants. But in her testimony in November 2015, Strydom said that 'everybody was waiting for this publication [the Naudé review] because we could not simply go ahead and make [a] statement about Prof. Noakes's hypothesis or diet without looking at the evidence'.

She essentially acknowledged that on 6 February 2014, when she laid the complaint, she had no evidence on which to base her claim that the LCHF diet was dangerous. When the Naudé review was finally published in June 2014, it failed to show that the LCHF diet was either more or less dangerous than the 'isoenergetic balanced diet'. Yet the HPCSA concluded that a negative study in adults provided definitive evidence that the LCHF diet must be harmful to infants.

Noakes's evidence took up the remainder of the February session. Adams adjourned the hearing to Monday 17 October 2016. Noakes concluded his presentation on the first day of the October session, and then spent four days under relentless cross-examination.

Bhoopchand was faced with several dilemmas when he eventually stood up to cross-examine Noakes. One was that he had to undermine the HPCSA's own witnesses' contention that LCHF did not actually conflict with official paediatric dietary guidelines. To do so, he frequently had to defend the indefensible. One was the cost of LCHF foods.

In his evidence, Noakes said that cereals and grains are a major contributor to the obesity epidemic and rising levels of T2DM in children as young as three. He referred witheringly to Vorster's stated rationale for including starchy foods in the dietary guidelines. 'We have to be realists and we have to realise that the poorer communities are eating maize,' she had said. Noakes and other public health experts found that advice shocking. 'These foods are bad for babies' brains,' he said. 'They have no place in diets for infant weaning.'

The Eat Better South Africa campaign has dispelled any notion that LCHF foods are expensive and beyond the reach of the poor, Noakes said. The campaign is an arm of The Noakes Foundation, which he established to do nutrition research independent of strangling vested interests.

When Bhoopchand challenged Noakes's evidence on the affordability of

LCHF foods, suggesting that the alternative was far cheaper, Noakes told him: 'Unfortunately, sir, you are forgetting that if you raise people on maize, there are costs to us, as taxpayers, because what you are producing is a population that is unhealthy. The rates of obesity and diabetes, cancer, hypertension, dementia are rising exponentially and we are paying those costs. Those costs are not included in what we provide to our poor people. If you were to do an analysis of what is the real cost of providing and weaning onto maize, you would discover, sir, that [the conventional LFHC diet] is an incredibly expensive diet.'

Noakes later suggested to me that the ADSA dietitians should perhaps review the ethics of their position. 'Surely our goal should be to ensure that the poor are provided with the best foods to allow their children to escape the poverty trap, and not just accept that it is good enough to provide high-carbohydrate foods to the children of the poor during the first two years of their lives when their greatest need is for a diet providing an abundance of fatty foods with sufficient protein?'

Bhoopchand tried and failed to get Noakes to concede that there was little or no research to show the safety of LCHF diets for infants. He painted himself into a scientific corner, because the same holds true for the safety of conventional LFHC diets. By calling into question the evidence for LCHF for infants, Bhoopchand put the spotlight back on LFHC and opened the door for Noakes to present significant evidence of the ill effects of the LFHC guidelines for infants.

Bhoopchand again tripped himself up trying to force Noakes to concede that he had contravened the HPCSA's rules on ethical conduct for medical professionals on Twitter. The HPCSA does not *have* rules for medical professionals on Twitter or any other social media platform. Bhoopchand even admitted to this, thereby undermining his own argument. He seemed oblivious to the obvious implication that Noakes was being charged with breaching rules that do not exist.

Bhoopchand read at length from the HPCSA's regulations relating to the practise of the health professions, in particular the norms and standards for medical practice. He read from Regulation 237, which contains the regulations defining the scope of the profession of medicine in terms of Section 33(1) of the Health Professions Act. The regulation deems an act pertaining to the medical profession to be 'on the basis of information provided by any person or obtained from him or her in any manner whatsoever, advising such person on his or her physical health status'. Bhoopchand suggested that 'any manner whatsoever' covered what was said on social media.

Noakes vigorously disputed this suggestion. He said that it would have serious implications for doctors and dietitians if everything they said on social media was deemed to be medical advice. It would change the nature of the way they communicated with the public, and would have implications for doctors not just on social media, but also when writing books and giving lectures.

To Bhoopchand's suggestion that he had no 'ethical restraint' in his tweeted communications, Noakes replied: 'Sir, I am a very ethical person and ethics drives what I do. I will follow the ethics that I believe are relevant. The reality is if you act unethically it does not matter if there are any rules, you broke them. Ethics is a way you live, it is a way you practise. You cannot make people ethical [just] by writing rules.'

He continued: 'I have lived my life as a highly ethical person in my medical career, in my scientific career. I have always been ethical and I will continue to be utterly ethical in whatever I do – including my interactions on Twitter. I would be absolutely disgusted with myself if I were to do anything unethical, and that includes anything that were to break the [HPCSA's] rules, whether or not I am practising as a medical doctor.'

Bhoopchand also tried and failed to get Noakes to concede that his tweet to Leenstra was medical advice, not information. Noakes dismissed the idea, saying that doctors and dietitians regularly give out information on and off social media. He argued that the real danger was a lack of information, not access to information. He said Twitter's 'natural democracy' meant that 'what works percolates to the top, what does not work falls to the bottom'.

The problem for Bhoopchand was that, like most of the HPCSA's expert witnesses, he is at best a 'Twitter virgin', at worst a 'Twitterphobe'. It didn't help that Noakes clearly has no fear of the medium. In his evidence, he described Twitter as a 'communication vehicle' that he uses specifically to learn information. For those who are clever about Twitter, it can be 'one of the most powerful ways' to get new scientific information, Noakes said. It is not possible for scientists to stay as up to date on the research as he is without being on Twitter. The future of medicine 'lies on the internet and on social media', he said. It is why the 'power of the anointed' is rapidly giving way to the 'wisdom of the crowds'. If he gave out any wrong or harmful information, social media would expose it within weeks, or even days. Crucially, Noakes said, social media is turning conventional advice into unconventional, incorrect advice. 'That's the key,' he said. The ultimate measure is not whether information is conventional or unconventional: 'It is whether it is right or wrong and the quality of the evidence that supports it.'

Bhoopchand tried changing tack, saying that Noakes, 'as a responsible human being', should have amplified the information he gave Leenstra. In other words, now he was suggesting that Noakes should have tweeted more, not less, information.

Noakes responded with barely disguised irritation: 'Sir, I am a very responsible human being. I am a teacher. I have spent my life, 40 years of it, educating people at my cost – answering emails, answering letters, writing articles, writing books. I have made essentially nothing out of it. I am here to help the public. That is my mission. I have dedicated my life to that. For you to say I am ... being unethical, badly behaved, breaking the ethics of medicine because I do not respond more to one question from this lady, I find that not very helpful, sir.'

Noakes threw the gauntlet back at the establishment: 'There are thousands of doctors and scientists around the world who believe exactly as I do, but that information is hidden and suppressed. The question is why that should be.'

He pointed out that he had been sharing his knowledge in lectures to the public and answering questions from interested people since 1972, without anyone claiming any harm or trying to silence him. 'I don't tell people what to do. I don't prescribe a diet for pregnant mothers or their babies. I simply talk about the biology of obesity, of insulin resistance, carbohydrate ingestion. I explain why a low-carbohydrate diet is the biologically proven diet to eat if one meets any of those other conditions.'

Bhoopchand then suggested that Noakes had brought the hearing on himself by not paying sufficient attention to his reply to Strydom's initial letter of complaint. He also suggested that Noakes wanted to be 'treated differently' because he considered himself to be 'special'.

Gone completely was the smile that usually played around Noakes's lips. 'That is just laughable,' he told Bhoopchand. He quoted from an email from Professor Amaboo Dhai, chair of the Fourth Preliminary Committee of Inquiry, to members of her committee, in which she called the hearing against Noakes a 'high-profile, celebrity case' and said that it should be expedited. The email had been in the file that the defence had obtained in November. It was clear that certain people in positions of power considered Noakes a 'celebrity' and demanded that he be prosecuted for it.

'It is the exact opposite of your suggestion,' Noakes told Bhoopchand.

Bhoopchand then asked Noakes if he was seeing conspiracy where none existed. Noakes said that he believed in truth, not conspiracy theories. Dhai spoke the truth in her email, he said. She used the word 'celebrity'. He asked why Dhai had not called him in to discuss Strydom's complaint. 'Is it a conspiracy? I do not know. I do not care. You used the word. So, I would just put the question back [to you], and say: Is it because I am a celebrity that I am here? That's the exact opposite of your question.'

Bhoopchand sensibly did not press the point any further.

Noakes was upbeat at the end of the cross-examination. Bhoopchand had not extracted a single major concession. Noakes, on the other hand, had presented robust evidence in his own defence. He had knocked down all the pillars of the HPCSA's case and highlighted instances of endemic bias and unfairness in its prosecution of him.

Noakes emphasised the implications of his case for scientists. He called for scientists to be protected, not prosecuted, for their opinions and research. He described himself lyrically as 'just one tiny ray of knowledge in a galaxy of billions of other humans who have their own experiences and their own know-ledge'. His focus, he said, is simply 'to get the people to see billions of bits of information out there and make their own decisions'.

13

The Angels

'Angels can fly directly into the heart of the matter.'
– Author unknown

The public had dubbed them 'Tim's Angels'. Although they weren't really celestial beings, there was something scientifically angelic about the three expert witnesses who flew into Cape Town from three different continents to defend Professor Tim Noakes in October 2016. British obesity researcher and public health nutrition specialist Dr Zoë Harcombe, US science journalist Nina Teicholz, and New Zealand–based nutrition academic Dr Caryn Zinn arrived in South Africa amid a hearing that was growing more Kafkaesque with each session.

In one report on the hearing, I described the Angels as all slender, gorgeous, glamorous women, highly intelligent and packing heavy scientific weaponry. The Twitter trolls didn't like that, and attacked me for being sexist, irresponsible, untrustworthy, unscientific, etc. I was simply stating the obvious. These women are the best advertisements for what they preach and practise – and the benefits of ignoring the conventional LFHC dietary guidelines.

All the Angels have impeccable scientific pedigrees. Harcombe is a Cambridge University graduate in mathematics and economics. She has spent years research-ing nutrition. Her doctoral thesis, on the evidence for the introduction of dietary fat recommendations in the US and the UK in 1977 and 1983 respectively, earned her a letter of commendation as well as a PhD. Her thesis is a fascinating nutrition science 'whodunnit', in which she looks at why the official dietary guidelines in the US, the UK and elsewhere are woefully inadequate, unscientific and yet still persist.

Harcombe co-authored a much-cited meta-analysis in the *BMJ*'s *Open Heart* in 2015, which showed that evidence from RCTs did not support the introduc-tion of the dietary guidelines in the US and the UK in the late 70s and early 80s. 'Dietary recommendations were introduced for 220 million US and 56 million UK citizens by 1983, in the absence of supporting evidence from RCTs,' the authors concluded.[1] Harcombe followed that meta-analysis with another in the *British Journal of Sports Medicine* in 2016, showing that evidence from prospective cohort studies does not support current dietary fat guidelines.[2] She has also authored many books, among them *The Obesity Epidemic.*

Teicholz took pre-med courses at both Yale and Stanford, graduating from the latter with a major in American studies. She also has an MPhil from Oxford University in the UK, and was the first journalist elected to Phi Tau Sigma, the elite American honour society for food science and technology. She is best known as the author of the international bestseller *The Big Fat Surprise: Why Butter, Meat and Cheese Belong in a Healthy Diet,* which is widely acknowledged by doctors and scientists as a seminal contribution to the understanding of nutrition and disease, and the politics of nutritional science. In her book, Teicholz documents the, personalities, politics and history of nutrition science, and shows how the belief that dietary fat, especially saturated fat, causes heart disease was enshrined in the public consciousness in English-speaking countries by health authorities. *The Big Fat Surprise* is the first mainstream publication to argue that saturated fats – found in dairy, meat and eggs – do not cause disease and can actually be considered healthy.

So influential has Teicholz become that in 2015 the Canadian senate invited her to give an hour of testimony on the findings of her book to its committee charged with overseeing the country's dietary guidelines. Some months later, the committee announced that the dietary guidelines would need a complete overhaul – a process that is now well underway. The USDA followed suit in 2016, inviting Teicholz to give testimony on how to improve nutrition policy. She also helped convince the United States Congress that it needed a formal peer review of America's dietary guidelines. The National Academy of Medicine began this review in 2016.

Zinn calls herself a 'proudly South African Kiwi'. She is a senior lecturer at the Auckland University of Technology Faculty of Health and Environmental Sciences and a registered dietitian and director of a private practice. She graduated from UCT with an honour's degree in nutrition and dietetics. She also has a master's degree in sports nutrition and a doctorate in weight loss from AUT. While she is an expert in sports nutrition and LCHF for optimum athletic performance, Zinn specialises in 'diabesity', a term coined by doctors for the twin global epidemics of diabetes and obesity.

With more than 21 years' experience as a nutritionist and registered dietitian, Zinn's views on diet have evolved alongside the research and science of nutrition. Many experts have 'got it all wrong with existing high-carb, low-fat guidelines', she says. Zinn is a 'whole-food' advocate. She believes that everyone can benefit from eating foods that are lower in carbohydrate and higher in healthy fat than the current guidelines recommend. She has done ground-breaking work on hyperinsulinaemia,[3] an under-recognised, poorly diagnosed but highly prevalent condition, which a low-carb diet can alleviate. She has also co-authored books on nutrition with New Zealand nutrition scientist Professor Grant Schofield, including *What The Fat? Fat's IN, Sugar's OUT*.

All of Tim's Angels had relevant expertise in all the issues pertaining to the case against Noakes. Despite this – or perhaps because of it – the HPCSA's legal team did its best to clip their wings and prevent them from appearing before the Professional Conduct Committee.

When I heard that the defence was applying to add Harcombe and Teicholz to their list of experts (Zinn had been on the list from the start), I emailed the HPCSA to ask if there would be an objection and on what grounds. As usual, they stayed resolutely mum. The instructing attorney, Katlego Mmuoe, politely declined to answer my questions. I wasn't all that surprised to learn later that Mmuoe had refused a written request from Noakes's legal team prior to the October session to allow the Angels to appear. Thus, when the hearing resumed on Monday 17 October, the HPCSA wasted most of that first day trying to block the defence's application.

Bhoopchand put up a spirited fight that added to the impression of ferocity with which the HPCSA was prosecuting Noakes. Up until now, the defence had called only one witness: Noakes himself. The HPCSA had called six. While Noakes did have 'two hats on', as Bhoopchand noted, giving both factual and expert testimony, he was still just one witness. One might reasonably have thought that, on the grounds of fairness alone, the HPCSA would have agreed to Tim's Angels beforehand. After all, six against four were still favourable odds, and there would have been some benefit in being seen to be reasonable for once. But perhaps the HPCSA realised just how big a threat the three women posed to its case.

In his vociferous objection to the inclusion of Harcombe and Teicholz, Bhoopchand used a shotgun approach to cover as much ground as he could. That included attempting to block any new evidence Noakes wanted to introduce (at this point, Noakes was still giving evidence). Bhoopchand's first major objection was procedural. He claimed that Noakes was introducing new and old evidence and witnesses too late in the proceedings. He said – ironically, given the HPCSA's well-documented delaying tactics and their own inclusion of last-minute witnesses – that this would 'cause delays' that would prejudice both Noakes and the HPCSA.

Bhoopchand likened Noakes's evidence to a 'deluge' and contended that the burden of evidence was so heavy that he would not be able to conduct a proper cross-examination. I didn't think it was so smart of Bhoopchand to suggest that he wasn't up to the job of cross-examining Noakes.

His major objection to Harcombe's and Teicholz's evidence had to do with relevance. The inclusion of Teicholz, in particular, rankled him. 'What my colleagues didn't tell me is that she's a *journalist*,' he said with emphasis, before adding with even heavier emphasis, '*an investigative journalist*.' She writes books about science 'in layman's terms', he observed. He completely ignored Teicholz's academic qualifications, as well as the acknowledged scientific content of her book, *The Big Fat Surprise*.

'Breathe deeply,' Van der Nest muttered audibly to himself as he rose to challenge Bhoopchand's objections. Portraying Teicholz as 'only a journalist' was an insult to a witness who had spent time at Yale, Stanford and Oxford, Van der Nest said. What was 'particularly egregious', however, was Bhoopchand's objection on the basis of relevance. He had clearly not read *The Big Fat Surprise* or Harcombe's doctoral thesis. 'I'll bet folding money on it,' Van der Nest said, adding, 'You can only say something is irrelevant if you have read it.' Bhoopchand remained silent at that suggestion.

Van der Nest also pointed out that the HPCSA's duty was 'not to secure a conviction', but rather to assist its Professional Conduct Committee in determining the truth. Hearing all relevant evidence was crucial to that process. Ramdass would later describe as 'unfathomable' Bhoopchand's argument that the evidence of Teicholz and Harcombe was irrelevant.

In the end, the Professional Conduct Committee agreed with the defence. The chair, Advocate Joan Adams, gave a short and concise ruling, using the HPCSA's own actions and statements in calling surprise witnesses to rebut their arguments. She pointed out that just as the HPCSA had argued for new evidence and new witnesses on the grounds of PAJA, so Noakes had the same right. '[He] is quite entitled to call witnesses, including expert witnesses, to submit background documentation and to lead evidence on certain documentation, in order to assist him to conduct a proper defence in this matter,' she said. 'This is his constitutional right and also his right in terms of [PAJA].' The committee then ruled unanimously that Noakes be allowed to call his Angels.

On the afternoon of Friday 21 October, with Noakes's evidence and relentless cross-examination now over, Zoë Harcombe embarked on the ritual slaughter of many nutrition sacred cows. She based the first part of her testimony on her PhD thesis, which focused on the lack of an evidence-base for the US and UK dietary guidelines. She pre-empted cross-examination by emphasising the direct relevance for South Africa, which closely follows the US guidelines.

Although the charge against Noakes made no mention of the guidelines, the HPCSA had made it clear that, in promoting LCHF, Noakes had gone against the country's guidelines and was therefore guilty of giving 'unconventional advice'. Harcombe said that she had researched South Africa's guidelines for all ages to see how closely they related to the US dietary guidelines. South Africa's paediatric guidelines, she said, are 'very good in relation to the rest of the adult guidelines'. She showed how Noakes's tweet aligned closely with South Africa's paediatric guidelines. The HPCSA's own expert witnesses had conceded as much under cross-examination, Harcombe said. Thus, his advice could not be considered unconventional, unprofessional or dangerous, as witnesses had suggested.

Keeping with the paediatric guidelines, Harcombe said they contained one problematic element in that they recommended starchy foods as key complementary foods for infants. 'Without that, it would be excellent advice for infants aged 12 to 36 months,' she said. In Harcombe's opinion, the introduction of starchy foods was unnecessary. Every time people eat starchy foods, she explained, they miss the opportunity to eat more nutrient-dense foods. And that exacerbates the risk of childhood obesity.

Harcombe spent much of her evidence on the currently unproven diet-heart hypothesis that saturated fat causes heart disease. In particular, she looked at South Africa's dietary fat guideline to determine if it still advises a total fat limit of no more than 30 per cent. It does. That advice still 'prevails across the world despite the fact that there has never been any evidence for that guideline'. She told the hearing that there is still extensive ignorance about cholesterol. Humans make cholesterol for good reason, she said. It is therefore 'probably not a good idea to be replacing it with a cholesterol that is intended for plants', as South Africa's guidelines recommend. Harcombe explained that there is a mechanism by which some plants can lower cholesterol, but commented: 'Please do not necessarily assume that to be a good thing.'

'Ignorance' is probably the best word to describe public opinion on dietary fat, Harcombe said. She gave the hearing a mini lecture on the composition of fats, explaining that there are three 'real' fats: saturated, monounsaturated and polyunsaturated. All foods that contain fat – olives, avocados, meat, fish, eggs, dairy, etc. – contain all three types, no exceptions. Only dairy products have more saturated than unsaturated fat – 'not that any real fat is better or worse than any other', she said. Ironically, red meat has far less saturated fat than oily fish and even olive oil, yet the experts still tell people to avoid eating red meat. They also regularly give messages that seem to suggest that it's possible to avoid saturated fat, for example, and increase consumption of polyunsaturated fat, Harcombe said. This is especially the case with recommendations to replace animal fats with vegetable oils or fats.

'It becomes a very complex exercise to try and swap some of them out,' Harcombe said. The only really hazardous fat that is truly unfit for human consumption is trans fat, she said. Trans fatty acids, or trans fats as they are more commonly known, are artificial industrial fats. They are created in a process that adds hydrogen to liquid vegetable oils to make them more solid (see Chapter 7).

Under cross-examination, Bhoopchand suggested that Harcombe had erred by not pointing out the fact that trans fats occur naturally in dairy and meat from grass-fed ruminants. Harcombe said that she took it for granted that experts would know that. She also drew attention to the important distinction between traces of naturally occurring trans fats in ruminants versus industrially produced trans fatty acids on a much larger scale, as she had previously clarified.

Harcombe gave another mini lecture on macro- and micronutrients and the constituents of nutrient-dense, 'real' foods. Real foods became a recurring theme in the Angels' evidence. There is only one food that is 100 per cent carbohydrate, Harcombe said, and that's sucrose (a type of sugar). Sucrose is arguably not even a food, as it has no nutritional value whatsoever. At the other extreme are foods that are 100 per cent fat, such as oils and lards. Every other food we come across, said Harcombe, has protein, whether it is of animal or plant origin.

'Nature makes foods either fat- or carbohydrate-based. Rarely does it put the two together,' she said. It is therefore unhelpful to set targets for macronutrients because, inevitably, when you set a limit of 30 per cent fat, you also set the recommendation of 55 per cent carbs. Instead, Harcombe said it would be more helpful if experts gave the same advice that Noakes gives: 'Just tell people to eat real food.'

Harcombe's armoury for undermining the evidence-base for 'conventional' dietary advice in South Africa was extensive. She used data from her meta-analysis published in *Open Heart* in 2015 to show that there was no evidence from RCTs at the time the US government introduced its guidelines to 264 million Americans.[4] There was still no evidence when the UK and most other English-speaking countries, including South Africa, slavishly followed suit. The UK essentially did a 'U-turn in dietary guidelines', Harcombe said. In 1969, the advice was to avoid fattening farinaceous (starchy) foods. In 1983, people were told to base their meals on these foods.

'So we move from the position of understanding starchy and sugary foods to be fattening to essentially "base your meal on starchy foods",' Harcombe said. She pointed out that this advice is a key theme running through the South African Food-based Dietary Guidelines for all ages. North-West University professor Hester Vorster, for example, admitted in her evidence that she wrote the guideline to 'make starchy foods the basis of all meals', but was unable to provide robust evidence for the recommendation.

The British and South African guidelines followed the American advice to restrict total fat intake to no more than 30 per cent of calorie intake, and saturated fat to no more than 10 per cent. The recommendation to increase carbohydrate content was an inevitable consequence of setting that dietary fat limitation, Harcombe argued. And the 'inevitable' negative consequences for health have been rising rates of obesity, diabetes and heart disease.

Harcombe looked at epidemiological evidence available when the dietary fat guidelines were introduced four decades ago. At the time, she said, research showed merely an *association* to indicate benefit. Some experts interpreted it according to the calories-in, calories-out model of obesity: that obesity is the result of gluttony and sloth, and that people just eat too much and move too little. Harcombe explained in detail why CICO is an inadequate model, not least because it contradicts one of the laws of thermodynamics. Tongue-in-cheek, she quoted US science writer Gary Taubes: 'We woke up somewhere around this point and decided to become greedy and lazy. We had managed to stay slim for three and a half million years, but suddenly 30 per cent of us became obese and almost 70 per cent of us overweight or obese.'

The reality, Harcombe said, is that since the guidelines were introduced, obesity has more than doubled and diabetes has increased sevenfold in the US. In the UK, obesity has increased almost tenfold, and diabetes four- to fivefold. Referring to South Africa's sky-rocketing obesity rates in the wake of the official dietary guidelines, Harcombe wrote at the end of her thesis that this 'at least deserves examination'.

'We are failing our populations if we do not look at the association between obesity and diabetes and the introduction of those dietary guidelines,' Harcombe told the hearing. If anyone is giving unconventional, unscientific advice, she said, it is not Noakes. It is more likely those who slavishly recommend the country's food-based dietary guidelines to people with obesity, diabetes, heart disease and other serious health issues.

Harcombe also raised the issue of compromising links between food industries and ADSA and its former president, registered dietitian Claire Julsing Strydom. Under cross-examination, Bhoopchand asked Harcombe for proof of her contention that ADSA was conflicted. Harcombe had evidence at her fingertips; she showed a slide of the association's long list of sponsors, which have included Nestlé, Unilever, the sugar industry and Coca-Cola. ADSA executives deny any influence from sponsors. Harcombe, Teicholz and many others have pointed out that – just like drug companies – food companies don't sponsor organisations that don't promote their products.

Harcombe went on to review and thoroughly undermine the Seven Countries Study, Dr Ancel Keys's seminal study underpinning the US dietary guidelines. Keys's own data did not support his conclusions about the link between dietary fat and coronary heart disease, Harcombe said. 'The dietary information in the Seven Countries Study is scant,' she noted. Keys also erred by not considering factors such as cigarette-smoking, sedentary behaviour, obesity and relative weight in people with CHD. Furthermore, the Seven Countries Study wasn't even a dietary study, although Keys presented it as such. And as an inter-country study it provided 'the lowest form of evidence'. Still, Keys concluded that saturated fat was linked to increased risk for heart disease.

The problem with Keys, Harcombe said, was his bias from the outset. One of the consequences of that bias was the statins industry. The diet-heart hypothesis created the conditions for statins to become the most prescribed drug in modern medicine, and earned the pharmaceutical companies that make them billions of dollars, despite compelling evidence of their inherent risks. In her testimony, Harcombe said that statins are 'one of the biggest crimes against humanity that the pharmaceutical industry has unleashed'.

Perhaps Harcombe's most startling contribution to Noakes's defence was her investigation into the Naudé review, which had concluded that low-carb diets were no better for weight loss than conventional, LFHC 'balanced' diets. Harcombe told the hearing that she and Noakes had done their own analysis of the Naudé review, due for publication in the *SAMJ* in December 2016.[5] They had found the review to be littered with errors, many of them material. While admittedly they had only re-examined one part of the Naudé review, given the amount of errors in that section alone, she and Noakes believed that it was unlikely that the conclusions were robust.

Noakes and Harcombe's findings raised troubling questions that continue to swirl around the Naudé review to this day. How is it possible that so many researchers from top South African universities could make so many mistakes in one study? Were these honest mistakes, or was there 'mischief' behind the errors?

Harcombe said that, among other errors, the researchers had included studies that failed their own inclusion criteria; used invalid and subjective meta-analysis sub-groupings; and repeatedly extracted data inaccurately. One instance of data extraction was so erroneous that Harcombe called it 'absurd', another 'inexplicable'.

A major limitation of the meta-analysis, Harcombe said, was that the authors claimed to have reviewed evidence for low-carb diets, but had not in fact done so. Put another way, she said, they could not judge low-carb diets because they did not study them. For example, the average dietary intake for 14 of the studies used was 35 per cent carbohydrate, 35 per cent fat and 30 per cent protein. That's very different from the 5 to 10 per cent carbohydrate and 80 to 85 per cent fat of an accepted, effective LCHF diet to treat or prevent obesity, diabetes and heart disease.

The Naudé review also set isocaloric (having similar caloric values) as a criterion. This negated the satiety advantage of low-carb diets. Satiety (the feeling of fullness) is a key effect of the low-carb diet despite a reduced energy intake. The researchers would therefore have had to restrict the caloric intake voluntarily of subjects on the control diet to match this effect.

In the background to the study, the review's authors referred to 'some weight loss diets widely promoted through the media', but named only one: the Atkins diet. They said that these diets 'recommend a regimen greatly restricting carbohydrates, with increased protein and unrestricted total and saturated fat intake'. This is simply untrue. Most low-carb diets don't advise unrestricted total and saturated fat intake; they cap it. 'It is plausible that these low CHO diets could be harmful, especially over the longer term,' the authors concluded in the background to the review. They gave references, but nothing that stood up to Harcombe and Noakes's independent scrutiny.

Harcombe said that, based on their own data, the researchers could just as easily have concluded that a 'balanced' (high-carb) diet was no better than a low-carb diet for producing weight loss. If the researchers were to redo their research properly, she said, without all the errors, they would have to draw a very different conclusion – namely, that the low-carb diet worked better than the (LFHC) control diet for weight loss.

Harcombe was scathing about the media's coverage of the Naudé review. While the review's authors made no mention of LCHF, Banting or Noakes, media reports quoting a press release claimed that the Naudé review effectively 'debunked the Banting diet' – and Noakes. Some reports personalised the message, referring to Noakes as a 'celebrity professor' and stating that the review proved that 'Noakes's low-carb diet is not healthier'. Others quoted HSFSA CEO Dr Vash Mungal-Singh saying: 'The current evidence means we cannot recommend a low-carbohydrate diet to the public.'

Harcombe said it was absurd, impactful and potentially harmful to claim that the review debunked Banting when it didn't even study Banting diets. In her opinion, the entire episode – the Naudé review, the accompanying press release and the media coverage that followed – was 'personal, unprofessional and, on examination, it was flawed'.

Noakes and Harcombe were not alone in raising questions about how the study got through peer review. Some said it signalled a deep rot in the process. Concerns about peer review are not new. In 2006, former *BMJ* editor Dr Richard Smith condemned the process in the *Journal of the Royal Society of Medicine*, saying that there is little evidence on the effectiveness of peer review, but considerable evidence on its defects. 'In addition to being poor at detecting gross defects and almost useless for detecting fraud,' he wrote, 'it is slow, expensive, profligate of academic time, highly subjective, something of a lottery, prone to bias, and easily abused.'[6]

In cross-examination, Bhoopchand attempted to undermine Harcombe's expertise. He suggested, for example, that she was not qualified to comment on statins, since she was neither a cardiologist nor any other kind of medical doctor. Harcombe easily deflected his objection, saying that part of the problem was that cardiologists and other doctors had little knowledge or training in nutrition. If they did, they would be better able to understand all the research pointing to the risks outweighing the benefits of statin use.

In particular, Bhoopchand tried to undermine the impact of Harcombe's devastating critique of the Naudé review, likely on instruction from Senekal, one of the study's co-authors and a consultant to the HPCSA in its case against

Noakes. Senekal was present through all the defence's evidence. When she wasn't staring stonily in Harcombe's direction, she was vigorously chewing gum and shaking her head. She scribbled notes throughout, which she passed to Bhoopchand, who referred to them repeatedly during cross-examination.

Bhoopchand's questions thus revealed what was probably Senekal's growing fury at Harcombe and Noakes. At one point, Bhoopchand asked Harcombe whether, as 'a question of collegiality', she had known that her critique of the Naudé review would cause 'some embarrassment to the University of Stellenbosch'. He seemed to be suggesting that the researchers' potential embarrassment should have stopped her and Noakes from going public with their findings. Bhoopchand asked Harcombe whether she should have 'at least elicited some response from at least the first author to that particular study'.

Harcombe responded that she was not aware that the authors had given Noakes the same privilege, prompting Bhoopchand to ask her if it was a case of 'an eye for an eye'. Looking him straight in the eye, Harcombe said: 'No, not at all, sir. I looked at the [Naudé review] and it was not robust. So I reported it as such.'

Harcombe made no major concessions under cross-examination on any issue, and especially not on her critique of the Naudé review. Yet in their first response to Noakes and Harcombe's re-analysis a week after its publication in December 2016, the review's authors claimed that all the 'numerous criticisms' had been 'addressed' during cross-examination at the hearing in October, and that Harcombe had 'conceded more than seven times' that the errors 'were in fact not material to the findings of [the] review'.[7]

It was as if they had attended a completely different hearing. I emailed the authors to suggest that someone must have given them the wrong information. They could look at the transcript to see for themselves, or they could ask Senekal for the facts, as she was present throughout. Celeste Naudé replied to say she was out of town and would get back to me. She never did, and I heard not a word from the other authors either.

In their official response to Noakes and Harcombe in the *SAMJ* in March 2017, Naudé and her co-authors basically rubbished the findings and suggested that Noakes and Harcombe had themselves erred and shown a 'lack of understanding of current methods in evidence synthesis'.[8] The Naudé-review authors appeared to have taken a leaf out of US President Donald Trump's strategy book. They were hiding behind alternative facts and creating fake news.

Noakes and Harcombe held nothing back in a rebuttal letter to the *SAMJ* in May 2017, titled 'Naude *et al.* avoid answering the essential question: Mistake or mischief?':

It is common cause that the Naude/Stellenbosch University/University of Cape Town meta-analysis played a decisive role in the multimillion rand prosecution of Prof. T Noakes by the Health Professions Council of South Africa ... Without the 'correct conclusion' from this meta-analysis, it is possible that the HPCSA trial against Noakes might never have happened. Therefore, the importance of the Naude et al. meta-analysis extends far beyond any role purely as a neutral scientific publication.

Had we realised the disproportionate consideration given to this ostensibly innocuous publication in the HPCSA trial, we would have examined it sooner.[9]

Noakes and Harcombe concluded: '... we may never receive an answer to our research question: was this mistake or mischief?' They were essentially accusing researchers from two of South Africa's top universities of scientific fraud and colluding with ADSA and the HPCSA to silence him. If that accusation is not shocking enough, the response of all the universities involved, and at the highest levels, has been even more surprising and telling. They have closed ranks and protected their academics.

Bhoopchand had nothing to say about Harcombe's vision of a way forward for public-health nutrition advice in future. She referred to the HPCSA's own 'Ethical rules of conduct for practitioners registered under the Health Professions Act, 1974'. Schedule 27A(d) states that a practitioner shall, at all times, 'provide *adequate information* about the patient's diagnosis, treatment options *and alternatives* ... and any other pertinent information to enable the patient to *exercise a choice* in terms of treatment and *informed decision-making* pertaining to his or her health and that of others' (Harcombe's emphasis).

This, Harcombe said, brings practitioners back to 'advising real food'. One obstacle is that many so-called experts still confuse saturated fatty acids with processed foods, she said, before listing the primary sources of saturated fat in the American diet as pizza, desserts, sweets, tacos and ready meals. These are not real foods, she said. If those preaching conventional 'wisdom' would just tell people not to eat processed, junk foods, 'we could find agreement. But call it what it is. Stop calling it saturated fat, because it is predominantly junk.'

Harcombe also stated that dietitians' associations globally should not have any compromising links with the food industry. 'It is difficult to embrace wholeheartedly the concept of real food when your sponsors include cereal companies and sugar companies and makers of polyunsaturated products,' she said. 'It is inevitably going to lead you towards demonising real food and favouring those processed foods. But if we can get that conflict out of the way, surely we can agree on real food, and the only-then valid nutritional debate the world should be having is, what should that real food be?'

Harcombe concluded by saying that health professionals in South Africa have an ethical and professional duty to share the fact that ADSA's advice is conflicted because of the association's links with the food and drug industries. They also have a responsibility to share the facts that the most nutritious foods are of animal origin, and are naturally low in carbohydrates and high in healthy fats. Health professionals act professionally and ethically when they give patients all relevant information and options so that they can make informed choices, Harcombe said.

Nina Teicholz was up next. Her mission: to explode as many fat bombs as possible. In the course of her evidence, she dispelled myths and misconceptions about the role of carbohydrates and fats – especially saturated fats – in a healthy diet. Like Harcombe before her, she effectively undermined the foundations of the HPCSA's charge against Noakes. Teicholz based her evidence on her ground-breaking book, *The Big Fat Surprise*, published in 2014. The fruits of nearly a decade of research into the surprisingly murky world of nutrition science, *The Economist* called it a 'nutrition thriller'. It is indeed a fascinating forensic journey into a field influenced by politics and corporations, and characterised by scientific one-upmanship. In the book, Teicholz analyses the last 50 years of nutrition policy in the US as it relates to dietary fat and cholesterol, and reveals how an idea about fat and health became official policy despite all the evidence contradicting it. She exposes the policies, personalities, politics and industries behind the construction, implementation and maintenance of the US dietary guidelines, which have been emulated the world over.

The Big Fat Surprise focuses on the pillar of those guidelines – and the case against Noakes: the diet-heart hypothesis that saturated fat and cholesterol cause heart disease. As we have seen, this hypothesis is at the heart of 'conventional' nutrition advice, not just for cardiovascular health, but also for the treatment and prevention of obesity, diabetes and a host of other illnesses. In the book, Teicholz demolishes the belief that saturated fat causes heart disease, and shows the opposite to be true. She presented evidence that low-fat diets actually increase the risk of cardiovascular disease. In her testimony, Teicholz thus sabotaged an important part of the HPCSA's case.

She also noted that the US Dietary Guidelines Advisory Committee had drawn attention to the harmful effects of the low-fat diet in its most recent report by warning that low-fat diets cause atherogenic dyslipidaemia (one of the major components of the metabolic syndrome, characterised by elevated levels of LDL and low levels of HDL cholesterol). The US dietary guidelines no longer include any official language about limiting total fat intake, and in the latest guidelines, cholesterol is 'no longer a nutrient of concern'.

'The low-fat diet is over,' Teicholz declared. Not only does this diet appear to cause heart disease, but in clinical trials on more than 52 000 people, the low-fat diet was shown to be 'ineffective in fighting any other kind of chronic disease', she said. Yet the demonisation of saturated fat in South Africa's official dietary guidelines continues.

Teicholz also presented evidence to show that low-fat diets deprive infants and children of the vital dietary fats needed to absorb vitamins and other nutrients during their most formative years. This effectively undermined the claim of the HPCSA's expert witnesses that Noakes's advice to a breastfeeding mother was potentially 'dangerous'. It wasn't difficult to work out who Teicholz believed was dishing out dangerous advice for infant weaning. She used robust science to finger the usual suspects, including Strydom, Vorster, Kruger and Dhansay.

Teicholz recounted for the hearing how her nutrition journey began: with an investigation into trans fats for food magazine *Gourmet* in 2004. This assignment introduced her to the 'world of fat', she said. 'Fat is what we obsess most about in nutrition – how much fat to eat, what fat, good fat, bad fat, low-fat, non-fat.' During her research, she began to realise that everything she thought she knew about dietary fat was wrong, and that US nutrition policy was 'completely upside down and backwards as to what we should be eating'. She demonstrated that the same is true of South Africa's official nutrition policy.

One of the strengths of her book, and thus of her evidence for Noakes, is that Teicholz did not rely on summary statements or review papers in her research. Instead, she went back to all the original papers, and sometimes to the original data. In many cases, she found that scientists had tried to hide their data, sometimes even publishing it in foreign-language publications to make it more difficult to access. Teicholz hunted those down too, and found professionals to translate them for her. She attended conferences and interviewed hundreds of top scientists from all over the world, as well as many leading food-industry executives.

Teicholz described how she was met with silence in unexpected places when asking certain questions. Interview subjects would say 'I can't talk about fat' and abruptly end the conversation. She said that sometimes experts were so reluctant to talk that she felt as if she were 'investigating the Mob'. The analogy is not inappropriate, as the case against Noakes has shown.

Besides showing the diet-heart hypothesis to be false, Teicholz's book addresses *how* it became enshrined as truth in the public consciousness. Like any idea, the diet-heart hypothesis was born in 'a moment in time', Teicholz said at the hearing. It began in the US in the 1950s, when there was 'rising panic over the increase in heart disease that had come from seemingly out of nowhere in the early 1900s'. Competing explanations for heart disease ranged from vitamin deficiency to vehicle exhaust fumes and an increasingly stressful lifestyle. Ancel Keys didn't buy into any of these.

There are various theories about how history unfolds, Teicholz said. One is that history is controlled by sociological forces ('guns, germs and steel'). Another, called the 'Great Man' theory, postulates that history is formed by powerful personalities. In the history of nutrition science, said Teicholz, Keys was one such person. As a man with a unique and forceful personality, an unwavering faith in his own beliefs and an 'indomitable will', Keys would virtually 'argue people to death'. In her characteristically measured style, Teicholz said it was fair to say that Keys was always 'more interested in being right than in being a good scientist'. Less diplomatic critics have called Keys a ruthless, arrogant bully.

By the mid-1950s, Keys was convinced that saturated fat caused heart disease. He believed that saturated fat and dietary cholesterol raised blood cholesterol levels, and that increased blood cholesterol clogged arteries, ultimately causing heart attacks. He called his theory the diet-heart hypothesis and endeavoured to make it a pillar of the US dietary guidelines. Teicholz described the circuitous route Keys took to get there. In 1950s America, the only group providing advice on lifestyle habits to avoid a heart attack was the American Heart Association. Fat did not feature among the foods to avoid. In fact, the AHA even warned against pulling the trigger on fat too soon, based on incomplete evidence.

In 1960, an AHA position paper castigated scientists – presumably Keys – for taking 'uncompromising stands based on evidence that does not stand up under critical examination'. Undeterred, Keys and a close colleague, Jeremiah Stamler, got themselves appointed to the AHA's nutrition committee. Within a year, through sheer force of personality, Keys had implanted his diet-heart hypothesis into the AHA, where it still beats strongly today, as it does in heart foundations all over the world, including in South Africa.

In 1961, the AHA began advising men not to eat saturated fat and dietary cholesterol. It was a world first, Teicholz said, telling people to avoid saturated fat and cholesterol in order to prevent heart attack. 'This was where it was all born.' From there, the advice spread around the globe. The AHA told people to reduce their consumption of meat, full-fat dairy and eggs; to switch to margarine instead of butter; and to use vegetable oils instead of ancient fats such as lard and tallow. It advised people to cut back on animal-based foods in general and to switch to plant-based foods, mainly grains.

This advice was hardly logical when one considered the trends in fat consumption at the time, Teicholz said. She showed how consumption of animal fat was already dropping in the US in the 1960s when the AHA made their pronouncements. At the same time, and since the early 1900s, the consumption of polyunsaturated vegetable oils had dramatically increased. This rise 'perfectly paralleled' the rising heart-disease rates, she said.

Teicholz challenged the validity of the conventional dietary recommendation that polyunsaturated vegetable oils, such as soybean, corn and sunflower oils, are beneficial for health. Strydom and the HPCSA's expert witnesses all actively promote vegetable oils as healthy components of a 'balanced' diet. Noakes and the Angels' evidence to the contrary suggested that this was another reason for the HPCSA's case against him. The vegetable-oil industry is a powerful and influential lobby worldwide. It isn't about to give up its lucrative cash cow without a fight.

Teicholz showed that these oils did not even exist as foodstuffs until 1911, the year in which industry introduced the first vegetable-oil food product. Consumers in the US knew it as Crisco, a hardened form of vegetable oil that was meant to replace lard. Research going back to the 1950s documents a long list of adverse health effects from these oils, including increased rates of cancer and inflammation. Still, Keys's beliefs about fats prevailed. In 1961, he even featured on the cover of *Time* magazine as 'the most important nutrition scientist of the 20th century'.

Teicholz spent much of her evidence describing how Keys came up with the diet-heart hypothesis and how he then needed research data to support it. As Harcombe had done, she showed how fatally flawed his Seven Countries Study was from the start, because he had cherry-picked the countries that were included. Good science, she said, requires randomisation – a way of selecting things randomly to avoid bias. In selecting countries for his study, Keys did not use randomisation. He deliberately avoided countries such as Switzerland, Germany and France, where he knew that people ate lots of saturated fat, yet had low rates of heart disease. These countries would have ruined his findings on saturated fat, Teicholz said. She once asked Keys's right-hand man, Henry Blackburn, why they had avoided those places. Blackburn said that Keys had 'just a personal aversion to being in those countries'. 'I think it is fair to say that the countries in the Seven Countries Study were cherry-picked,' Teicholz told the hearing.

Other problems with the study included data 'inconsistencies' that Keys could not resolve. One error is particularly 'emblematic', said Teicholz. Keys studied men on the island of Crete who seemed to eat very little saturated fat and had very low rates of heart disease. Yet of the three study periods during which Keys collected data on the island, one fell during the month of Lent, when the islanders would have been religiously avoiding all meat, dairy, eggs and even fish. 'The Greek orthodox fast is a strict one,' Teicholz said. Keys would have therefore under-counted the amount of saturated fat the Cretans actually ate. He knew of this problem, but dismissed it without explanation. What he 'found' became the foundation for the Mediterranean diet as we know it today. This was just another in a litany of unscientific practices Keys used to ensure that the results of the study would demonstrate what he wanted.

Despite all its flaws, the Seven Countries Study became 'extremely influential' and is still widely cited today, Teicholz said. But while large and seemingly persuasive, it is still only observational. 'It's a basic principle of science that observational studies can only show association but not causation,' she said. Causation requires clinical trials, preferably RCTs. Teicholz described how governments around the world undertook large, multicentre RCTs on the diet-heart hypothesis throughout the 1960s and 1970s. They replaced animal foods with inferior food items, such as faux meat, margarine and soy-filled cheese. The US National Institutes of Health alone spent billions of dollars on these studies, trying – and ultimately failing – to prove Keys's hypothesis. The NIH trials were 'remarkably special' in that they were conducted in highly controlled, in-patient environments where researchers served all meals to participants.

Additionally, almost all of the NIH studies had 'hard endpoints', Teicholz said. Hard endpoints refer to 'indisputable outcomes', such as death, which cannot be contested. The diagnosis of a heart attack is another endpoint, but is 'a little more disputable', she explained, given the range in diagnoses among doctors. Many studies today use far less reliable, softer, intermediary endpoints, such as lipid markers like LDL and HDL cholesterol. There is disagreement about which of these best predicts heart-attack risk, said Teicholz. The early large, well-controlled RCTs looking at hard endpoints are therefore a valuable source of data.

Altogether, the NIH-funded trials on the diet-heart hypothesis included more than 75 000 subjects, mostly men. They showed that while restricting saturated fats did successfully reduce total blood cholesterol, there was no impact on the ultimate outcome – whether people died of a heart attack – and mortality rates overall. For decades, those in positions of power and influence suppressed and ignored this data, said Teicholz.

In recent years, researchers around the world have gone back to examine the data and there are now more than a dozen published meta-analyses and systematic reviews of the evidence, she said. Nearly all have concluded that saturated fat and dietary cholesterol do not cause death from heart disease. Yet if you read 10 000 nutrition papers, as Teicholz has done, you will find that they all telescope back to the Seven Countries Study. Keys's research was thus the 'Big Bang of modern nutrition studies'.

Teicholz introduced – and demolished – another key element in the case against Noakes: the role of sugar and other carbohydrates in a healthy diet. Alessandro Menotti, one of Keys's fellow project leaders, headed up the Italian part of the Seven Countries Study. Years later, in 1999, Menotti went back to re-analyse the dietary data. He found that the food that best correlated with heart disease was not saturated fat, but 'sweets', Teicholz said. She interviewed Menotti to ask how that finding had escaped Keys. He told her that the Seven Countries Study leaders 'did not know how to treat [sugar]. We reported the facts and had some difficulty explaining our findings.'

Keys clearly understood that any hypothesis associating heart disease with sugar would compete with his own, Teicholz said. He also knew that only one was likely to be right. He therefore did what he always had when faced with inconvenient data: he ignored it and went on the attack, suggesting that all those who promoted the idea that sugar caused heart disease were financially motivated. Or 'just plain wrong'.

Teicholz described how British physiologist and nutritionist Dr John Yudkin, one of the most prominent proponents of the sugar hypothesis in the 1970s, fell afoul of Keys. Yudkin was a professor at Imperial College, London, and author of *Pure, White and Deadly: How Sugar Is Killing Us and What We Can Do to Stop It*. Keys dismissed Yudkin's theory as 'a mountain of nonsense' and accused him of being motivated by unnamed financial backers. Yudkin eventually paid a heavy price for going head to head with Keys. As Ian Leslie noted in *The Guardian* in 2016: 'Prominent nutritionists combined with the food industry to destroy his reputation, and his career never recovered. He died, in 1995, a disappointed, largely forgotten man.'[10] (Big Sugar loomed large in the wings of the case against Noakes, as Russ Greene's 2017 exposé showed.[11])

Teicholz noted that Yudkin's experience was not uncommon. Others who challenged establishment dogma faced similar vilification. The whole scientific community, not just Keys, tried to diminish critics by calling them names, dismissing the quality of their work, exaggerating errors, and denigrating their opinions as strange or bizarre.

Teicholz drew parallels with the HPCSA's prosecution of Noakes. 'You can't walk down a half block with Professor Noakes without someone calling out "20 kilograms, Professor", "15 kilograms, Professor", she said. Many people have lost weight on the Noakes diet, she pointed out, and there is a 'whole body of research' that supports his advice.

'What, then, is the response by experts?' she asked rhetorically. 'To deny his work, to make fun of him, to pretend his work is full of errors, instead of reckoning with him and saying: "Okay, here are a number of observations that our hypothesis does not explain. We need to explain it."' The latter is what one expects of good science, said Teicholz, but it does not happen in nutrition science. That's due mostly to the hostile and aggressive way in which contesting views are treated. It's an attitude that goes back to the formative days of the field, to Keys and his colleagues. The bullying and denials have prevailed for decades, Teicholz said, with the result that few know that Keys's diet-heart hypothesis is 'the most tested hypothesis in the history of nutrition and disease', and that 'the results were all null'.

The consequences for public health have been nothing short of tragic, Teicholz said. It's quite likely, she argued, that by shifting towards a greater consumption of grains and other carbohydrates, the US guidelines have been a major contributor to the pandemics of obesity, diabetes and heart disease.

Teicholz also presented evidence on the safety and efficacy of low-carb diets. There have been more than 74 RCTs, virtually all on Western populations, including at least 32 that lasted six months or longer, and three that lasted two years.

(RCTs are considered the gold standard when it comes to judging whether there are any adverse side effects.) These trials have all established the efficacy of the low-carb diet for fighting obesity, diabetes and heart disease. Some official bodies are now in fact taking notice of the risks of low-fat diets, Teicholz said. In 2015, for example, the Heart and Stroke Foundation of Canada lifted the cap (as a percentage of calories) on saturated fats.

Teicholz also addressed common criticisms of low-carb diets. One is that certain ancient civilisations ate high-carb diets, yet did not have high rates of obesity and diabetes. These included the Japanese, who ate rice, and the Egyptians, who ate lots of bread. The criticism is reasonable enough, Teicholz observed. Experts don't know exactly why carbohydrates are now driving disease more than they did in the past. 'We do not know if it is some combination of total carbohydrates plus sugar that has an especially negative metabolic effect,' she said. 'We do not know if it is that we have changed the way we produce wheat. We do not know if it is something about food processing, or if it is vegetable oils plus carbohydrates … We really do not know. All we know is that if you restrict carbohydrates, you see benefit.'

Bhoopchand seemed almost overwhelmed by the sheer volume of Teicholz's evidence. His cross-examination was uncharacteristically brief. Apart from a couple of questions, he left the bulk of her evidence unchallenged. He made a valiant attempt to undermine Teicholz on South Africa's paediatric guidelines by suggesting that her expertise related only to the US dietary guidelines and not to those of the World Health Organization or to paediatric advice in South Africa. Teicholz dismissed that out of hand. The US dietary guidelines are considered the global gold standard, she said. They have been 'exported, imitated and copied all over the world' by nearly all Western countries and also by the WHO. 'You will find that most guidelines internationally mirror the US dietary guidelines,' she told Bhoopchand.

Bhoopchand then tried to interpret her evidence and personal views on nutrition as contradicting Noakes's tweeted advice. 'What I will not stay away from asking,' he said, 'is that [in] your evidence you do not personally recommend a diet high in meat and fat, do you recall that?' In reply, Teicholz said that she is not a nutritionist and does not make recommendations, but rather talks about what the evidence supports. When Bhoopchand then suggested that she avoids meat and high fat in her own diet, Teicholz told him that her diet is 'generally low in carbohydrates, and higher in fat'. He pushed her to concede that while her diet is 'higher in fat', it is not high fat. Teicholz responded that 'high fat' could mean anywhere from 40 to 90 per cent fat. 'I am in that range,' she said.

With that, Bhoopchand said that he was done. It surprised everyone, especially Adams, who thought that she had misheard him. 'I was just stunned for a moment,' Adams remarked once he had taken his seat. Teicholz was equally surprised when, after having dismissed *The Big Fat Surprise* as the work of 'a mere journalist' just a few days earlier, Bhoopchand asked her to autograph his copy.

Caryn Zinn gave her evidence on the final day of the hearing, 26 October. As a practising dietitian and a nutrition academic, Zinn was able to provide a two-pronged perspective. Like Harcombe and Teicholz before her, she aimed her evidence at the pillars of the charge against Noakes, and effectively undermined them without making a single major concession under cross-examination.

Zinn told the hearing that three things embarrass her these days: as a university student, she never questioned what any of her lecturers told her about the benefits of diet and nutrition; then, as a university lecturer, she told her students that low-carb diets were dangerous; and later, in her private practice, she prescribed low-fat diets to adults and children for 15 years.

For the past five years, she has used LCHF in her practice for adults and children with no adverse side effects. Zinn said that she prefers to talk about low-carb, healthy-fat – rather than high-fat – foods. LCHF is about eating 'real' food, she said. Like Noakes, Harcombe and Teicholz, she believes that when people eat real food, they tend naturally to eat fewer carbohydrates and more fats.

Zinn said that she had been loyal to the conventional LFHC dietary guidelines until she experienced her own 'Damascene moment' in 2011. That was when an AUT colleague, Professor Grant Schofield, asked her opinion on LCHF research, some of which she had not come across before. Zinn thought she would easily 'set [Schofield] straight' with research that refuted any benefits of LCHF. She expected to be able to tell him to 'take your low-carb diet and go somewhere else. I am the dietitian and I know because my lecturers taught in my dietetics degree that this [LFHC] is how it is.'

At the time, Zinn believed that dietitians were best placed to give dietary advice. She was therefore 'flabbergasted' to discover that most of what she had learnt and thought she knew about diet and nutrition was wrong. 'The evidence that led to mainstream dietary guidelines was largely observational, correlation-based research,' Zinn said. 'From a quality viewpoint, it did not compare to the solid, randomised controlled trials that were available to support low-carb, high-fat diets.'

Zinn began to realise that there was good reason why patients in her own practice were battling to lose weight and keep it off: they were constantly hungry because they were eating too many carbohydrates and too little fat. In the face of this realisation, Zinn made what she described as 'a logical, biological and scientific leap to LCHF'.

Her research over the last five years has focused almost exclusively on the LCHF paradigm in public health for all ages. She and her postgraduate students have led studies on hyperinsulinaemia that demonstrate how a substantial subset of the population with normal glucose curves (supposedly healthy) have elevated insulin levels. This could be the start of chronic disease, she said.

In her review of the literature around LCHF research, Zinn said that she uncovered some 'staggering outcomes'. One RCT in particular compared a low-carb, high-fat diet with a low-fat diet, and found that LCHF outperformed low fat in all metabolic parameters, including weight loss, HDL cholesterol and triglycerides (blood fats). Especially relevant was the fact that the LCHF diet contained triple the amount of saturated fat compared with the low-fat diet. 'Even more staggering' was that LCHF showed a substantial reduction in all inflammatory markers, while the low-fat diet showed an increase in some of them. 'When you are in practice and you read this kind of research, you start thinking about your own ethics and morals,' Zinn said. She now believes that for dietitians to be ethical, they must include all evidence-based dietary options in their advice to patients, not just the ones they believe to be true based on what they have been taught.

The HPCSA's expert witnesses had made it clear that one of the reasons for charging Noakes with giving 'unconventional advice' was because he did not promote cereals as good first foods for infant weaning. Zinn argued that there is no evidence whatsoever that cereals are good first foods for infants. She also dismissed the HPCSA experts' contention that cereals fortified with iron are beneficial for infant weaning. She argued that the advice to make starchy foods the basis of a child's main meals could, in fact, cause malnutrition. That's because phytates (antioxidant compounds found in wholegrains, legumes, nuts and seeds, and that bind to certain dietary minerals) reduce the bioavailability of important nutrients, such as iron, zinc and the B vitamins.

Zinn admitted that in the past she had 'unthinkingly' advised parents to feed infants cereals fortified with iron. 'It never occurred to me to ask why infants would need cereals fortified with iron when meat is available and a very good source of iron,' she said. 'Anthropologically, we have done fine for millions of years without giving infants cereals with added iron.'

She agreed with the HPCSA expert witnesses that LCHF 'aligns easily with South Africa's paediatric dietary guidelines'. So did Noakes's tweeted advice, Zinn said. The problem is that there is 'a disconnect' when dietitians implement the guidelines on a practical level, she said, because of the insistence on including cereals as part of complementary feeding for infant weaning.

Under cross-examination, Zinn agreed with Bhoopchand that she was not against starchy foods 'per se'. She did not, however, agree with the official dietary guideline that starches 'should form the basis of most meals' for children and adults. Bhoopchand introduced the issue of 'nutrition transition' from rural to urban populations in South Africa. Nutrition transition refers to the shift in diet that coincides with economic, demographic and epidemiological changes.

Vorster had raised this as proof that Noakes's advice was 'unconventional'. Bhoopchand told Zinn that she should be aware of 'the stark reality of poverty' and 'aspects like under-nutrition and over-nutrition amongst the children in this country'. He referred to a public-health principle: 'To establish what your population that you are working in actually eats,' he said.

He focused on mieliepap, a porridge made from ground maize that is a staple in South Africa's poor communities. He suggested that it is unrealistic not to expect poor people to feed it to their infants. Zinn responded by saying that it is 'not necessarily best practice' to tell people to eat something just because they have done so historically, or because it is cheap. She endorsed Noakes and Harcombe's view that it is not right to recommend a food on the grounds of affordability alone, especially when it is a carbohydrate food that is not essential to the infant's diet.

Zinn dismissed the HPCSA witnesses' claim that LCHF could cause nutrient deficiencies in infants. An abiding myth about the diet is that it is low in nutrients, she said. 'In fact, a well-formulated LCHF diet provides even better nutrients and more fibre than a mainstream low-fat diet.' Harking back to what she had said previously about starchy foods and phytates, she argued that there is a far higher risk of micronutrient deficiency in infants raised on baby cereals and carbohydrate-based foods, because the phytates in these foods compromise infants' levels of essential vitamins and minerals.

Zinn addressed another issue that the HPCSA experts had flagged as a potential problem with LCHF: possible vitamin A toxicity from excessive liver consumption. She showed that this concern is irrational. Vorster herself had said that South Africa follows the WHO's paediatric guidelines, which advise 'fish, meat, eggs, liver every day and as much as possible'. Liver is one of the best food sources of bioavailable iron and vitamin A, but you'd have to eat enormous amounts of liver daily to suffer vitamin A toxicity, Zinn said. And because liver is 'not the sexiest food ... you usually have to combine it with meat to make it palatable, especially for infants'.

If vitamin A toxicity occurs at all, it is usually from dietary supplements (synthetic vitamin A), not real food sources, Zinn said. She knew of only one reported case of infant death due to vitamin A toxicity. It involved a synthetic preparation of 90 000 international units given daily for 11 days to a month-old infant weighing 2.25 kilograms. Vitamin A deficiency, not toxicity, is a far greater problem in the South African population.

Zinn also destroyed the link the HPCSA's witnesses had tried to make between Noakes's tweet and ketogenic diets. His tweet wasn't even close to being about a ketogenic diet, she said. Through her research she had come to realise that fears about low-carbohydrate and ketogenic diets are 'just scaremongering'. Zinn told the hearing that she is now embarrassed to say that she used to teach her students that low-carb diets were bad because ketosis was dangerous. This was largely due to confusion around nutritional ketosis and ketoacidosis. The latter is a condition that mostly affects type-1 diabetics. It is very different from nutritional ketosis. Zinn said that she had not even heard about nutritional ketosis until she looked at the biology and the evidence. What she found led her to change her mind and her practice.

'Ketones occur naturally in the body and are safe,' she said. 'Infants default into a state of ketosis when they are born. They need ketones for optimum brain development in their early years.' And while ketogenic diets could be 'extreme both for adults and for children', nutritional ketosis is 'not something that you can reach easily at all'.

Zinn agreed under cross-examination that she is not an expert on ketosis or neonate nutrition, but said that she has never claimed to be one. She has, however, done extensive and ongoing research into ketogenic diets for sports performance. In one study of the ketogenic diet for multisport athletes, while data showed a drop in performance in the short term, all athletes experienced substantial improvements in health outcomes and inflammatory conditions that convinced them to continue eating LCHF after the study was over, with only minor adjustments. In another study of low-carb diets for power-lifters gearing up for competition, Zinn's team found that athletes could drop body fat without compromising strength in the lead-up phase.

Zinn also addressed society's fear of fat. For too long, she said, people 'feared fat' because the experts had drummed it into their heads that 'fat is bad'. These days, when she lectures to students, her message is simple: 'Don't believe me. This is a university. Here is the evidence for both sides. Go and read widely through a critical lens and make up your own mind.'

This last remark was clearly aimed at the HPCSA's witnesses. All the Angels emphasised that good science requires looking at all the evidence, not just the bits that suit a cherished belief. The subtext was that if the HPCSA and its willing cohort of experts had bothered to look at all the evidence, the hearing might never have happened. The HPCSA might not have foolishly rushed in where angels fear to tread. The HPCSA would have found that Noakes's advice was neither unconventional nor dangerous.

There's a proverb that says: 'Angels speak to those who silence their minds long enough to hear.' The HPCSA's legal team, witnesses and consultants did not appear willing or able to silence their minds long enough to hear the compelling scientific evidence presented by Tim's Angels. As the final day of the hearing drew to a close, Noakes and his supporters could only hope that the members of the Professional Conduct Committee had heard loudly and clearly.

14

Closing Arguments

'I was taught that a lawyer was supposed to be a
custodian of the community's legal and ethical sense.'
– Joe Jamail, American attorney and billionaire

There were many factors that made the HPCSA's prosecution of Professor Tim Noakes seem suspect. One was the ferocity with which the statutory body went after him. Another was the unbridled enthusiasm with which the HPCSA, which is meant to represent all its members, argued so vociferously on behalf of the dietitians who had allied against him. Yet another was the HPCSA's disingenuous habit of changing tack or simply moving the goalposts whenever it failed to prove an element of its case, which was often. This legally and ethically questionable tactic, however, led to some spectacular own goals. One example was a press release the HPCSA put out on Friday 28 October 2016, two days after the hearing adjourned. In it, the HPCSA mistakenly announced to the world that it had found Noakes guilty of unprofessional conduct. The HPCSA admitted its error, but only six hours later. By then, extensive damage had already been done as the libel spread rapidly across social media. While the HPCSA ended up with legal and ethical egg on its face, no heads rolled over the matter.

The HPCSA's conduct has led me to describe the case against Noakes variously as a bizarre theatre of the absurd, a sojourn down the rabbit hole into Wonderland, and Kafkaesque. Noakes's lawyers deliberately called his prosecution 'a persecution'. Their reasoning became apparent during closing arguments on 4 and 5 April 2017.

Unsurprisingly, there was tension in the air when the hearing reconvened at the Belmont Square Conference Centre in Rondebosch, Cape Town. The HPCSA's legal team was present: HPCSA prosecutor Meshack Mapholisa and two external lawyers, instructing attorney Katlego Mmuoe and counsel Dr Ajay Bhoopchand. Assisting them as usual was UCT nutrition professor Marjanne Senekal. Many people saw Senekal's involvement in the case as inappropriate for an academic of her status and position. After all, Noakes was a colleague and her superior at UCT. From the outset, she would not engage with him on the science for LCHF.

Seated next to Senekal was Cape Town paediatrician Dr Muhammad Ali Dhansay. Dhansay's continued presence, even after he had given his evidence as an expert witness for the HPCSA, was noteworthy. His links to the ILSI had by now caught up with him. In February 2017, Russ Greene had revealed that the SAMRC was investigating Dhansay's ties to the sugar and soft-drink industries.[1]

Claire Julsing Strydom, the 'complainant' in the case, was once again conspicuous by her absence.

Noakes and his legal team, comprising instructing attorney Adam Pike, senior counsel Michael van der Nest and counsel Dr Ravin 'Rocky' Ramdass, settled in as Bhoopchand began his lengthy closing argument. He took more than 104 000 words to make his case. It ended up circuitous, contradictory and rambling, a lesson in sophistry. Bhoopchand began by acknowledging Noakes as 'an extraordinary South African', but then went straight for the jugular. Employing mixed metaphors, he attacked Noakes's character, questioning his trustworthiness, reliability, integrity and credibility as a scientist. He suggested that Noakes had brought 'the blade of the guillotine' down on himself.

In the course of the hearing, the HPCSA had unambiguously built its case on three pillars:
1. Noakes had a doctor–patient relationship with Leenstra.
2. He had breached the HPCSA's norms and standards for medical professionals.
3. He had tweeted unconventional 'medical advice' that was not evidence-based, and which was therefore dangerous and could have caused harm.

The first pillar had proved particularly challenging for the prosecution lawyers. Bhoopchand now argued that the HPCSA did not need to prove a doctor–patient relationship; that the charge against Noakes was 'independent of whether a doctor–patient relationship had formed'. The provisions of the Health Professions Act that govern the HPCSA do not require proof of a doctor–patient relationship, he said, or even the existence of 'a contractual nexus'. Bhoopchand argued that the onus was now on the defence to prove that there was no doctor–patient relationship. At the same time, he claimed that it was irrelevant whether Leenstra was Noakes's patient, for anyone reading his tweet could be considered a patient. Thus, Bhoopchand argued, even if Leenstra were not Noakes's patient, he had still acted unprofessionally in giving unconventional medical advice on a public platform. Bhoopchand seemed oblivious to the absurdity of his claims.

Using Noakes's written reply to Strydom's complaint, Bhoopchand tried to show that Noakes had knowingly tweeted as a doctor, not as a scientist. 'Which hat was the respondent wearing when he answered the initial tweet?' Bhoopchand asked. 'That of a scientist or that of a medical practitioner? This is a question of fact and the answer lies in the nature of the question asked, the nature of the reply and the content of the letter of reply ... The pro forma [the HPCSA] submits that the tweets point conclusively to clinical material and the replying tweet was a clinical answer. The content of the letter of reply indicates that the respondent was responding to the complaint that he had given medical advice and that he was protecting his reputation as a medical professional. The pro forma argues that in the absence of a contemporaneous denial from the respondent that he acted as a scientist when he tweeted the replying tweet to Ms Leenstra, and with the content of his letter of reply suggesting that he acted as a medical practitioner, any allegation to the contrary smacks of a retrospective reconstruction of the evidence to evade the charge.'

Bhoopchand was essentially accusing Noakes of some sort of deliberate sin of omission. He faced similar problems with the second pillar of the HPCSA's case: that Noakes had breached the norms and standards for medical professionals with his tweet. The HPCSA does not have any norms and standards for doctors on social media. Bhoopchand called this the 'elephant in the room', but then said that the elephant didn't really matter. 'The current guidelines indicate that they cannot be construed as a complete set of rules of conduct,' he argued. 'The HPCSA is empowered to deal with any complaint of unprofessional conduct referred to it. Practitioners are implored to apply the set of ethical guidelines in Booklet 1 to any situation that is not covered by the guidelines.' The implication is that the provisions of the Act and the various HPCSA guideline booklets bring activity on social media into the ambit of HPCSA norms and standards.

The third pillar was two-pronged and represented the real meat of the case against Noakes: that his tweet constituted medical advice, not information; and that this 'advice' was unconventional, not evidence-based and therefore dangerous. Bhoopchand focused much of his argument on the claim of harm. He said that according to Noakes's own evidence, there is no globally accepted definition of LCHF. Without consensus on a definition, the tweet could not be considered conventional advice. And in the HPCSA lexicon, unconventional is a synonym for harmful or, at the very least, potentially harmful. None of the HPCSA's witnesses had produced any evidence of harm from Noakes's tweet. But, Bhoopchand said, the HPCSA did not need to prove any harm. All it had to prove was the potential for harm. There went those goalposts again.

Bhoopchand argued that LCHF is not 'globally known as a complementary feeding diet', and that the WHO and health bodies in Canada, America, Australia and Europe all consider advising LCHF for babies to be unconventional. He also argued that LCHF is more widely known for weight loss. It therefore made no sense to recommend a diet 'related to losing weight' for an infant. Furthermore, a 'reasonable person' could have interpreted Noakes's tweet as advising a 'dangerous' ketogenic diet, Bhoopchand said. Besides the fact that the HPCSA had not charged Noakes with advising a ketogenic diet, like all his expert witnesses, Bhoopchand was wrongly conflating LCHF with ketosis, and ketosis with ketoacidosis.

Bhoopchand also tried to dismiss all of the evidence Noakes had presented by saying that the charge was 'narrow' and related to infant nutrition only, and expressing 'surprise' that the defence had interpreted it broadly to include adults. In a clear swipe at the Angels, and Teicholz in particular, he said that Noakes had placed a 'burden' of superfluous evidence on the 'jury', and that Adams and her committee would have to dismiss most of it.

What was perhaps most surprising was how glibly Bhoopchand glossed over glaring contradictions in his own arguments. Most of the evidence presented by the HPCSA's witnesses related to adult, not infant, nutrition. Even the Vorster report, commissioned by the HPCSA's Fourth Preliminary Committee of Inquiry and used to charge Noakes, was based on evidence related to adult nutrition. The Naudé review and the so-called UCT professors' letter, both of which that committee relied on to make its decision, also looked at adult nutrition, and said nothing about infant nutrition. Bhoopchand himself, perhaps taking a cue from his witnesses, drew extensively on *The Real Meal Revolution*, which Noakes had co-authored. This despite the fact that the book deals with adult nutrition.

Bhoopchand also tried to dismiss Noakes's evidence on the grounds that he had worn 'two hats', as both a factual and an expert witness in his own defence. Bhoopchand attempted to argue that this represented a conflict of interest. Adams and her committee should consider Noakes's evidence through a 'lens', he said, to detect any bias. He further accused Noakes of being 'evasive' and 'untruthful', and of contradicting his own evidence on the role of carbohydrates in the diet. Where he got that from is anyone's guess. Aside from his about-turn on the benefits of high-carb diets in 2010, Noakes has made no material changes to his stance on carbohydrates since.

Perhaps unsurprisingly, Bhoopchand made it clear that it was not so much what Noakes had said in his tweet as what he did *not* say that led to his prosecution. Enter cereals as supposedly good first foods for babies. The fact that Noakes did not advocate cereals and starchy foods in his tweet went to the heart of the charge that his 'advice' was dangerous. Cereals and grains feature prominently in South Africa's dietary guidelines for all ages, but no one was able to present any proof of their benefits during the hearing. On the contrary, Noakes and his witnesses provided compelling evidence that cereals and grains do more harm than good, and that the recommendation to base meals around them is the real 'dangerous advice'.

Undeterred by yet another weakness in his case, Bhoopchand concluded his argument by saying that the HPCSA had proved the charge against Noakes on a 'balance of probability'. He believed the committee would have to find the professor guilty of unprofessional conduct.

Van der Nest and Ramdass were up next. The eloquence with which they made their submissions contrasted starkly with Bhoopchand. At just over 42 000 words, their closing argument was elegant and succinct by comparison. With legal precision, they forensically eviscerated the HPCSA's case, labelling it an 'unprecedented prosecution and persecution of one of South Africa's eminent scientists' simply for his opinions on nutrition. Van der Nest argued that the HPCSA had shown bias and had treated Noakes unfairly and unjustly, with double standards and hypocrisy, from the outset. The HPCSA appeared to have issued its legal team with a 'win at all costs' order, he said. In altering the charge against Noakes to suit its crumbling case, the HPCSA had created 'schizophrenic moments'. One example was the attempt to dismiss all the evidence that Noakes and his experts presented on the science for LCHF.

Ramdass easily undermined a key aspect of the charge against Noakes: that there was no robust science to support his tweet. The HPCSA had demanded that Noakes provide evidence to support his tweet, yet when he did so, they had gone to extraordinary lengths to dismiss it all. Ramdass pointed out the irrationality and manifest unfairness of this response. All of the evidence presented by the defence was scientifically relevant, he said. Noakes himself had spoken for almost 40 hours, showing 1163 slides and citing 354 publications and other materials, from RCTs to anecdotal evidence. Ramdass broke it down: Noakes had drawn on 47 RCTs; 28 intervention trials/laboratory experiments; 11 meta-analyses; 77 observational studies; 78 review articles; 24 editorials; 15 books; 48 newspaper articles/media reports/blogs; 14 position stands/statements; 8 letters; 3 videos; and a PhD thesis. In contrast, the HPCSA's witnesses had come up with little more than a single meta-analysis, the flawed Naudé review.

Ramdass also undermined the suggestion that Noakes's advice was dangerous and life-threatening because it was unconventional. As a family physician, Ramdass has seen first-hand the effects on people's health of the so-called conventional nutrition 'wisdom'. He argued that this conventional advice is based on the South African Food-based Dietary Guidelines, which themselves are unscientific and wrong in material respects. They are also 'umbilically linked' to the Dietary Guidelines for Americans, which are based on the diet-heart hypothesis that saturated fat causes heart disease. There is currently no evidence to support this proposition, Ramdass said. Conversely, recent evidence-based teaching has it that a high fat intake is actively beneficial, as it reduces the complications of IR T2DM.

Furthermore, evidence shows that carbohydrates cause serious health problems, Ramdass argued, among them non-alcoholic fatty liver disease. NAFLD has been reliably shown to cause a condition known as atherogenic dyslipidaemia, which leads to arterial damage over time, and eventually cardiovascular disease and cerebrovascular disease. In other words, a low-fat diet actually *increases* the risk of fatal heart disease, Ramdass said.

It is concerning that Strydom and ADSA still promote the low-fat diet despite all the evidence to the contrary, Ramdass noted. Dr Zoë Harcombe's observation that it is 'unethical and unprofessional that ADSA is promoting a low-fat diet despite that there is no evidence to limit fat to 30 per cent' was both 'poignant and ironical', he said.

Harcombe's evidence on the flawed Naudé review was also critical, Ramdass said. She had found at least 14 errors in the meta-analysis, all of which favoured the conventional, 'balanced' diet. Correcting for these errors had shown that the low-carbohydrate diet was superior to the conventional, low-fat diet. The HPCSA had not convincingly contested this finding, Ramdass noted. Its charge that Noakes had given unconventional advice that was not evidence-based was, therefore, 'ill-conceived and bereft of scientific justification'.

Ramdass also argued that South Africa's dietary guidelines – and dietary guidelines worldwide – failed to consider the pervasive influence of industry on their formulation. He referred to the evidence presented by Noakes and his Angels that multinationals with vested commercial interests exert significant influence on the guidelines. It was telling that the HPCSA had been unable to answer these allegations, Ramdass said, and that it had failed to address the significant conflicts of interest of its witnesses. Strydom, Vorster and Kruger are all members of ADSA, which has been, and in some cases still is, sponsored by Kellogg's, Nestlé, Unilever and several other food companies, including Coca-Cola.

In summary, Ramdass submitted that 'conventional' dietary advice:

- is based on poor or non-existent science;
- has no scientific validity;
- is the antithesis of what is good;
- has contributed to the diabetes and obesity epidemics;
- is disease-causing rather than disease-preventing; and
- requires moving from the conventional towards a new conventional.

The totality of currently available evidence shows that Noakes is scientifically correct, Ramdass concluded. Strydom, ADSA and the doctors who promote 'conventional' dietary advice are wrong. The conventional diet is 'a recipe for disaster', and so they are the ones giving dangerous, unconventional advice.

Van der Nest argued that the case against Noakes was never about a tweet or his conduct as a medical doctor. One of many ironies of the case was that it was not a patient or even a member of the public who initiated proceedings. Rather, it was healthcare professionals who had a scientific disagreement with Noakes who launched the prosecution.

'Their gripe was about his views and the fact that the public seemed to be listening to him and not to them,' Van der Nest said. 'The problem was never his conduct as a medical doctor.' Instead, Noakes's innocuous tweet was 'the perfect pretext' for a prosecution and persecution. It was ominous that Strydom had somehow, 'miraculously', managed to get the HPCSA to prosecute him seemingly on a whim. At heart, the case was a 'wholly objectionable' invasion of Noakes's right to freedom of speech and expression, Van der Nest argued.

Starting with the formulation of the charge, Van der Nest said that the HPCSA had faltered at the very first hurdle. It defined unprofessional conduct as 'improper or disgraceful or dishonourable or unworthy'. Those were serious words dealing with serious conduct, Van der Nest said. Thus, the question that Adams and the committee had to answer was whether the evidence showed that Noakes's conduct as a medical doctor had been improper, disgraceful, dishonourable or unworthy.

A key pillar of the HPCSA's charge of unprofessional conduct was the claim that a doctor–patient relationship existed. That was 'always nonsense and guaranteed to fail', Van der Nest said. It should have been obvious that the prosecution was not, 'in truth and reality', about how Noakes had acted as a medical doctor. It was, after all, common cause that Noakes had not practised clinical medicine for more than 15 years.

Leenstra had addressed an abstract, non-confidential question on an extremely public forum to Noakes and one of his co-authors of the bestselling book, *The Real Meal Revolution*. It was clear from the outset that she was speaking to them as authors, Van der Nest said. She was not seeking a free medical opinion from a doctor she didn't know. Understanding this, Noakes had clearly answered her question in his capacity as an author and a scientist. Soon thereafter, Ellmer and Strydom tweeted their responses, expressing their opposing views. Van der Nest pointed out that both are dietitians and thus healthcare professionals. If it were indeed true that Noakes gave 'medical advice', then it followed (and the HPCSA's own expert witness, Professor Willie Pienaar, had conceded) that both Ellmer and Strydom also gave 'medical advice'.

Of course, Ellmer and Strydom were entitled to differ with Noakes, Van der Nest said. However, the obvious question was why the HPCSA had prosecuted Noakes for expressing his views on Twitter, but not the dietitians. They had given 'medical advice' to the same person, in the same way, on the same social media platform as Noakes. Why were they entitled to give 'medical advice', but he was not? Who said that Noakes, a scientist with a rare A1 rating in both sports science and nutrition, was wrong and should be silenced, and that the dietitians were right and thus permitted to speak freely?

Van der Nest raised other uncomfortable questions for the HPCSA: 'Is that even how we approach freedom of expression? And are the millions who are active on Twitter not entitled to hear all sides of a diet debate and make up their own minds?'

The HPCSA's response to its failure to prove a doctor–patient relationship spoke volumes. Van der Nest said that the HPCSA had created yet another schizophrenic moment by refusing to accept the failure as proof that it had no case. Instead, it had changed tack, with Bhoopchand claiming in his closing argument that the doctor–patient relationship was, in fact, irrelevant, and that Noakes had acted unprofessionally in circumstances where Leenstra was *not* his patient. The HPCSA's claim that the onus was now on the defence to prove that there was no doctor–patient relationship was never a tenable position, Van der Nest said. Raising a defence did not lead to a reverse onus. Nor did it excuse the prosecution from having to prove the pillars that supported its case.

Van der Nest showed other instances where the HPCSA had significantly shifted the basis of its case. According to Bhoopchand's closing argument, Noakes was now guilty of unprofessional conduct merely for saying something on Twitter. The HPCSA claimed that Noakes's tweet fell within the 'scope of the profession of medicine' and was an 'act pertaining to the medical profession'. Citing Regulation 237 of the Health Professions Act, they tried to argue that instead of giving advice to a single patient, Noakes had tweeted an 'unconventional public health message' to the world. This was another nonsensical claim, Van der Nest said.

He similarly dispatched the claim that Noakes had breached the norms and standards of his profession with his tweet. In acknowledging the 'elephant in the room' – the lack of norms and standards for medical professionals on social media – the HPCSA should have realised that it had no case. Without saying so directly, Van der Nest made it clear that the elephant had trampled the HPCSA's case to death. The statutory body had it 'back to front', he said. It should have written up rules first, *before* prosecuting Noakes. The HPCSA had 'hopelessly lost its way' in its 'win-at-all-costs' approach.

Van der Nest continued to systematically demolish another crucial pillar of the HPCSA's case: that Noakes gave 'medical advice', as opposed to information, in his tweet. Van der Nest argued that there was 'a very big difference between medical advice and information'. For starters, liability assumed that a doctor could only give medical advice, conventional or otherwise, to a patient. Absent a patient, that argument fell away, or so any reasonable person would assume. Noakes had made it clear from the outset that Leenstra was not his patient, and that he had answered a scientific question as a scientist and an author. Moreover, Leenstra's tweeted question was neither clinical nor medical.

Twitter is well known as a large, information-sharing, public platform, Van der Nest said. It is not a place where doctors and patients go for one-on-one consultations, because there is no privacy and confidentiality. Leenstra was not Noakes's patient. She was simply a consumer of the information he and others tweeted. She was free to do whatever she liked with that information.

Giving information on Twitter is no different from writing it in a book or delivering it from a stage, Van der Nest argued. If the HPCSA believed its own argument that Noakes gave medical advice by expressing an opinion on Twitter, then the same could be said of his books and public talks. It could also be said of any other author who gives information related to nutrition or health. Thus, if the HPCSA found Noakes guilty of giving medical advice on Twitter, it would have to prosecute all health professionals who wrote diet books or said anything that irritated Strydom or ADSA. Dietitians would only need to label views as dangerous or life-threatening to have the HPCSA prosecute those who disseminated them in public, Van der Nest said. The dietitians would not even have to show any harm. The massive invasion of freedom of expression was obvious, he said.

In charging Noakes with tweeting unconventional advice, the HPCSA was also legally obliged to define what it meant by 'unconventional'. In providing further details of the charge, the HPCSA had told Noakes that 'the key consideration' was that recommended 'medical nutrition therapy' should be 'grounded in evidence-based best practice, which in this case would be the evidence-based dietary guidelines'. In other words, the HPCSA defined conventional advice as evidence-based advice that followed South Africa's nutritional guidelines for breastfeeding and complementary feeding. Yet both Vorster and Kruger had conceded that LCHF, in fact, aligns with these guidelines.

Another major weakness in the HPCSA's case was that it could not define LCHF. 'If you prosecute someone with giving unconventional advice, you must be able to say what the unconventional content of that advice is,' Van der Net said. 'If you, as the prosecutor, can't say what it is, then it means that you cannot show that the advice is unconventional. You cannot prove your case.' The moment the HPCSA said that it did not know what LCHF was – and that no one knew – its case went 'out the window'.

Another bizarre element of the HPCSA's case – probably tied to its limited understanding of LCHF – was its experts' insistence that Noakes had somehow advised a 'dangerous' ketogenic diet for babies. Van der Nest pointed out that the HPCSA had not charged Noakes with advising ketogenic diets for infants, and that nowhere in his tweet had he made any reference to ketogenic diets. Noakes and his experts gave extensive evidence to show that he had not advised such a diet for infants. They also showed that ketogenic diets are not dangerous when used appropriately. The HPCSA was unable to challenge their evidence, yet ketogenic diets remained an obsessive red herring.

Van der Nest also highlighted the irony behind the HPCSA's charge that Noakes's advice was unconventional. Ordinarily, a charge of unprofessional conduct meant disgraceful, unworthy or improper conduct by a medical practitioner, he said. Yet how could it be disgraceful, unworthy or improper to give unconventional advice that was not harmful? 'Do we really prosecute people for being unconventional, without doing any harm?' Van der Nest asked.

This brought him to the 'most objectionable part' of the HPCSA's case against

Noakes: that he had been prosecuted in the complete absence of a patient and in an 'absolute vacuum of harm'. More than three years after the tweet, the HPCSA had still not provided a shred of evidence to show harm from an LCHF diet, Van der Nest said. It had not shown any evidence of harm from Noakes's tweet or from any of the other 29 000 tweets he had sent up till then. One of the HPCSA's own witnesses, Professor Salome Kruger, had even acknowledged that LCHF 'is not harmful'. Noakes and the Angels had also testified in detail about the safety and efficacy of LCHF. The HPCSA had been unable to challenge or answer their evidence. And when it could not prove harm, Van der Nest said, the HPCSA did what it does best: it changed tack once again. After having made it clear from the beginning that harm was crucial to the charge of unconventional advice, Bhoopchand now said in closing that the HPCSA did not have to show harm. That's because there was no harm, Van der Nest remarked. 'When one tries to determine why this has happened [a prosecution in the absence of any harm], the answer lies, at least in part, in the fact that this case has revealed gross unfairness and injustice on the part of the HPCSA.'

In fact, the HPCSA had demonstrated significant bias against Noakes even before it decided to prosecute him, Van der Nest argued. It started with instances of 'highly irregular', inappropriate and biased conduct on the part of members of the HPCSA's Fourth Preliminary Committee of Inquiry. The committee's primary function was to decide whether there should be a hearing and, if so, to formulate points of inquiry against Noakes. After that, committee members should have hung up their HPCSA hats and returned to their day jobs. As the incriminating email chain in the prosecution's file showed, that's not what happened.

The preliminary inquiry committee became personally vested in the prosecution of Noakes, Van der Nest said. Before they charge anyone with unprofessional conduct, committee members should 'perhaps look at their own conduct', he observed drily.

Returning to the topic of Noakes's scientific views being 'unconventional', Van der Nest said that history is replete with examples of pioneers who furthered medical science, yet who were considered unconventional at the time. By way of example, Van der Nest cited Australian physician Dr Barry Marshall, who infected himself with *Helicobacter pylori* to prove his hypothesis that peptic ulcers were caused by the bacterium, and not by acid, stress and spicy foods, as the conventional view held. When he developed an ulcer and treated it with an antibiotic, he won the Nobel Prize. 'That was the end of the conventional way of treating such ulcers,' Van der Nest said.

Galileo was another who was relentlessly prosecuted and persecuted for his views. People called him a heretic for saying that the earth revolved around the sun. 'Have we learnt so little about prosecuting scientists in the past 300 years?' Van der Nest asked.

The HPCSA appeared not to understand the fluid nature of scientific research and that 'what is unconventional today easily becomes tomorrow's conventional', he said. Credible scientists and doctors could easily be unconventional without being dishonourable. They could be 'incorrect without being unworthy'. They could also express unconventional views in public to a person who was not their patient without being disgraceful or improper.

For medicine to develop, scientists and doctors must challenge conventional frontiers, Van der Nest said. 'The HPCSA should have no sway over what scientists and authors believe and say.' This holds true, no matter the nature of the forum scientists and authors use to express their views. Every South African should 'recoil when a scientist [or doctor] is prosecuted for his scientific opinions'.

'Sometimes we all need to hear why the earth might not be flat and why the sun does not revolve around the earth,' Van der Nest said. But most importantly, he said, South Africans should not stand for the use of statutory bodies to bully into submission those with whom other academics, scientists, doctors and dietitians may disagree. Therefore, he concluded, the HPCSA's Professional Conduct Committee should find Noakes innocent of all charges.

15

The Verdict

'... in our reasonings concerning matter of fact, there are all imaginable
degrees of assurance, from the highest certainty to the lowest species of
moral evidence. A wise man, therefore, proportions his belief to the evidence.'
– David Hume, Scottish philosopher[1]

Tensions and emotions were running high on the morning of Friday 21 April 2017.
The sixth and final session of the HPCSA hearing into the conduct of Professor
Tim Noakes was due to begin, and Professional Conduct Committee chair Joan
Adams was expected to deliver the long-awaited verdict. The HPCSA had wisely
chosen a chair with extensive legal knowledge, more than a decade's worth of
experience in medical law, an enviable reputation for credibility and integrity,
and a fiercely independent spirit. Advocate Adams had negotiated the medico-
legal, scientific and ethical landmines that the HPCSA had set with consummate
skill, humour and humanity.

It was now more than three years since Noakes had sent the tweet that started
it all. Seated in the by-now familiar Cape Town conference room, I watched as
the various key players in the case arrived. Lawyers for both sides bustled about,
shuffled papers on the tables in front of them and spoke to one another in
hushed tones. It was a seminal day for all involved. What should have been a
simple, impartial, non-adversarial hearing by a statutory body had ballooned
into a full-blown trial of Noakes and the LCHF diet he advocated.

The session started late because the stenographer was missing. He had forgotten that Adams had agreed to start an hour earlier, at 9 a.m. instead of the usual
10 a.m. Members of the committee offered to negotiate Cape Town's notorious,
early-morning, peak-hour traffic to collect him. The hearing eventually got
underway just before 10 a.m.

Adams began by placing on the record the names of all present, including her
fellow committee members: Dr Janet Giddy, Dr Haroon Saloojee, Dr Alfred Liddle
and Mr Joel Vogel. After indicating that she had a lengthy judgment to read out,
thus dashing any hopes of a quick verdict, Adams stated that her five-member
committee was required to reach a majority decision only, not necessarily a

unanimous one, and that the majority decision would be binding. The committee, she stated, had reached a majority decision: four members to one. She would read out the binding, majority decision, after which Dr Liddle, the lone dissenter, would read out his minority judgment.

Referring to Noakes as the 'respondent' and the HPCSA's legal team as the 'pro-forma complainant', Adams reminded those present that Noakes is a medical doctor who has not practised clinical medicine since 2005. She then went through the events leading up to the hearing, starting with the complaint laid by dietitian Claire Julsing Strydom on 6 February 2014, and referring back to Pippa Leenstra's original tweet and the various responses from Noakes, paediatric dietitian Marlene Ellmer, Strydom and others.

Adams quoted extensively from the pro-forma complainant's arguments. She said that the HPCSA's legal team bore the onus of proof on a balance of probabilities, compared with the stricter requirement of proof beyond reasonable doubt required in a criminal trial. This was an important point. Bhoopchand had sought more than once in his closing argument to shift the burden of proof from the HPCSA onto the defence, especially with regard to the claim that Noakes had a doctor–patient relationship with Leenstra.

Adams paid particular attention to the evidence of Stellenbosch psychiatry professor Willie Pienaar. Pienaar was the only one of the HPCSA's six witnesses who was called to testify solely on ethics and the existence of a doctor–patient relationship. The relationship was a pillar of the charge against Noakes.

As to the charge that Noakes had been unprofessional in giving advice that could have caused harm, Adams stated: 'The maxim *res ipsa loquitur* [the principle that the occurrence of an accident implies negligence] has no application in South African law to matters involving alleged medical negligence or unprofessional conduct.' Citing case law, she said, 'courts have repeatedly cautioned that it should not be readily accepted that a professional person such as for example an advocate or a medical practitioner would act in an unprofessional manner'. She added that 'there is a very real danger of measuring the reasonable practitioner against too high a standard or judging him too strictly and that should be guarded against'.

Her committee had to judge Noakes's conduct as a medical professional by the standard of reasonableness in terms of South African law, Adams said. She quoted *S v Burger*, 1975 (4) SA 817 (A), page 879:

> One does not expect of a reasonable man any extreme, such as Solomonic wisdom, prophetic foresight, chameleonic caution, headlong haste, nervous timidity or the trained reflexes of a racing driver. In short, a reasonable man treads life's pathway with moderation and prudent common sense.

And *Minister of Police v Skosana*, 1977 (1) SA 31 (A), page 32:

> The reasonable man is presumed to be free from both over-apprehension and over-confidence.

'This committee is obliged to avoid adopting the approach of the armchair critic when judging the conduct of the respondent [Noakes],' Adams said. 'It is trite that after the event even a fool is wise.' She cited the judgment in *Van Wyk v Lewis*, 1924 (AD), pages 461–462:

> We cannot determine in the abstract whether a surgeon has or has not exhibited reasonable skill and care. We must place ourselves as nearly as possible in the exact position in which the surgeon found himself.

'Equally applicable to this case we have to place ourselves in the exact position in which the respondent ... found himself,' Adams noted.

Adams adjourned the hearing mid-morning for a 15-minute coffee break. When it resumed, she came out firing on all cylinders. 'This Committee is bound by the Health Professions Act and its various regulations,' she said. 'For this reason, various collateral issues raised during argument will not and cannot be canvassed here. To do so would entail this committee exceeding its statutory mandate. It also deserves mention that this committee's purpose and mandate is not to set nutritional or dietary standards for the world. So that counts for all babies.'

Adams thus signalled that her ruling would cover Noakes's conduct as a medical doctor only. It would not be any kind of endorsement of the science for or against LCHF or the conventional, LFHC diet on which South Africa's dietary guidelines are based.

Adams said that her committee was bound by the 'four corners of the charge':
- That Noakes had a doctor–patient relationship with Leenstra.
- That he had breached the norms and standards of his profession on social media.
- That he gave medical advice.
- That he gave advice that was unconventional, as it was not evidence-based.

This was a crucial legal point. The HPCSA's lawyers had often diverged from the four corners in what appeared to be an overzealous attempt to secure a guilty verdict. Their peculiar strategy of 'changing tack', as Van der Nest described it, every time they failed to prove a pillar of the charge had clearly not escaped Adams and her committee.

The committee had been tasked with a 'unique set of facts and circumstances', Adams said. Firstly, and to the best of her knowledge, the case was the first of its kind at the HPCSA involving the use of social media. It was also 'one of the first of its kind in South Africa involving social media in general'. Secondly, the use of social media platforms by healthcare professionals is not directly regulated by HPCSA legislation, regulations, ethical rules or guidelines. 'As an aside, the HPCSA would appear to be seriously lagging in this regard,' Adams noted.

On the subject of admissibility of evidence, Adams was quite clear. 'There is no case law or legislation in South African law prohibiting the respondent from giving expert testimony,' she said. 'From the manner in which the charge has been couched it would in any event not have been reasonable or fair and neither constitutional towards a respondent as a scientist with expertise in sports nutrition to prohibit him from giving expert evidence. It, however, deserves mention that this committee is not a rubberstamp and is not obliged to follow all opinions or expert opinions which witnesses may have expressed in this matter, especially on aspects which this committee is quite capable of deciding without an expert.'

The committee had to establish the facts and make a finding based on those facts. This required scrutiny of Leenstra's tweet and Noakes's response, not in a vacuum, but in the context of Twitter as a social media platform and the entire tweeted conversation. 'To do otherwise would result in a gross injustice,' Adams said. Consideration also had to be given to all the surrounding circumstances prevailing at the time.

'From the manner in which the charge sheet was formulated, read with the further particulars, it cannot without further ado simply be said that the matter concerns only infant nutrition and that all evidence in respect of adult nutrition is irrelevant,' Adams announced. This was another crucial point. Bhoopchand had tried repeatedly to dismiss most of the evidence presented by Noakes and his expert witnesses. Adams made it clear that his tactic had not worked. 'For one, this is not common cause but vehemently contested and in dispute,' she said. 'Secondly, the tweet concerned the diet of breastfeeding mothers. It deserves mention that breastfeeding mothers are also adults with the same rights, duties, obligations and freedom of choice as all adults, including matters concerning their nutrition and that of their babies. After all, it is not babies and infants who are tweeting, reading tweets or deciding which diet to follow amidst a confusing minefield of information and divergent opinions, it is their adult mothers. Thirdly, the pro forma conceded that adult nutrition is not totally unrelated to infant nutrition, and fourthly, on all the expert evidence tendered the relationship between infant and adult nutrition would appear to be somewhat controversial.'

This was putting it mildly.

With a forensic toothcomb, Adams proceeded to unpick all the elements of the HPCSA's case against Noakes. Leenstra's first question was general and the HPCSA had made far too much of her words, Adams said. 'One must not assume something short of a medical emergency by Ms Leenstra's use of the word "worried" in her initial tweet and neither read into baby winds more than that, namely a relatively normal bodily function of babies and humans in general for that matter. Baby winds are not an illness,' said Adams. 'People use all types of words, exaggerations, emotions and subjective expressions in their communications with others. Social media is certainly no exception. One must not assume the worst or anything nail-biting by the mere use of the word "worried". Worry is a subjective state of mind.'

If Leenstra were genuinely concerned about any kind of medical emergency with her infant, she would 'in all probability not have been wasting precious time on Twitter', Adams said. Leenstra was far more likely to have used the time to consult a medical practitioner, paediatrician, or the casualty or trauma unit of her nearest hospital or clinic if she really suspected that her child was ill.

Adams further said that it was not possible to impute a doctor–patient relationship to either Leenstra as the patient or Noakes as the doctor given the available evidence. 'There is no evidence of such a relationship,' she said. 'In fact, the circumstantial evidence proves exactly the opposite.'

It was also not reasonable to assume that Leenstra 'was some unenlightened or uninformed vulnerable and helpless consumer who happened to stumble upon Twitter by chance'. 'The tweet thread begs the opposite,' Adams stated unequivocally.

The HPCSA could also 'not assume in this day and age of technology that the general public using Twitter or reading Twitter comments, including breastfeeding mums and Ms Pippa Leenstra, are ignorant and vulnerable users in need of protection from themselves and others,' Adams said. 'Indeed, with the information technology explosion the general public is far more enlightened and informed than it has ever been in the past.'

About the worst that Adams had to say to Noakes was that his tweet was ambiguous, as the HPCSA's witnesses had claimed. 'However, the law does not and cannot protect every user in cyberspace from themselves, their ignorance or downright absurd behaviour,' she said. 'If anyone had wanted more information, they could simply have tweeted and asked and hoped for a timeous intelligible and unambiguous response, for nothing is guaranteed. They could also have Googled, blogged or used other internet and/or also social media platforms or not. They could have likewise made appointments and consulted with dietitians, medical practitioners and other healthcare practitioners in a traditional professional setting or not.'

Those who randomly follow cyber advice or information out of context, without a clear understanding of the nature of the advice or information, do so at their own peril, Adams said. After all, 'Dr Google can vacillate between a diagnosis of a mild headache to clinically dead with a few clicks of a mouse.'

Adams disagreed with the HPCSA's expert witnesses who said that Noakes had diluted the breastfeeding message with his tweet. 'In fact,' she said, 'if anything, [Noakes] would appear to be very supportive of, and not at all undermining of, breast milk based on his praise thereof in a tweet. There is nothing to suggest that he was advocating immediate cessation of breastfeeding, discouraging breastfeeding or had a problem with breast milk. Even Prof. Kruger commended him in this regard during her testimony.'

Adams spent much of the final section of her ruling on the implications for modern medicine in the information age and on social networks in particular. 'Information sharing, media and social media is no longer what it was,' she said. Not so long ago, few could have envisaged the social media explosion of today. And for those who did, it was 'considered to be the figment of a very disturbed imagination'.

'It is not unheard of that conventional science in medicine may become bad and even mad science or medicine,' she said. 'Something initially considered outrageous may on the other hand subsequently become established practice. History is indeed riddled with examples, some rather extreme.'

Adams cited the example of Hungarian physician Dr Ignaz Semmelweis, an early pioneer of antiseptic procedures. 'He introduced hand disinfection standards in obstetrical clinics,' said Adams. 'He was severely ostracised by his peers and society even after he had proven how he could prevent infant mortality. He spent his last days in an asylum at a relatively young age.' Today it is established medical practice for health professionals to follow the protocols developed by Semmelweis so as to prevent the spread of germs.

Adams reflected on what it means to be unconventional. 'We live in a dynamic, not static environment,' she said. 'Humans are ever evolving, as is knowledge related to medicine, science and technology. Unconventional does not equate per se to unprofessional. It would depend on the facts in a particular case.'

She then moved on to another key pillar of the charge against Noakes: that his advice or information was not evidence-based. 'On the evidence before this committee it cannot be found that the pro forma has proven on a balance of probabilities that the respondent gave advice or information on Twitter which was not evidence-based,' Adams stated.

On the contrary, she said that based on the facts and all the expert evidence, it appeared that Noakes's advice was 'sufficiently aligned to prevailing South African paediatric dietary guidelines at the time, such that the only reasonable inference to be drawn is not that the advice was or could be deemed to be unconventional'. In any event, said Adams, whether or not the advice or information was conventional was really only relevant if the committee found on the facts that Noakes was indeed acting in his capacity as a medical practitioner. The majority of the committee had found no evidence that he had acted as such, and therefore any information he gave could not be construed as medical advice, conventional or otherwise.

Adams was careful not to endorse or write off LCHF. She stated simply: 'After hearing all the expert evidence it is clear that the issue of the LCHF diet is complex and an evolving field of science and nutrition.'

She also said that her committee would make no 'credibility finding' as far as any of the nutrition experts was concerned. However, she did say that in terms of case law relating to expert testimony, 'on the totality of all the expert evidence presented before this committee it cannot be said that the testimony of the respondent and his witnesses does not also have a logical basis'.

Adams then proceeded to deliver the death blow to the HPCSA's case. 'The majority of this committee, being four of the five votes, find the following on the facts,' she began, before launching into a final 10-point summary:

1. The HPCSA had not proven that Noakes 'was acting in his capacity as a medical practitioner or in any dual or multiple capacity, which included the capacity of a medical practitioner, when he tweeted Ms Leenstra on 5 February 2014';
2. Noakes had acted 'as an author and proponent of the LCHF diet';
3. The HPCSA had not proven that Noakes 'gave medical and/or clinical and/or medical nutritional advice and/or medical nutrition therapy when he tweeted Ms Leenstra';
4. Noakes had 'provided information to Ms Leenstra as an author and proponent of the LCHF diet. At best his response was ambiguous and not a direct response to her query. At worst, the response, without clarification, may be interpreted as confusing or unclear. To understand the response properly and in the context of the LCHF diet there would have had to have been meaningful dialogue between Ms Leenstra and the respondent. It is common cause there simply was none';
5. The HPCSA had 'not proven the existence of a doctor–patient relationship on a balance of probabilities';
6. 'On the facts and probabilities there was indeed no doctor–patient relationship';
7. The HPCSA had not proven that Noakes had 'contravened any law, regulation or ethical rule. It has certainly not proven on a balance of probabilities a contravention of Regulation R237 of 6 March 2009 in that this committee could not find on the facts that the respondent advised or diagnosed anyone or any baby on his or her physical health status';
8. The HPCSA had not proven that Noakes 'gave unconventional advice or advice which was not evidence-based';

9. On the facts, 'no actual or potential harm was proven, neither that any information provided on Twitter by the respondent, whether unsolicited or not, was dangerous or life-threatening'; and

10. The HPCSA had not proven that Noakes 'as a medical practitioner acted unprofessionally and in a manner that is not in accordance with the standards and norms of the medical profession'.

At that moment, the silence in the conference room felt stifling. Adams stopped shuffling her papers and looked directly at Noakes. The professional legal mask she had maintained throughout slipped. With a smile that stretched from ear to ear, she slowly and deliberately delivered her verdict, emphasising the last two words: 'Professor Noakes, on the charge of unprofessional conduct, the majority of this committee find you *not guilty*.'

The room erupted. People rose to their feet, cheering, applauding and hugging. Noakes remained seated. He dropped his head into his hands, but only for a moment. He later told me that he thought he would cry. Instead, he lifted his head, raised both arms and punched the air with clenched fists in victory, shouting, 'Yes!' His lawyers were equally jubilant, reaching over and embracing him and one another, their relief etched on their faces.

The ruling was as thorough a vindication as Noakes could have hoped for, under the circumstances.

Liddle's dissenting opinion was anticlimactic. He prefaced it by saying that he could not presume 'to profess a judgment'. Then he broke down and sobbed, saying that all he 'sort of wanted to do' was to give his reasons for voting against the rest of the committee. Liddle said that Noakes had given 'advice' that was 'unconventional in the extreme'. He echoed Pienaar: the absence of any recorded harm from Noakes's tweet was 'a fortunate consequence and not an indication of innocence'. It did not exclude 'unreported and presently unknown evidence of harm'. In essence, Liddle believed that the HPCSA had proved its case.

In his first interview after the verdict, Noakes said that the outcome of the hearing 'could not have been better'. However, he looked forward to the day when the HPCSA investigated the veracity of the evidence-base on which universities train dietitians. He also said that he hoped to see the HPCSA investigate the effects of orthodox advice on the obesity and diabetes epidemics, which are crippling the health of populations in South Africa and elsewhere.

In her newsletter announcing the verdict, Dr Zoë Harcombe praised Adams, calling her the 'magnificent Chair'. She said that Adams and her committee had 'the emotional intelligence and decency to put themselves in [Noakes's] shoes'. These were qualities that Strydom and the HPCSA 'demonstrably lacked'.

It quickly became clear that the dietitians involved in prosecuting Noakes were not about to let go of their fight to silence him. Immediately after the ruling,

ADSA president Maryke Gallagher said in a TV interview that her organisation would not change its advice to the public. Claiming that her association gave evidence-based dietary advice, Gallagher signalled that while Noakes had won a significant battle, ADSA's war with him was still alive and well.

The HPCSA was also not ready to let go of its prosecution. It had 21 days to decide whether to appeal its committee's decision. Eighteen days after the ruling, it did just that, shocking Noakes's detractors as much as his lawyers and supporters. In announcing its decision, the HPCSA gave no reasons for lodging the appeal. All that was apparent was its continuing desire – or obsession, as some were calling it – to find him guilty.

PART III

THE SCIENCE

16

Once We Were Healthy

'Human health depends above all on sound nutrition; sound nutrition
means growing food and using it in accordance with nature's laws;
of all foods made "unnatural" by industrial processing the commonest
are refined sugar, refined flour and certain processed vegetable oils.
I know of no research that refutes this simple concept.'
– Dr Walter Yellowlees, *A Doctor in the Wilderness*[1]

My 'trial' was a unique event in the history of modern medicine. By placing
my fate in the hands of a legal process, I challenged ADSA and the HPCSA to
prove that the 'unconventional' nutritional ideas that I promote are not evidence-
based.

In presenting their case, the prosecution produced just one 'scientific' paper,
the disputed Naudé review. Importantly, that study had nothing to do with infant
nutrition. Neither did the UCT professors' letter and Hester Vorster's secret
report, both of which the Fourth Preliminary Committee of Inquiry had used,
along with the Naudé review, to charge me.

That is why, over the prosecution's protestations, my three expert witnesses
and I focused our scientific defence on both adult and infant nutrition. Over
12 days of testimony, we argued that obesity and T2DM begin during pregnancy.
If the mother eats a high-carbohydrate diet during pregnancy, and if she then
weans her infant onto conventional, high-carbohydrate, rice- or maize-based
'complementary foods', the probability that her infant will develop all the scourges
of insulin resistance as an adolescent or young adult is greatly increased.

Crucially, despite all the resources at its disposal, including an apparently
unrestrained budget of between R7 million and R10 million, the prosecution
failed to contest any of the facts that we presented. They were thus unable to prove
that our 'unconventional' dietary advice is not evidence-based.

The sole conclusion I can draw is that the LCHF dietary model I propose is
currently, in my opinion, the best evidence-based model of modern human
nutrition. Conversely, the LFHC, 'prudent', 'balanced' diet promoted by ADSA,
the CDE, the HSFSA and the HPCSA, and religiously taught at all South African

medical schools, is at best not evidence-based, at worst completely wrong and extremely harmful, not least because it is has caused the obesity/T2DM epidemic. Hence, those who advocate the LFHC diet are promoting practices that are 'unconventional'.

What this effectively means is that after 12h32 on Friday 21 April 2017, when Advocate Joan Adams completed her final judgment, all those South African dietitians and medical doctors who prescribe the LFHC diet are potentially liable for practising unconventional medicine/dietetics. What is more, because the HPCSA is responsible for the education of all South African doctors and dietitians, its top priority after 21 April 2017 should be to ensure that all present and future health practitioners are educated appropriately to provide only that dietary advice that is evidence-based, beginning with the scientific material that we presented during the trial and some of which is now in this book.

When Marika and I decided to write *Lore of Nutrition*, we soon realised that if we were to include ALL the scientific evidence supporting the prescription of the LCHF/Banting diet, the book would simply be too overwhelming for the vast majority of readers. Instead, we agreed that to supplement the science in the preceding chapters, I would write a couple of chapters at the end outlining the key themes underpinning the evidence that the three Angels and I presented at the trial. And to save the more complex details for a second book – a supplement to this one, as it were – for doctors, dietitians and others interested in the complete evidence that supports our promotion of the LCHF eating plan.

Modern humans evolved from herbivorous primates
Our story begins about six million years ago. Africa is the home of the great apes. Climate change beginning about eight million years prior has caused significant alterations in the immediate environment. Progressive global cooling with the formation of the large permanent ice sheet on Antarctica has reduced the amount of rain falling at the equator, causing a gradual but relentless replacement of the equatorial jungles and forests – the natural habitat of the great apes – with more open savannah. Some of the great apes living on the edge of the retreating forests decide to leave the safety of their natural habitat and venture forth into the unknown, where they must either change what they eat or face extinction.

Others decide to remain in the jungle, eating the foods they have always eaten. Modern gorillas are their descendants. They have eaten the same diet for the past six million years, comprising, for the most part, plant stems and leaves with a small contribution from fruit.

But the challenge posed for all mammals eating a plant-based diet is that no mammals, and only some species of anaerobic bacteria, have the capacity to digest the cellulose that forms the cell lining of all plants. Mammals that survive exclusively on plant material have had to develop a symbiotic relationship with anaerobic bacteria. Billions of anaerobic bacteria are given safe residence in specifically adapted intestinal organs, where they busily ferment ingested cellulose into usable mammalian food. In gorillas, this special organ is a voluminous large bowel (colon), making gorillas 'hindgut fermenters', a feature they share with horses, pigs, zebras, elephants, warthogs, rhinoceroses, rabbits and other rodents. In other grass-eating ruminants, including cattle, sheep, antelope and gazelles, the special fermenting organ is a four-chambered stomach in the foregut. Hence 'foregut fermenters'.

The basis for this symbiosis is that in exchange for an environment where they can safely reproduce, the bacteria convert the cellulose into a form of saturated fat called volatile fatty acids, on which the host mammal bases its existence.[2] So this is the important point: grass-eating ruminants convert a 100 per cent nutrient-poor carbohydrate food – grass – into energy-dense saturated fatty acids that are essential for their survival.

In truth, the specifically adapted fore- and hindguts of these herbivores can rightly be labelled super-specialised organs for manufacturing saturated fats.

Equally remarkable, the proteins in the bodies of those same bacteria become the source of the proteins that these mammals need to build their own bodies. Thus the protein in the meat that humans eat is derived from the bodies of the symbiotic bacteria.

In this way, all plant-eating mammals use cellulose as the growth medium for the bacteria in their intestines. These bacteria then produce the fatty acids and proteins that are missing in the nutrient-poor grass, roots, fruits and shoots on which these mammals must survive.

The point is that simply by looking at the intestinal anatomy of any mammal, one can determine the foods for which that animal is designed – either carnivory or herbivory. An important but unanswered question is whether one can be a bit of both – an omnivore eating both plants and animal produce. The assumption is that since humans eat both it must be possible. But is it ideal?

Figure 16.1 on page 310 shows that the key difference between humans and the great apes is that humans have much shorter colons (large bowels).[3] As a result, the percentage of the total gut length taken up by the colon is much greater in all great apes than it is in humans. This confirms that these apes are hindgut fermenters. And all the biological and social features of these mammals follow from that: their small brains; their need to spend most of their waking hours eating (nutrient-poor plants); their production of copious faeces, 20 to 40 times a day; their lower levels of physical vigour (gorillas especially); and their relatively simple social structures. All are the result of their nutrient-poor diets.

For example, a study of fossil bones found on the shores of Lake Turkana in northern Kenya showed that as far back as two million years ago, 'hominins,

Figure 16.1

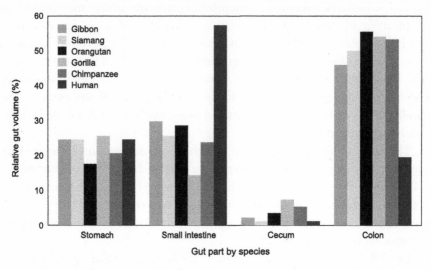

Relative volumes of the stomach, small intestine, caecum and colon in five species of primates compared to humans. Note that in all the primates, the small intestine comprises about 30 per cent of the total intestinal volume, whereas in humans it is ~60 per cent. In contrast, the colon comprises ~50 per cent of the total intestinal volume of the primates, but less than 20 per cent in humans. These features indicate that the primates are hindgut fermenters, whereas humans have evolved the intestinal features of carnivores. Redrawn from K. Mu, 'What are chimpanzee digestive systems like compared to humans?'[4]

predating *Homo erectus*, enjoyed access to carcasses of terrestrial and aquatic animals that they butchered in a well-watered habitat'.[5] Included in this fossil record were the bones of elephants, rhinoceroses, crocodiles and many species of antelope. The authors drew attention to 'the inclusion of various aquatic animals including turtles, crocodiles, and fish, which are rich sources of specific nutrients needed in human brain growth'. It is the eating of foods rich in these nutrients – protein, essential polyunsaturated fats (specifically docosahexaenoic acid), iron, zinc, copper, iodine, selenium, vitamin A, choline and folate[6] – that some argue explains why human brain size began to increase progressively about two million years ago, before a second rapid acceleration about 200 000 years ago.[7] This latter acceleration may have been triggered when our immediate ancestors at Pinnacle Point in the Southern Cape, South Africa, began to incorporate even more fish products into their diets.[8]

In contrast, humans share the typical features of a carnivore's gut dimensions – think lions, wolves and wild dogs, animals that eat only meat. The key is that the digestion of nutrient-dense foods does not require the intervention of anaerobic bacteria in an extensive large bowel, but rather can be done very effectively within the confines of a relatively short small bowel. Table 16.1 includes all the other evidence showing that humans are designed for carnivory.

Figure 16.2

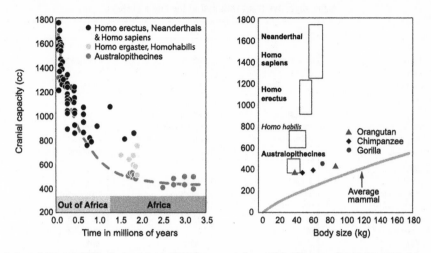

Left panel: Increase of brain size (cranial capacity) in humans over the past 3.5 million years. Note that human brain size begins to increase about 1.75 million years ago, with a rapid increase over the past 200 000 years. Right panel: Relationship between brain size and body weight in fossil hominids. Note that brain sizes are disproportionately large for body size in all hominids. Redrawn from http://www.indiana.edu/~brainevo/publications/dissertation/Dissertationch2.htm[9]

The conclusion from Figure 16.1 and Table 16.1 on page 312 is unambiguous. Humans are primarily carnivores designed to eat animal products. This irrefutable anatomical evidence fits well with the record of what our hominin ancestors ate.

There is also a growing body of evidence showing that our ancestors specifically chose to hunt animals that would provide the most fat. Surprisingly, these were the larger, healthier animals. In the Levant, this meant hunting elephants.[10] Why was this, when logic suggests that 'feeble' humans would surely choose to hunt the weakest animals they could find? There is a constraint in the human ability to metabolise protein to energy.[11] As a result, humans are unable to eat a diet in which more than about 40 per cent of their daily calorie intake is provided by protein; accordingly, the remaining 60 per cent of the energy must come from carbohydrate or fat. There is strong evidence that early humans specifically chose those animal species, and indeed individuals within those species, whose bodies contained the most fat.

Thus, 'fat, not meat, was the essential food for survival to hunting and gathering cultures';[12] 'it therefore must be fat rather than protein that drives the desire for meat in many foraging societies';[13] and 'fat, not protein, seemed to play a very prominent role in the hunters' decisions about what animals (male vs. female) to kill and which body parts to discard or take away'.[14]

Table 16.1 Function and structural comparison of man's digestive tract with that of the dog and sheep

	MAN	DOG	SHEEP
TEETH			
Incisors	both jaws	both jaws	lower jaw only
Molars	ridged	ridged	flat
Canines	small	large	absent
JAW			
Movements	vertical	vertical	rotary
Function	tearing, crushing	tearing, crushing	grinding
Mastication	unimportant	unimportant	vital function
Rumination	never	never	vital function
STOMACH			
Capacity	2 quarts	2 quarts	8.5 gallons
Emptying time	3 hours	3 hours	never empties
Interdigestive rest	yes	yes	no
Bacteria present	no	no	yes – vital
Protozoa present	no	no	yes – vital
Gastric acidity	strong	strong	weak
Cellulose digestion	none	none	70% – vital
Digestive activity	weak	weak	vital function
Food absorbed from	no	no	vital function
COLON AND CAECUM			
Size of colon	short, small	short, small	long, capacious
Size of caecum	tiny	tiny	long, capacious
Function of caecum	none	none	vital function
Appendix	vestigial	absent	caecum
Rectum	small	small	capacious
Digestive activity	none	none	vital function
Cellulose digestion	none	none	30% – vital
Bacterial flora	putrefactive	putrefactive	fermentative
Food absorbed from	none	none	vital function
Volume of faeces	small, firm	small, firm	voluminous
Gross food in faeces	rare	rare	large amount
GALL BLADDER			
Size	well developed	well developed	often absent
Function	strong	strong	weak or absent
DIGESTIVE ACTIVITY			
From pancreas	solely	solely	partial
From bacteria	none	none	partial
From protozoa	none	none	partial
Digestive efficiency	100%	100%	50% or less
FEEDING HABITS			
Frequency	intermittent	intermittent	continuous
SURVIVAL WITHOUT			
Stomach	possible	possible	impossible
Colon and caecum	possible	possible	impossible
Microorganisms	possible	possible	impossible
Plant foods	possible	possible	impossible
Animal protein	impossible	impossible	possible
RATIO OF BODY LENGTH TO			
Entire digestive tract	1:5	1:7	1:27
Small intestine	1:4	1:6	1:25

Reproduced from W.L. Voegtlin, *The Stone Age Diet*, New York: Vantage Press, 1975, pp. 44–45

The benefit of hunting large (but more dangerous) mammals like elephant, rhinoceros, hippopotamus, buffalo and eland is then more easily understood. Miki Ben-Dor has calculated that the body of an eland – the revered prey of the !Kung San – provides the same amount of fat as 24 impalas, even though the body weight of an eland is only 10 times greater than that of an impala. A single hippopotamus provides the fat equivalent of 75 impalas.[15]

My conclusion is that humans evolved as obligate fat-eaters, and our biology is dependent on eating diets high in fat and moderate in protein, with carbohydrates providing only that balance of calories that cannot be obtained from readily available fat and protein sources.

All this evidence demonstrates that fish and animal produce are essential to optimise human brain development. Only fish and animal produce contain the necessary brain-specific nutrients[16] in high concentrations; these nutrients are not present in appropriate concentrations in cereals and grains. That is why meat and fish – and not cereals and grains, however much they might be 'fortified' – are the only suitable complementary foods.

This raises the next key question: If humans are big-brained mammals, when in our life cycle do our big brains develop?

Logically, one might think it occurs in the womb, i.e. before birth. But if this were the case, the diameter of the female pelvis would have had to increase proportionally to allow the passage of a large-brained foetus. And wide-hipped humans would have been less efficient runners, preventing effective persistence hunting in midday heat, another key to our evolution as a species.[17] So a better solution had to be found. And this was to concentrate the period of greatest growth of the human brain to within the first 1 000 days of life.

But there was still one other critical problem that had to be overcome.

The human brain comprises 60 per cent fat, over 25 per cent of which is cholesterol. The presence of a blood–brain barrier that prevents the passage of large molecules (such as dangerous bacteria or viruses) directly from the bloodstream to the brain also means that any large molecules needed to construct those fats cannot reach the brain directly. The solution that human evolution conferred was to use ketone bodies for this purpose.

Ketone bodies are produced by the liver whenever blood insulin concentrations are low, and fat, not carbohydrate, is being used as the principal energy fuel. Ketones are small, water-soluble molecules that can cross the blood–brain barrier and be used to build the complex fat molecules (like cholesterol) that comprise a large proportion of the human brain. In this way, 'Humans co-opted a trait that was previously an adaptation to cope with periods of starvation, into our default metabolism to support brain growth in particular, but also to meet the brain's ongoing energy requirements.'[18]

Figure 16.3

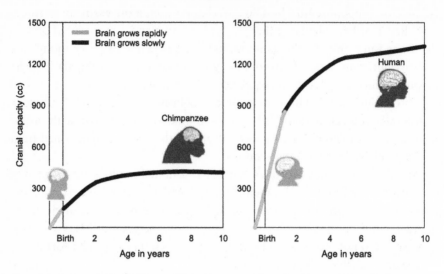

Change in brain size during the first 10 years of life in chimpanzees (left panel) and humans (right panel). Note that most of the increase in brain size (cranial capacity) in humans occurs during the first four years after birth, but especially during the first two years of life. Crucial to my HPCSA trial was my argument that, during this period, infants need to be weaned onto foods that are high in brain-specific nutrients – namely, animal- and fish-based foods. Reproduced from Amber O'Hearn, 'Optimal weaning from an evolutionary perspective'[19]

Blood-borne ketone bodies are thus essential for human survival and brain growth, a fact that none of the HPCSA's expert witnesses seemed to understand. Instead, all expressed the false belief that ketones are harmful because of their association with diabetic ketoacidosis, a condition with which each 'expert' seemed to have a shallow acquaintance. It is clear that doctors and dietitians in South Africa are not taught that ketosis is healthy and the natural state of the newborn, and crucial for the full development of the large human brain.

It follows that during the first 1000 days of life, the infant must be fed a diet that is rich in brain-essential nutrients. In addition, the diet must ensure that sufficient ketone bodies are produced to fuel this period of rapid brain growth. As I argued in both *Raising Superheroes* and the HPCSA trial, brain-essential nutrients are **not** found in maize and other cereals onto which South Africans are encouraged to wean their babies. In *Raising Superheroes* I also presented evidence that the human newborn has a high capacity to both produce and metabolise ketone bodies, perhaps even better than fat-adapted adults.

For Claire Julsing Strydom to suggest that ketosis is dangerous for newborns and might even be 'life-threatening', and for the HPCSA then to prosecute me on that basis, exposes a very worrying level of ignorance in the South African medical and dietetics professions.

In summary, we can conclude that two million years ago our hominin ances-

A foregut fermenter that has adapted to carnivory; a carnivore that has failed to adapt to herbivory

Two mammals show that it is easier for the mammalian intestine to convert from herbivory to carnivory than to do the reverse. Dolphins are sea-living, fish-eating carnivores whose closest relatives are thought to be land mammals, specifically the hippopotamuses and other hoofed ruminants, including camels, pigs and giraffes, from whom they diverged about 50 million years ago when some enterprising dolphin ancestor decided she would prefer to live in the sea. While modern dolphins retain anatomical evidence of a four-chambered (ruminant) stomach, it no longer operates as a fermenting vat filled with anaerobic bacteria. Instead, the dolphins' herbivore-like stomach now works exactly as do the stomachs of other carnivores such as wolves, lions and humans.

Contrast this to the experience of the panda bear. Bears have the digestive tract of carnivores, although most bears (other than polar bears) are omnivores. Lacking a long large bowel specifically designed for fermentation, the omnivorous bears compensate by eating more plant material and supplementing with meat and fish when available. For the past two million years or so, however, panda bears have lived in an environment in which bamboo makes up 99 per cent of their diet. Yet in that time, the panda has not adapted in any way to herbivory.

In particular, the gut of the panda bear does not contain the cellulose-digesting bacteria present in abundance in the intestines of fermenting herbivores. Instead, 'the giant panda appears not to have evolved a gut microbiota compatible with its newly adopted diet, which may adversely influence the co-evolutionary fitness of this herbivore'.[20] So 'the giant panda still retains a gastrointestinal tract typical of carnivores. The animals also do not have the genes for plant-digesting enzymes in their own genome. This combined scenario may have increased their risk for extinction.'[21] Scientists speculate that it was the unfortunate loss of one of the genes driving meat-eating – the umami taste receptor – that may have converted pandas to herbivory.

As a result of this failure to adapt to herbivory, pandas must spend up to 14 hours a day eating up to 13 kilograms of leaves and stems of which they digest only about 17 per cent. Because so little of this material is digested, pandas must pass voluminous faeces – as many as 40 times per day. In addition, they are prone to develop irritable bowel syndrome: 'They get stomach cramps, go off their food and lie in a heap for a few days.'[22]

Their nutritionally poor diet explains why panda bears reproduce so poorly – female pandas ovulate only once a year and are fertile for about three days; why they limit their social interactions; why they must spend up to 12 hours a day sleeping; and why they avoid walking up steeply sloping terrain. Their somnolence gives 'the impression of an animal that eats purely to have enough energy to carry on eating'.[23]

This is the natural consequence of eating a nutrient-poor, exclusively plant-based diet.

tors had already mastered the art of killing and eating large mammals on the African savannah, with little more than stone implements. These skills were essential for the conversion of humans from herbivory to carnivory. In the process, they evolved from small- to large-brained mammals capable of prodigious mental achievements.

By leaving behind the security of the forests and jungles, our hominin ancestors embarked on the journey that would ultimately lead to us, *Homo sapiens*.

When humans began their conversion to carnivory two to three million years ago, they no longer needed bacteria to enhance the quality of the nutrient-poor, plant-based diet they had eaten in the past. Perhaps our ancestors realised that rather than eating a nutrient-poor diet and having to eat and defecate all day, it would be much more efficient to leave that to the experts – cellulose-fermenting herbivores – and then simply catch and eat those experts.

The change to a nutrient-dense diet removed the need for a long and volumin-ous fermenting large bowel, producing humans with a much-reduced abdominal cavity. As a result, our hips became narrower, allowing more efficient running (as our knees were closer together). With time and additional adaptations, as described in my book *Waterlogged*,[24] humans became the perfect two-legged running mammal, able to chase even four-legged ruminants to their exhaustion in midday heat. In time, the development of highly mobile shoulders allowed humans to become adept throwers of spears and other stone implements, so that running in the heat became a less important method of hunting. The end result was that the more nutrient-dense foods our human ancestors ate, the larger our energy-demanding brains became.

I argue that these anatomical changes – but most especially our conversion from hindgut fermenting hominins to carnivorous *Homo sapiens* dependent only on a functioning small bowel for the digestion and absorption of our nutrient-dense, predominantly animal-based diet – adequately explain why the obesity/T2DM epidemic was bound to happen when modern humans switched to a diet that derives most of its energy from carbohydrates.

And that is exactly what happened after 1977 when we were told that, to pro-tect ourselves from heart attack, we had to replace most of the fat in our diet with carbohydrates.

Unfortunately, those who advised us to undertake this disastrous experiment failed to understand that the carnivore's digestive tract is simply not designed to cope with a high-carbohydrate diet. And it was not as if we had not already been warned by the first disastrous human dietary experiment, courtesy of the agri-cultural revolution.

The agricultural revolution

Beginning about 12 000 years ago, humans living in the Fertile Crescent in Western Asia, including the areas surrounding the Tigris, Euphrates and Nile rivers, began to domesticate animals and cultivate grains for the first time. The addition of cereals and grains to the human diet reduced our reliance on hunting, fishing and gathering. A secure source of storable, year-round food allowed the growth of stable communities living together in towns and villages.

Jared Diamond suggests that, for the future of the earth and the human spe-cies, agriculture was 'the worst mistake in the history of the human race'.[25] According to him, the adoption of farming produced a number of serious disad-

Figure 16.4

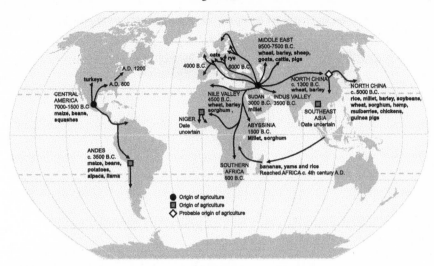

The spread of agriculture since 8 000 BC. Dates indicate achievement of food production by some people in the region. Arrows show movement of imported domesticated food products. Note that wheat and barley were first domesticated in the Fertile Crescent, whereas maize, beans, potatoes and squashes come from Central and South America. Rice, millet, soybeans, sorghum and hemp are from North China. Redrawn from 'Agriculture slowly spreads'[26]

vantages, including starvation, epidemic diseases and malnutrition. By 3 000 BC, humans living on cereals and grains had lost at least five inches in height; some peoples, the Greeks and Turks in particular, have still to regain the average heights of their pre-agricultural relatives. But perhaps worst of all, agriculture produced deep class divisions, as it allowed some to accumulate wealth by storing food.

Similarly, in his book *Sapiens*, Yuval Noah Harari devotes an entire chapter to the agricultural revolution, which he calls 'history's biggest fraud'. He argues that wheat domesticated humans, not the reverse (to wheat's, not humans', advantage), so that: 'This is the essence of the Agricultural Revolution: the ability to keep more people alive under worse conditions.'[27]

The precise reason why humans turned to cereals and grains as a food source after millions of years of hunting is contested, and at least three separate theories have been advanced. The first is that human hunters were so successful that they exterminated the once-plentiful animals on which they lived, especially those with the highest body-fat contents.[28] Thus they had to find an alternative source of energy to compensate for the 'fat gap' in their daily energy intakes. The second is that humans fell for some or other addictive chemicals present in grains. This is compatible with Harari's idea that grains domesticated humans, rather than the other way around. The third theory is that cereals and grains were grown to entice wild animals so that they could be more easily captured.

With time, the cultivation of cereals spread east and west (see Figure 16.4), in

Figure 16.5

Landmasses covered by ice during the last ice age (114 000–10 000 years ago)

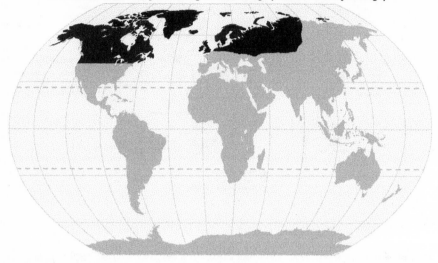

The last ice age lasted from 114 000 to about 10 000 years ago, during which much of North America, Europe, including most of the British Isles, and Asia were under sheets of ice up to a mile thick. Redrawn from A. Watts, '90% of the last million years, the normal state of the Earth's climate has been an ice age'[29]

part because cultivation destroyed the soil of the Fertile Crescent so that new, still-fertile lands had to be found.

So for people like myself, with Western European ancestry, the first exposure of our ancestors to dietary cereals and grains can only have occurred within the last 10 000 years. Until then, our (Western) European ancestors most likely lived mainly on the woolly mammoths, whose distribution matched almost perfectly the distribution of the ice cap,[30] but which were hunted to extinction as recently as 4 000 years ago.

As described in *The Real Meal Revolution*, the Egyptians were one of the first to adopt wheat as a dietary staple, to the extent that they were nicknamed 'artophagoi', meaning eaters of bread. Comprising primarily carbohydrates (bread, fruits, vegetables, honey), oils (olive, flaxseed, safflower, sesame), goat's milk and cheese, fish, waterfowl and occasional red meat, their diet was an almost perfect example of the kind – low in saturated fat and cholesterol – that would be prescribed as ideal in the 1977 US dietary guidelines.

As Dr Michael Eades points out, if such is the ultimately healthy diet, then the 'ancient Egyptians should have lived forever or at least should have lived long, healthy lives and died of old age in their beds. But did they?'[31]

Eades provides evidence to answer his own question: 'So, a picture begins to emerge of an Egyptian populace, rife with disabling dental problems, fat bellies and crippling heart disease … sounds a lot like the afflictions of millions of

Figure 16.6

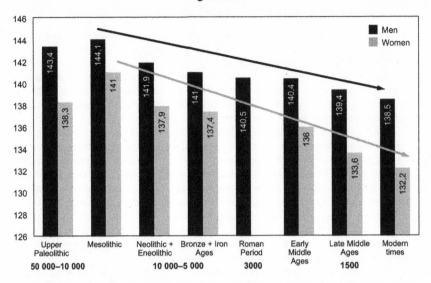

Fossil evidence showing a reduction in human skull size in the past 10 000 years. Redrawn from M. Henneberg, 'Decrease of human skull size in the Holocene'[32]

people in America today, doesn't it? The Egyptians didn't eat much fat, had no refined carbohydrates ... and ate almost nothing but whole grains, fresh fruits and vegetables, and fish and fowl, yet were beset with all the same diseases that afflict modern man. Modern man, who is exhorted to eat lots of whole grains, fresh fruits and vegetables, to prevent or reverse these diseases.' Eades concludes that this historical evidence might suggest that 'there are some real problems with the low-fat, high carbohydrate diet'.[33]

Interestingly, this grain-based diet did not prevent the development of arterial disease. In a treatise published in 1911, Sir Marc Armand Ruffer wrote: 'I cannot therefore at present give any reason why arterial disease should have been so prevalent in ancient Egypt. I think, however, that it is interesting to find that it was common, and that three thousand years ago it represented the same anatomical characteristics as it does now.'[34]

Another cost of adopting a cereal-based diet may be that human brain size has decreased progressively in the past 10 000 years. The decline began at precisely the moment when humans began to raise their children on cereals and grains and less animal produce. This possibility should be of interest to those involved in my HPCSA trial, as should the story of how maize, a nutrient-poor food that does not contain all the brain-specific nutrients, became the staple 'complementary food' for infant weaning in South Africa.

The special place of maize in the traditional South African diet

Maize has a special place in the South African diet and formed a key ingredient in the debate over whether or not I had acted unprofessionally by suggesting that LCHF foods are the ideal complementary foods for weaning.

As shown in Figure 16.4, maize is a Central American, not a traditional African, cereal. It was introduced to the east coast of South Africa by Portuguese sailors in the 1500s,[35] and was adopted as an agricultural crop by local Xhosa-speaking persistence farmers, but not to any great extent by European settlers.

The discovery of diamonds in the north-eastern Cape in 1867 and gold in the Witwatersrand in 1886 dramatically increased the number of people attracted to the South African interior. Their requirements for food, especially for the mineworkers, rapidly outstripped local production. The solution was to import maize from Lesotho. But beginning in the 1930s, South African farmers began to invest in maize production, especially in what would become known as the Maize Triangle, extending from the North West province in the west to Swaziland in the north-east and to the northern borders of Lesotho in the south. At the end of the Second World War, government subsidies to these farmers caused a boom in maize production, so that today locally grown maize accounts for 40 per cent of South Africans' dietary energy intake,[36] the seventh highest in the world.

Interestingly, Hester Vorster and Salome Kruger, two of the HPCSA's expert witnesses, are from North-West University, which sits comfortably within the Maize Triangle. The university is actively involved in maize-based research.

Under cross-examination in the hearing, Vorster argued that the reason why the South African paediatric nutritional guidelines do not mention that carbohydrates are an essential dietary element for infants between 6 and 12 months was because it was obvious – the majority of South Africans just know that maize is the complementary food of choice for infant weaning.

But maize can never be a complementary food, because it does not complement breast milk by adding that which breast milk lacks. Even when fortified, maize lacks decent amounts of brain-essential nutrients. And where are the RCTs confirming the effectiveness of maize as a complementary food for weaning? Neither Vorster nor Kruger produced any such evidence.

If maize only entered our food chain very recently (about 1930), what did South Africans eat before?

This raises a further question, one for which I have struggled to find an answer: What did the Nguni tribes, who entered South Africa from the north between AD 600 and 1400, and who gave rise to all current ethnic groups in South Africa – specifically the Zulu, Xhosa, Ndebele and Swazi peoples – eat?

It is clear that until the last century, cattle (and perhaps goats) played a central role in Nguni culture. Zulu-speaking South Africans in KwaZulu-Natal revered the Nguni cattle. By 1824, for example, Shaka Zulu's royal cattle pen contained 7000 pure white Nguni cattle.[37] Similarly, when the original pioneers arrived in Zimbabwe (then Rhodesia), they reported that the country was 'teeming with cattle that were, apparently, in good health and were immune to local diseases'.[38]

In *The Abundant Herds*, Marguerite Poland writes:

Before 1850, there were an estimated four to five million Nguni cattle in what is now KwaZulu-Natal. Indeed it could have been said that, so immense was the number of cattle, *idaka liye lahlaba ezulwini* (the kraal-mud was splashed up to heaven), but war, disease, political unrest and the introduction by whites of their own cattle, led to a decline in numbers so that a decade ago only about 100 000 pure Ngunis remained. In 1879, at the close of the Anglo-Zulu War, in which the power of the Zulu Kingdom was broken, Sir Garnet Wolseley ensured the end of the Zulu royal herds by slaughtering and confiscating what remained.[39]

There is also ample evidence that cattle were critically important to the health of Xhosa-speaking South Africans living in the Eastern Cape (then British Kaffraria).

In 1856, on the basis of a spiritual encounter, the AmaGcaleka prophetess Nongqawuse informed her uncle that to rid their people of the oppressive British colonial influence, the AmaGcaleka had to slaughter all their cattle. At the time, many of their herds were plagued with 'lung sickness', possibly introduced by European cattle. In return, Nongqawuse prophesied, the spirits would sweep the British settlers into the sea, and the AmaGcaleka would be able to replenish their granaries and fill their kraals with more beautiful and healthier cattle. Nongqawuse's uncle duly informed Paramount Chief Sarhili of his niece's prophecy.

Historians estimate that the AmaGcaleka killed between 300 000 and 400 000 head of cattle between 1857 and 1858. In the aftermath of the crisis, the population of British Kaffraria dropped from 105 000 to fewer than 27 000 due to the resulting famine. If cattle and dairy produce had not been a key food of the AmaGcaleka, this famine would not have happened.

Another event proving the importance of cattle to Xhosa- and Zulu-speaking South Africans was the destruction caused by the rinderpest virus that swept through Southern Africa between 1896 and 1897, killing an estimated 2.5 million cattle. So catastrophic was the event that, in December 1896, the German physician Robert Koch, considered the father of modern bacteriology, arrived in Cape Town, where he worked for three months perfecting a cure.[40]

The effects of this disease on the future health of South Africans would, in retrospect, prove catastrophic. As historian Charles van Onselen notes:

> The loss of large numbers of cattle caused considerable social and economic distress in African communities. With the disappearance of the source of meat and milk, Africans experienced considerable hardship and, in some cases, starvation ... the impoverishment of Africans caused by rinderpest contributed to the growing proletarianisation of Africans and the process of labour migration.[41]

The end result was a tragic repeat of what befell the Plains Indians* of North America, who lived exclusively on bison and who, in the early 1800s, were among the world's tallest and healthiest humans.[42] In 1877, Lieutenant Scott, a US cavalry scout, wrote about the Cheyenne scouts, who had led to the defeat of General Custer at the Battle of the Little Bighorn in 1876:

> ... they were all keen, athletic young men, tall and lean and brave, and I admired them as real specimens of manhood more than any body of men I have ever seen before or since. They were perfectly adapted to their environment, and knew just what to do in every emergency and when to do it, without any confusion or lost motion. Their poise and dignity were superb; no royal person ever had more assured manners. I watched their every movement and learned lessons from them that later saved my life many times on the prairie.[43]

Scott also noted that the Crow, the enemies of the Cheyenne, hunted bison once a week from large herds and that their camp 'was full of meat drying everywhere. Everybody was carefree and joyous.'[44]

Others reported that the American Indians were free of the diseases that afflicted European settlers, including diabetes, cancer, heart disease and most infectious diseases: 'It is rare to see a sick body amongst them'; they are 'unacquainted with a great many diseases that afflict the Europeans such as gout, gravel and dropsy, etc'; 'While cancer is occasionally met with in primitive [sic] races, it occurs so seldom among the American Indians for instance, that this race may be considered practically immune from this disease'; and 'In bodily proportions, color, gesture, dignity of bearing, the race is incomparable. It was free from our infectious scourges, tuberculosis and syphilis ... probably free from leprosy, scrofula and cancer, and it is safe to say that nervous prostration was unknown to the [American] Indian.'[45]

The expansion of the settlers west of the Mississippi after 1860 foretold the end of the Plains Indians' free and healthy existence, for the settlers exterminated the bison, replacing the carnivorous diet of the Plains Indians with the modern industrial diet. As a result, diabetes and obesity are now rampant among their

---

* Much of the research of obesity and diabetes in Native Americans has focused on the Pima Indians, who were subsistence farmers with a higher-carbohydrate intake. Pima obesity began when their water supply was cut off with the building of the Hoover Dam in Colorado and they were no longer able to farm. As a result, the conclusion has been drawn that Native Americans became obese when they began to eat a higher-fat diet, conveniently exonerating the 1977 US dietary guidelines of any blame. But the opposite has occurred in the Plains Indians, whose obesity is clearly associated with the adoption of the modern industrial diet, which contains less fat and protein than their historic carnivorous diet of bison. For some reason, the cause of obesity in the Plains Indians is almost never discussed or researched. This raises many questions.

descendants.[46] Essentially the same has happened in Southern Africa, and for the same reasons.

In South Africa, the rinderpest epidemic drove rural South Africans to the cities, where they invariably got work on the mines. The wealth generated by their work was used to fund the production of maize, which then became the staple diet particularly of those living and working on the mines in the Maize Triangle.

My conclusion is that if we travel far enough back in the history of the Nguni peoples, who entered Southern Africa in the last 1 000 years, we will find that animal produce constituted a significant proportion of their diet. And why not? The countryside teemed with wild game, even before the Nguni domesticated their cattle. Since the development of mining, which led to the industrialisation of South Africa over the last 100 years or so, that diet has been replaced by one in which maize is the single most important contributor. I would, therefore, argue that the ill health of so many South Africans can be traced directly to these historical events.

But in my trial, I learnt that those responsible for drawing up the South African dietary guidelines have little interest in exploring these facts. Which raises the question: Why? The answer can be found in the fact that humans were very healthy before they began eating the modern industrial diet with its high amounts of sugar, refined grains, trans fats and vegetable oils.

The health of the mid-Victorians living in England between 1850 and 1880
The mid-Victorian period between 1850 and 1880 is now recognised as the golden era of British health. According to P. Clayton and J. Rowbotham,[47] this was entirely due to the mid-Victorians' superior diet. Farm-produced real foods were available in such surplus that even the working-class poor were eating highly nutritious foods in abundance. As a result, life expectancy in 1875 was equal to, or even better, than it is in modern Britain, especially for men (by about three years). In addition, the profile of diseases was quite different when compared to Britain today.

The authors conclude:

> [This] shows that medical advances allied to the pharmaceutical industry's output have done little more than change the manner of our dying. The Victorians died rapidly of infection and/or trauma, whereas we die slowly of degenerative disease. It reveals that with the exception of family planning, the vast edifice of twentieth century healthcare has not enabled us to live longer but has in the main merely supplied methods of suppressing the symptoms of degenerative disease which have emerged due to our failure to maintain mid-Victorian nutritional standards.[48]

Figure 16.7

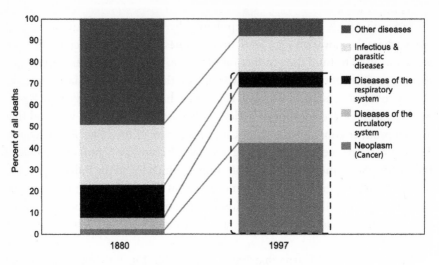

Comparison of causes of death in mid-Victorians living in England and Wales in 1880 compared with modern data from 1997. Note the large increases in deaths from cancers and diseases of the circulatory system, with reductions in deaths from infections, and parasitic and 'other' diseases. Redrawn from P. Clayton and J. Rowbotham, 'How the mid-Victorians worked, ate and died'[49]

This mid-Victorians' healthy diet included freely available and cheap vegetables such as onions, carrots, turnips, cabbage, broccoli, peas and beans; fresh and dried fruit, including apples; legumes and nuts, especially chestnuts, walnuts and hazelnuts; fish, including herring, haddock and John Dory; other seafood, including oysters, mussels and whelks; meat – which was considered 'a mark of a good diet' so that 'its complete absence was rare' – sourced from free-range animals, especially pork, and including offal such as brain, heart, pancreas (sweetbreads), liver, kidneys, lungs and intestine; eggs from hens that were kept by most urban households; and hard cheeses.

Their healthy diet was therefore low in cereals, grains, sugar, trans fats and refined flour, and high in fibre, phytonutrients and omega-3 polyunsaturated fatty acids, entirely compatible with the modern Paleo or LCHF diets.

This period of nutritional paradise changed suddenly after 1875, when cheap imports of white flour, tinned meat, sugar, canned fruits and condensed milk became more readily available. The results were immediately noticeable. By 1883, the British infantry was forced to lower its minimum height for recruits by three inches; and by 1900, 50 per cent of British volunteers for the Boer War had to be rejected because of undernutrition. The changes would have been associated with an alteration in disease patterns in these populations, as described by Yellowlees (Chapter 2).

The health of traditional societies eating their traditional foods

India

Major General Sir Robert McCarrison, who died in 1960, is remembered as one of the very first to understand the essential role of proper nutrition in human health.[50] He wrote that 'the greatest single factor in the acquisition and maintenance of good health is perfectly constituted food':

> I know of nothing so potent in maintaining good health in laboratory animals as perfectly constituted food; I know of nothing so potent in producing ill health as improperly constituted food. This, too, is the experience of stockbreeders. Is man an exception to a rule so universally applied to the higher animals?[51]

'So it is,' he continued, 'that research has provided, or is providing, an explanation of the fundamental fact that a diet composed of natural foodstuffs, in proper proportion one to another, is the **paramount influence in the maintenance of health** [my emphasis].'[52]

This statement is profound; so profound that it has yet to make any impact on the teachings and practices of modern (allopathic) medicine, which, aside from the obvious nutritional deficiency diseases like scurvy and pellagra, ignores the role of nutrition in ill health, preferring rather the use of pharmacologically active agents to suppress disease symptoms, seldom producing cures.

McCarrison was the first to study the effects of nutritionally deficient diets in different animal models, establishing how particular nutritional deficiencies caused specific medical conditions, including goitre, cretinism and beriberi. On the advice of 1932 Nobel laureate Sir Charles Sherrington, McCarrison spent the bulk of his medical career as Director of Nutritional Research in India. There, as Sherrington had suggested, he set about studying the diets and health of the different Indian peoples.

He wished to understand how different dietary patterns across the Indian continent produced peoples with different body shapes, physical abilities and disease patterns, and the possible role of nutritional deficiencies in determining these characteristics. 'Indeed, nothing could be more striking than the contrast between the manly, stalwart and resolute races of the north – the Pathans, Baluchis, Sikhs, Punjabis, Rajputs and Maharattas – and the poorly developed, toneless and supine people of the east and south: Bengalis, Madrassis, Kanarese and Travancorians,' he wrote.[53]

McCarrison noted that the Pathans are meat-eaters, whereas the Bengalis, Madrassis and Kanarese are, for the most part, vegetarians:

As we pass from the north to the east, south-east, south-west and south of India, there is thus a gradual fall in the nutritive value of cereal grains forming the staples of the national diet, this fall reaching the lowest limit amongst the rice-eaters of the east and south. There is also a gradual fall in the amount of animal protein, animal fats and vitamins entering into these diets.[54]

He concluded:

The poorer classes, according to the degree of their poverty, drop out, in part or in whole, the more expensive or less easily obtainable items: milk, milk products, animal fats, legumes, fruit and vegetables. So that as the people are poorer and poorer their diets are more and more cereal in nature, more and more imbalanced, more and more depleted of animal protein, animal fats, vitamins and essential nutrients.[55]

A key weakness of this poor diet, he observed, 'takes the form of an excessive richness of the food in carbohydrates'.[56]

McCarrison's key conclusion was that differences in physical appearance and physical vigour between the different Indian populations could be explained by the extent to which their diets were nutritionally adequate, especially in terms of animal proteins and fats. The overriding problem was not gross dietary deficiencies ('complete want of certain food factors'), but rather the 'combinations of such insufficiencies'.[57]

What is so remarkable is that the LFHC nutrient-poor diet of the rice-eating southern Indians that McCarrison described is not too dissimilar to the 'prudent' diet advocated by the US dietary guidelines. Should we really be so surprised that our health has deteriorated so dramatically since we adopted a diet that more closely resembles that of the poorer Indian peoples?

McCarrison concluded the following overall:

The newer knowledge of nutrition has revealed, and reveals the more with every addition to it, that a chief cause of the physiological decay of organs and tissues of the body is faulty food, wherein deficiencies of some essentials are often combined with excess of others. It is reasonable, then, to assume that dietetic malnutrition is a chief cause of many degenerative diseases of mankind. However this may be, it seems clear that the habitual use of a diet made up of natural foodstuffs, in proper proportions one to another, and produced on soils that are not impoverished is an essential condition for the efficient exercise of the function of nutrition on which the maintenance of health depends. This, combined with the proper exercise of the body and of its adaptive functions, is mankind's main defense against degenerative diseases:

a bulwark, too, against those of infectious origin. Such, at least, is the conclusion to which my own studies in deficiency disease have led me.[58]

Another forgotten Indian nutrition researcher, S.L. Malhotra, was the chief medical officer of Western Railway in Mumbai (formerly Bombay). From that office, he studied the rates of hospital admission of railway employees in different regions of India. He showed that the incidence of acute heart attacks was seven times higher in the rice-eating Indians living in the south than among the Punjabis in the north, who ate 8 to 19 times more fat, chiefly of animal origin, and about 9 times more sugar.[59]

Malhotra also noted that the fats ingested by the two populations differed: in the north, the preponderant fat was saturated fat mainly from milk and fermented milk products, whereas in the south, vegetable fats dominated. Naturally, he concluded that his data did 'not fit the hypothesis that low ratios of poly-unsaturated to saturated fatty acids in food, or even an excess of sugar in food, contribute to an increased incidence of ischaemic heart disease'.[60]

Malhotra also compared rates of gallstone formation (cholelithiasis) – seven times higher in the north than in the south;[61] peptic ulceration,[62] including the effects of wheat or rice diets in recovery;[63] gastrointestinal cancers[64] – more stomach and colon cancers in the south, more liver and gallbladder cancers in the north; and varicose veins, which were more common in those living in the south.[65]

Africa

One of the first observations made by early medical missionaries in Africa was the apparent absence of cases of cancer. Albert Schweitzer, who worked as a physician in Gabon for 41 years, wrote:

> On my arrival in Gabon in 1913, I was astonished to encounter no case of cancer … I cannot, of course, say positively that there was no cancer at all, but like other frontier doctors, I can only say that if such cases existed they must have been quite rare. In the course of the years, we have seen cases of cancer in growing numbers in our region. My observation inclines me to attribute this to the fact that the natives were living more and more after the manner of the whites.'[66]

Denis Burkitt, considered the father of the dietary-fibre hypothesis, spent 24 years in Uganda during and after the Second World War. He wrote that 44 hospitals he surveyed had never seen a case of colon cancer, heart disease, diverticulitis or appendicitis.[67]

Africa also includes ethnic groupings that chose to eat different diets either predominantly carnivorous or plant-based. In 1931, J.B. Orr and J.L. Gilks compared the health and physical attributes of the Akikuyu, a 'vegetarian tribe' eating predominantly cereals supplemented with roots and fruits, with the 'largely carnivorous' Masai, whose diet comprised milk, meat and raw blood. Compared to adult Akikuyu, adult Masai were about five inches taller, 23 pounds (10 kilograms) heavier, and 50 per cent stronger when tested with a hand dynamometer. In addition, bony deformities, dental caries, anaemia, pulmonary conditions and tropical ulcers were much more prevalent in the Akikuyu, whereas rheumatoid arthritis and 'intestinal stasis' were more common in the Masai.[68]

When the diet-heart hypothesis began to attract serious attention in the 1960s, some scientists wondered about the health of the carnivorous Masai and Samburu tribes of Tanzania and northern Kenya. If the diet-heart and lipid hypotheses were true, these groups would exhibit high blood cholesterol concentrations and rampant rates of heart disease. But neither proved true: both tribes had low to normal blood cholesterol concentrations and an apparent absence of coronary heart disease, although, interestingly, the Masai did have 'extensive atherosclerosis but very few complicated lesions'.[69] Complicated lesions occur when the arterial plaque ruptures. Thus, the apparent immunity to heart disease in the Masai must be because their diet and lifestyle protect them from coronary artery plaque rupture, not from atherosclerosis.

Another nomadic population eating the same diet as the Masai and Samburu, the Anagamba of eastern Niger, also had low blood cholesterol concentrations despite eating a diet comprising 73 per cent fat.[70] Interestingly, and seemingly forgotten, the Anagamba's blood cholesterol concentrations were no higher than those of the Kanouri, who ate an LFHC diet of millet and sorghum, and deriving just 9 per cent of calories from fat.

Multiple populations studied by Dr Weston Price

Perhaps the person who has made the greatest contribution to our understanding of how dietary changes influence human health is Dr Weston Price, a dental surgeon from Cleveland, Ohio. In 1931, Price and his wife, Florence, embarked on an epic medical journey to discover why the prevalence of dental caries in patients treated in his dental practice had suddenly increased so dramatically.[71]

Price's thinking would have been influenced by a 1928 paper that reported the serendipitous finding that children with T1DM treated with insulin and a LCHF diet, as was the practice in the 1920s, showed reversal of their dental caries.[72] The diet was made up of milk, cream, butter, eggs, meat, cod liver oil, bulky vegetables and fruit. It seems that before he left on his world tour, Price tested this theory for himself. He showed that feeding one meal a day high in fat-soluble vitamins to a group of 30 children with active dental caries prevented the progression of dental decay.[73]

In the course of his investigations, Price had also discovered South African fossil evidence showing that dental caries were not present in prehistoric humans;[74] thus, by the time he left Cleveland, he must have strongly suspected that dental decay had a purely nutritional cause. But to prove this hypothesis, the Prices realised that they had to measure the prevalence of dental caries in populations still eating a 'control diet', i.e. populations that have continued to eat the same foods their forefathers ate before the agricultural revolution and the more recent introduction of industrial, processed foods.

Over the next decade, the Prices examined the teeth and general health of the Swiss inhabitants of the Lötschental Valley; of Scottish families living on the Outer and Inner Hebrides; of the Inuit (Eskimos) of Alaska; of the Indians of north, west and central Canada, the western United States and Florida; of the Melanesians and Polynesians inhabiting eight archipelagos of the Southern Pacific; of six tribes in eastern and central Africa, including the Masai; of the Aborigines of Australia; of Malay tribes living on islands north of Australia; of the Maori of New Zealand; and of South Americans in Peru and the Amazon Basin. Wherever possible, the health of those continuing to eat the traditional foods was compared with others in the area who had begun to eat the imported diet of processed foods.

Without exception, the findings in all these populations were the same. Specifically, those who continued to eat the foods of their ancestors showed:
- an almost total absence of tooth decay;
- broad faces, wide nostrils and perfect dental arches;
- superior immunity, demonstrated by an absence of tuberculosis in some communities (such as the Swiss of the Lötschental Valley); and
- an absence of most of the modern 'chronic diseases of lifestyle', including cancer, rheumatic diseases and other autoimmune diseases.

Yet dental decay and the other 'chronic diseases of lifestyle' started to appear in the first generation of those who began to eat what Price called the 'displacing foods of modern commerce', including 'chiefly white flour, sugar, polished rice, vegetable fats and canned goods'. To which Price should perhaps have added other sources of sugar, such as confectionery and soft drinks.

Price concluded that

> the diets of the primitive groups which have shown a very high immunity to dental caries and freedom from other degenerative processes have all provided a nutrition containing at least four times these minimum requirements; whereas the displacing nutrition of commerce ... have invariably failed to provide even the minimum requirements. In other words the foods of the native Eskimos contained 5.4 times as much calcium as the displacing foods of the white man, five times as much phosphorus, 1.5 times as much iron, 7.9 times

as much magnesium, 1.8 times as much copper, 49.0 times as much iodine, and at least ten times the number of fat-soluble vitamins.'[75]

Price also noted: 'As yet I have not found a single group of primitive racial stock which was building and maintaining excellent bodies by living entirely on plant foods.'[76] In part, he thought this might be because vegetables do not contain vitamin D (or the most usable form of vitamin A).

Price's overriding conclusion is perhaps that traditional diets produce robust health by providing a high intake of minerals together with 'known and unknown vitamins particularly the fat-soluble'.[77] In essence, he concluded that the diet that prevents dental caries promotes optimum health. Or, stated in the converse: any diet that promotes dental caries, promotes chronic ill health.

According to Ron Schmid,[78] Price uncovered that peoples immune to the modern 'diseases of civilization' valued nutrient-dense animal fats: organ meats, especially liver (often eaten raw), bone marrow, fish oils and roe, egg yolks, lard and butter. They also considered foods from one or more of six different groups to be absolutely essential:
1. Seafood: fish and shellfish, fish organs, fish liver oils and fish eggs.
2. Organ meats from wild animals or grass-fed domestic animals.
3. Insects.
4. Fats of certain birds and single-stomached animals, such as sea mammals, guinea pigs, bears and hogs.
5. Egg yolks from pastured chickens and other birds.
6. Whole milk, cheese and butter from grass-fed animals.

Price believed that fat-soluble vitamins acted as 'catalysts' or 'activators', optimising the assimilation of all other nutrients – proteins, minerals (especially phosphorus and calcium) and fats. We now know that the fat-soluble vitamins – D, E, A and K, and perhaps especially vitamin K2 – serve these functions, as Price concluded. So 'it is possible to starve for minerals that are abundant in the foods eaten because they cannot be utilized without an adequate quantity of fat-soluble activators'.[79]

A subsequent study that has also been lost to time confirmed that a diet high in fat and essential vitamins, especially vitamin D, could prevent or reverse dental decay. M. Mellanby and C.L. Pattison compared the effects of eight different diets, given for six months, on the progression of dental caries in five-and-a-half-year-olds. They showed that a diet high in calcium and vitamin D, and free of cereals, 'almost eliminated' the 'initiation and spread of caries'.[80]

It is perhaps not surprising that these studies, showing that dental caries can be prevented by high-quality diets, have been essentially forgotten or, perhaps, actively suppressed.

Figure 16.8

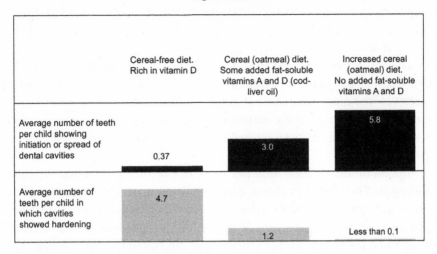

Mellanby and Pattison found that, whereas a cereal-free diet rich in vitamin D reduced the initiation of dental cavities (caries) and produced 'hardening' of established cavities (left columns), a diet high in oatmeal without added fat-soluble vitamins A and D was associated with an increased number of dental cavities and little evidence of hardening of established cavities (right columns)

Reading Price's book should be sufficient to convince even the most wary sceptic that basing a diet on the 'displacing foods of modern commerce', as current dietary guidelines would have us do, is not a particularly clever decision. Rather, it appears to be the single cause of the devastating 'chronic (modern) diseases of lifestyle'.

The Inuit

Price studied the Inuit of Alaska and described them as 'an example of physical excellence and dental perfection such as has seldom been excelled by any race in the past or present', and as 'robust, muscular and active, inclining rather to sparseness than corpulence, presenting a markedly healthy appearance. The expression of the countenance is one of habitual good humor. The physical constitution of both sexes is strong.'[81]

Harvard biologist Vilhjalmur Stefansson wrote a number of books describing his experiences of living with the Inuit for many years eating a very low- or no-carbohydrate diet.[82] His observations match those of Price. When he returned to New York, Stefansson chose to subject himself to a year-long experiment during which he and a friend ate only meat.[83] He wished to prove that it was possible to survive without developing scurvy if one ate lightly cooked meat daily (which contains just enough vitamin C to prevent scurvy). If anything, their health improved over the period of the experiment.

In a fourth book, Stefansson, who observed no evidence of cancer in the Inuit, postulated that cancer is a disease of modern civilization.[84] Schmid includes quotes from three doctors who worked among the Inuit, all of whom confirmed that 'cancer was unknown' there. But once the Inuit adopted the industrial diet, cancer 'frequently occurred', as did tuberculosis.[85]

The absence of cancer in mummies from Egypt and South America[86] led one study to propose: 'In industrialised societies, cancer is second only to cardiovascular disease as a cause of death. But in ancient times, it was extremely rare. There is nothing in the natural environment that can cause cancer. So it has to be a man-made disease, down to pollution and changes to our diet and lifestyle.'[87]

Studies of less-isolated Inuit like those in Greenland show that they have undergone a major dietary change over the past 150 years. The intake of sugar by Greenland Inuit increased thirtyfold, and refined carbohydrates five- to seven-fold, between 1855 and the 1970s.[88] As a result, carbohydrate intake increased from 2 to 8 per cent to 40 per cent of daily calories in the same period. This increase in carbohydrate intake and fall in fat intake is associated with the dramatic appearance of ill health and the chronic diseases of insulin resistance. Samuel Hutton noted: 'I have seen how the natives degenerate when they take to European food. They lose their natural coating of fat to a great extent, and need more clothing to withstand the cold; they become less robust, less able to endure fatigue, and their children are puny.'[89] It is as Weston Price wrote: 'Like the Indian, the Eskimo thrived as long as he was not blighted by the touch of modern civilization, but with it, like all primitives, he withers and dies.'[90]

Today, cancer is the leading cause of death among the Inuit in Alaska. Tuberculosis is rife, T2DM is considered to be an epidemic, and the Inuit's life expectancy is 11 years less than the Canadian average. In addition, the mental health of the Inuit has declined.[91] These outcomes are the precise opposite of the predictions of Keys's diet-heart hypothesis.

The Australian Aborigines

Weston Price reserved special praise for the health and physical abilities of those Australian Aborigines who continued to live according to their traditional ways, yet he also saw that, like the Inuit and the American Indians, Aboriginal health deteriorated catastrophically once they adopted the white man's ways:

> While these evidences of superior physical development demand our most profound admiration, their ability to build superb bodies and maintain them in excellent condition in so difficult an environment commands our genuine respect. It is a supreme test of human efficiency. It is doubtful if many places in the world can demonstrate so great a contrast in physical development and perfection of body as that which exists between the primitive Aborigines of

Australia who have been the sole arbiters of their fate, and those Aborigines who have been under the influence of the white man. The white man has deprived them of their original habitats and is now feeding them in reservations whilst using them as laborers in modern industrial pursuits.[92]

As a result, Price noted, their health was now as poor as that of Caucasian Australians. Today, it is much worse.

Urbanised Australian Aborigines have rates of T2DM that are four to six times higher than Caucasian Australians.[93] With high rates of obesity, 40 per cent of those over 55 years are now diabetic. There is good evidence that Aborigines are genetically insulin resistant,[94] so that some of their metabolic traits 'are associated with being Aboriginal (mild impairment of glucose tolerance, hyperinsulinemia and elevated total and VLDL [very low density lipoprotein] triglycerides)'.[95] In such a population, replacing ancestral food choices with the 'displacing foods of modern commerce' must predictably lead to high rates of T2DM.

In one remarkable study that has also gone 'missing', Kerin O'Dea returned 10 urbanised Aborigines with T2DM to their traditional hunting grounds in north-western Australia, where for seven weeks they reverted to eating the foods of their ancestors. The results were perhaps predictable – the biochemical markers of T2DM were either 'greatly improved or completely normalized'.[96]

Yet the Australian Dietary Guidelines continue to dictate that urbanised Aborigines must eat low-fat diets deriving 45 to 65 per cent of their energy from carbohydrates.

The saccharine diseases
In the course of his career as a naval surgeon travelling the world, Captain T.L. Cleave,[97] together with South African physician G.D. Campbell, formulated the hypothesis that a variety of medical conditions – including dental caries and associated periodontal disease, peptic ulcers, obesity, diabetes, colonic stasis 'and its complications of varicose veins and haemorrhoids', heart attack (coronary thrombosis) and certain gut infections – are caused by diets high in sugar and refined carbohydrates, and should therefore be termed the 'saccharine diseases'. As a result, 'in any disease in man due to alterations in his food from the natural state, the refined carbohydrates, both on account of the magnitude and the recentness of the alterations, are always the foods most likely to be at fault; *and not the fats*'.[98]

Cleave and Campbell built their hypothesis on the evidence that global sugar consumption began to increase exponentially after 1850, increasing fivefold within the next century, reaching 110 pounds per individual per year in the UK by 1950. They next compared the health and diets of Indians living in India with those in South Africa. Despite eating less carbohydrate and more protein and fat, the South African Indians had much higher rates of T2DM, which Cleave and

Campbell concluded must be due to the roughly 10-times higher consumption of sugar (110 vs 12 pounds) by Indians living in South Africa.

Next they showed that urbanised Zulu-speaking South Africans in Durban also ate more sugar than their rural compatriots and developed high rates of T2DM after living in the city for 20 or more years. This became known as the Rule of Twenty Years, as it takes 20 years of exposure to a high-sugar diet before T2DM develops.[99]

Cleave and Campbell also confirmed my suggestion that 'until the disastrous rinderpest of 70 years ago the Zulus have been predominantly meat-eaters', so that they wondered if 'the more carnivorous peoples of the world are more vulnerable to the diabetogenic effects of the consumption of refined carbohydrates than are the more vegetarian peoples, or are they less vulnerable?'[100] The studies of O'Dea clearly establish that Australian Aborigines show this very obviously, as they are insulin resistant even when eating a low-carbohydrate diet. I suspect that this can perhaps be generalised to all populations traditionally eating carnivorous diets.

Cleave and Campbell next presented evidence that T2DM is more common in countries that eat more sugar. Like Weston Price, they argued that the rising incidence of T2DM in American Indians, the Inuit, the Icelanders, the 'Black Jews' who moved to Israel from Yemen, and the Pacific Islanders coincided with the adoption of the high-sugar Western diet. Interestingly, Cleave and Campbell understood that 'obesity is not due to diabetes, nor diabetes to obesity, but both arise from a common cause'.[101]

The work of Professor John Yudkin

The final nutrition scientist who has until very recently been written out of history is John Yudkin, formerly professor of nutrition and dietetics at the University of London from 1954 to 1971. Yudkin's error was to provide answers to the question he posed in the introduction to his classic book *Pure, White and Deadly*: 'I am often asked why we don't hear very much about the dangers of sugar, while we are constantly being told we have too much fat in our diet and not enough fibre. I suggest that you will find at least part of the answer in the last chapter of this book.'[102] Perhaps unwisely, he concluded the opening chapter of his book with the statement: 'I hope that when you have read this book, I shall have convinced you that sugar is really dangerous. At the very least, I hope I shall have persuaded you that it might be dangerous ... If as a result you now give up all or most of your sugar eating ... I shall not have wasted my time in writing the book, and more importantly you will not have wasted your time in reading it.'[103]

Yudkin's thesis is essentially the same as that of Cleave and Campbell, specifically:

The diet of early man contained little carbohydrate. With the discovery of agriculture, the amount of carbohydrate increased, and the amounts of protein and fat decreased ... Increasing prosperity, both between countries and within a country, leads to an increasing proportion of sugar being bought in manufactured foods, rather than as household sugar. It is suggested that the effect of this is that wealthier countries, and the wealthier section of a national population, tend to have a higher intake of calories from the accompanying flour, chocolate, fat and other ingredients of these manufactured foods ... one of the effects of this contribution of calories from sugar-containing foods is to reduce the consumption of nutritionally desirable foods, such as fruit and meat ... In the wealthier countries, there is evidence that sugar and sugar-containing foods contribute to several diseases, including obesity, dental caries, diabetes mellitus and myocardial infarction ... the known association of the prevalence of diabetes and of myocardial infarction with the level of fat intake is fortuitous and secondary. It is more likely that the primary association is with levels of sugar intake, which I have shown are, in turn, closely related to levels of fat intake.[104]

For suggesting this hypothesis and for devoting the latter part of his scientific career to the study of the medical consequences of ingesting sugar, Yudkin was demonised and ultimately excommunicated from the research community, losing all his research funding. He was pretty certain who was behind it:

It is difficult to avoid the conclusion that this is the result of the vigorous, continuing and expanding activities of the sugar industry. Their product is pure and white; it would be difficult to use these adjectives for the behavior of the product and distributors and their intermediates ... The result is such a compact nucleus of power that, like a magnet surrounded by a strong induction coil, it produces a field of influence that invisibly affects many of those not in direct contact with the centre.[105]

In 2009, paediatric endocrinologist Robert Lustig released a YouTube video titled *Sugar: The Bitter Truth*, in which he highlighted the (now) established dangers of sugar and high-fructose corn syrup.[106] The video has been viewed more than seven million times to date. In 2013, Lustig published *Fat Chance: Beating the Odds Against Sugar, Processed Food, Obesity and Disease*, in which he fully vindicated Yudkin.[107] Three years later, Gary Taubes would do the same in *The Case Against Sugar*.[108] In 2012, on the 40th anniversary of its first publication, Yudkin's *Pure, White and Deadly* was re-published with a foreword by Lustig.

Another significant modern contributor to this science is Professor Richard J. Johnson, now of the Department of Medicine at the University of Colorado,

Denver. Johnson was interested in discovering the metabolic 'switch' that hibernating animals, such as bears and squirrels, use to gain weight by storing fat in the autumn prior to hibernation. He discovered that the key lies in the production of uric acid by an enzyme called AMP deaminase, which is present in all cells, but is of particular importance in the liver.[109] He then found that fructose activates this enzyme.

Thus, Johnson's theory is that the fructose in sugar increases uric acid production, which switches susceptible humans into hibernation mode, producing hyperphagia (overeating due to increased hunger), IR, and elevated blood glucose, insulin and triglyceride concentrations, leading to fat accumulation in the liver and fat cells. He believes that it is the increase in sugar consumption over the past 50 to 100 years that is the single most important driver of the IR/metabolic syndrome/obesity/T2DM epidemics.

The case against sugar, begun by Cleave, Campbell and Yudkin, has now become mainstream.

Summary
It seems to me that in this series of books and articles that are never discussed or presented to modern medical students, a group of highly inquisitive scientists have clearly established that humans are not designed to be unhealthy. Instead, we are the survivors of a biological arms race that we entered four to six million years ago when our puny and highly vulnerable hominin ancestors left the safety of the jungles and forests to become savannah dwellers – they survived by eating the fat of other animals specifically to fuel our enlarging, metabolically expensive brains.[110] As a result, humans have a strong preference for high-fat foods, including the capacity to determine the fat content and food reward of different foods within milliseconds.[111]

Over the course of the next four million years, we became remarkably robust and healthy. Only when we began to eat cereals at the start of the agricultural revolution, and most especially when our ancestral food choices were displaced by the 'displacing foods of modern commerce', did the 'modern diseases of lifestyle' begin to emerge in ever-increasing numbers.[112]

The key point is that these diseases are not 'of lifestyle'. Rather, they are caused by the 'displacing foods' that industry wishes us to eat.

In the next chapter, I explain how this degrading of human health was accelerated largely by the efforts of one man, Dr Ancel Keys, who, ignoring the work of McCarrison, Price, Cleave, Campbell and Yudkin, plunged the world into the worst health crisis in history. Keys was the father of what will be judged, in time, as the greatest mistake in modern medicine/science: the acceptance of the diet-heart and lipid hypotheses without adequate evidence.

17

The Worst Mistake
in the History of Medicine

'But biology does not readjust to accommodate the false theories of scientists ...'
– James le Fanu, British physician[1]

The agricultural revolution initiated *Homo sapiens*' ruinous move away from carnivory to diets dominated by cereals, grains, vegetable oils and sugar. But it was the second great dietary disaster, the adoption of the 1977 Dietary Guidelines for Americans, that initiated the devastating obesity/T2DM epidemic that has swept across the globe since the 1980s.

The US dietary guidelines were the first ever to inform the general public about what should **not** be eaten. Specifically, we were told to avoid fat, especially saturated fat, and to replace dietary saturated fats with carbohydrates and polyunsaturated 'vegetable' (actually seed) oils. Failure to do so, we were warned, would cause us all to die of heart attacks, because cholesterol, we were told, causes coronary heart disease. Instead, the advice drove us down the road to obesity and the much more severe form of arterial disease caused by T2DM.

Some have described this monumental error as the greatest scam in the history of modern medicine. The fallout has produced some very big 'winners', specifically those pharmaceutical companies that have benefited from the sale of the largely ineffective statin drugs, and the processed-food industry, dominated by 10 companies that produce the 'displacing foods of modern commerce' (see Figure 17.1 on page 338).

So how did this all come about?

In 1955, US president Dwight D. Eisenhower suffered a heart attack while in office. This event focused national attention on an apparently dramatically rising rate of heart attacks in the US. On the advice of his attending cardiologist, Dr Paul Dudley White, during his illness Eisenhower received dietary advice from Dr Ancel Keys, a biologist at the University of Minnesota. Although Keys was

Figure 17.1

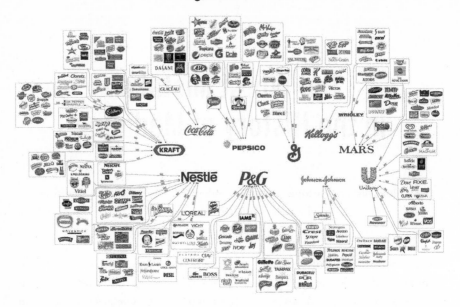

The 10 companies that control almost every large food and beverage brand in the world

still in the process of developing a model to explain how specific foods cause heart disease, he was sufficiently certain to prescribe the completely unproven low-fat diet to the most powerful politician in the world. Unfortunately, Keys's untested diet was largely ineffective, possibly even harmful.

On the low-fat diet, Eisenhower complained that he was always hungry; his blood cholesterol concentration rose progressively; he became increasingly irritable; and he suffered a further six heart attacks before dying from heart disease at age 78 in 1969.[2] Not a great advert for Keys's dietary approach.

At the time, there were essentially three competing possibilities to explain the rising incidence of heart disease: saturated fat intake; cigarette-smoking, which was Eisenhower's vice and which had increased dramatically during and after the First World War (see Figure 4.1 on page 64); and sugar, the global consumption of which took off at about the same time (Figure 17.2 on the following page). A fourth possibility – an increased intake of trans fats produced in the production of margarines, hydrogenated vegetable oils and shortening – would only be revealed some years later, largely because of the persistence of two pioneers: Dr Mary Enig[3] and Dr Fred Kummerow.[4]

Whereas cigarette-smoking and sugar intake had clearly increased steeply to match the increase in heart disease, at that time there was no data showing changes in saturated fat intake in the US over the same period. Even today, this information is difficult to find.

Figure 17.2

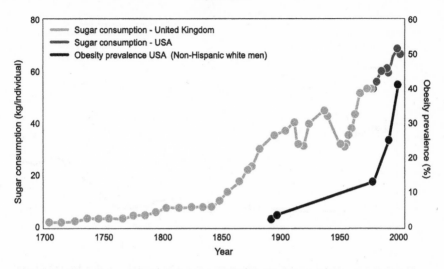

The change in sugar intake in the UK from 1700 to 1978, and in the US from 1975 to 2000 (upper line). The change in obesity rates in non-Hispanic white males aged 60–69 is also shown (lower line). Redrawn from R.J. Johnson *et al*, 'Potential role of sugar (fructose) in the epidemic of hypertension, obesity and the metabolic syndrome, diabetes, kidney disease, and cardiovascular disease'[5]

What we do know is that consumption of the three main sources of saturated fat in the US diet – red meat, full-cream milk and all dairy produce (including cheese) – either did not change much (red meat) or fell steeply (milk and consequently all dairy produce, by 15 per cent).[6] The result is that saturated fat intake in the US appears to have fallen since 1935, with the greatest fall since 1967.[7]

In contrast, Enig *et al*. estimate that the intake of trans fatty acids in the US diet increased almost threefold, from 4.4 grams per day in 1910 to 12.1 grams per day in 1972, comprising 8 per cent of the total daily fat intake. The main contributors to trans fatty acid consumption in 1972 were commercial vegetable oils containing 17 per cent of fat as trans fats, margarines containing 47 per cent as trans fats, and vegetable shortening containing up to 58 per cent as trans fats.[8]

Today, few would argue that of the four, cigarette-smoking is the most likely leading culprit, with trans fatty acids a close second. Figure 4.1 on page 64 shows a remarkably good fit for an (associational) relationship between the rise and fall of cigarette consumption and the rise and subsequent fall of US heart-disease rates. However, the rise and fall of trans fatty acid consumption follows a similar pattern, because, after 1968, the Institute of Shortening and Edible Oils, responding to the suggestion of Fred Kummerow,[9] began to increase the essential fatty acid content of margarine and shortening and to lower the trans fat content of these products.[10] As we know, heart-disease death rates began to fall quite dramatically after 1968 (Figure 4.1).

Figure 17.3

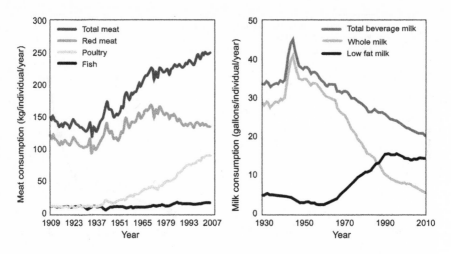

Left panel: change in total meat, red meat, poultry and fish consumption in the US from 1909 to 2007. Note that red meat consumption is the same in 2007 as it was in 1909, but has fallen progressively since 1965, whereas the consumption of poultry increased substantially during the same period. Redrawn from C.R. Daniel *et al.*, 'Trends in meat consumption in the USA'.[11] Right panel: change in total, whole-milk and lower-fat milk intakes in the US between 1930 and 2010. Source: USDA, Economic Research Service, Food Availability Data, redrawn from USDA *Agriculture Fact Book 2001–2002*[12]

But Keys ignored these known relationships, as well as the fact that sugar consumption had also risen during the same period. Instead, he stuck with his personal theory that it was an increased intake of saturated fats from animals that was causing the heart-disease 'epidemic'. This allowed him to ignore any potential role of polyunsaturated 'vegetable' oils, margarine and shortening with their high contents of trans fatty acids, the intakes of which had exponentially increased, or were about to, thanks to the promotion of his theory by, among others, the American Heart Association. We now understand that it was the chemical extraction of polyunsaturated 'vegetable' oils from cotton, soy, sunflower and safflower seeds that produced trans fats, which increased the risk of heart disease and perhaps cancer, as argued earlier and in Chapter 7.

Furthermore, Keys ignored the finding that there was a very close relationship between the intake of fat and sugar in most countries, making it impossible to differentiate between sugar and saturated fat as the cause of heart disease.

In 1970, Keys wrote a memorandum that was later published in the journal *Atherosclerosis*. In it he criticised the theory that sugar is the main dietary factor causing heart disease.[13] According to Yudkin, Keys ended his memorandum 'triumphantly pointing out that both sugar and fat intakes are related to heart disease, but that the cause must be fat, not sugar, because he had found in 1970 that fat intake and sugar intake are themselves closely linked'.[14] It was a relationship that Yudkin himself had already shown in 1964.[15]

Figure 17.4

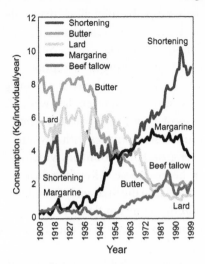
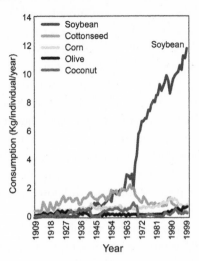

Left panel: changes in US consumption of butter, shortening, lard, margarine and beef tallow from 1909 to 1999. Note that consumption of butter and lard fell steeply, whereas intakes of shortening and margarine increased dramatically beginning in the 1940s. Right panel: changes in US consumption of 'vegetable' oils from 1909 to 1999. Note that the promotion of the diet-heart hypothesis by the AHA produced an astronomical increase in soybean consumption beginning after 1961. Redrawn from T.L Blasbalg *et al.*, 'Changes in consumption of omega-3 and omega-6 fatty acids in the United States during the 20th century'[16]

Keys devoted the rest of his life to convincing the world of his diet-lipid-heart hypotheses – that a diet high in fat, especially saturated fat, raises blood cholesterol concentrations, clogging arteries and causing heart attacks and strokes. He also taught the world to fear fat, giving rise to the chronic lipophobia that still exists today.

As described fully in *The Real Meal Revolution*, Keys performed two associational studies to show a relationship between the total amount of fat consumed by the citizens of first six[17] and then seven countries[18] and their rates of heart disease. He showed that the more fat eaten in a particular country, the higher that country's death rate from 'degenerative heart disease'.

The problem with such research is that it attempts to identify causative factors on the basis of associational studies. This is pseudo-science. Associational studies can only ever develop hypotheses, which must then be tested using RCTs in which the single factor of interest – in this case total fat or saturated fat intake – is manipulated and the health outcomes monitored in a large number of humans for at least eight years, as was done in the WHI trial (see Chapter 4).

When comparing populations in different countries, the most obvious problem is that they do not differ solely in what they eat. To suggest that differences in heart-attack rates between citizens in the US and Japan can be explained solely on the grounds that the former eat more saturated fat is patently absurd.

It ignores a host of other ways in which the citizens of the US and Japan differ. Only those who have already convinced themselves that diet alone determines heart-attack rates would ever fall for such trickery. For more than 60 years – perhaps until the publication of Nina Teicholz's book *The Big Fat Surprise* in 2014 – Keys successfully hoodwinked the world into sharing his deception.

Keys has been heavily criticised for the way in which he selected the countries for his analyses, in particular his choice of just six or seven when data was available for 22 countries.[19] A subsequent analysis of 21 of the 22 countries showed that they fell into two distinct groups: a group of six countries with low rates of both fat intake and heart disease, and another group of 15 countries with higher rates of fat intake but very variable rates of heart disease.[20] Keys's inclusion of mostly those countries with low rates of fat intake into the final analysis dramatically increased the probability that he would detect a significant relationship; a relationship that was absent when almost any combination of countries with higher rates of fat consumption was analysed.

Accordingly, P.D.P. Woods concluded: 'It seems probable therefore that the Seven Countries study suffered from a selection effect of some magnitude. It is prudent whenever very small samples are offered as evidence in support of a hypothesis to make sure that they are fully representative of the population from which they were drawn.'[21]

For there to be definitive evidence that cholesterol is the direct cause of heart disease, all the strands of evidence must point in the same direction. We now know that all the evidence does indeed point in one direction, but it is the opposite of what is required for Keys's hypothesis. This evidence was superbly presented by Nina Teicholz and Dr Zoë Harcombe in my trial (see Chapter 13), and was not contested by the complainant's legal team.

I now briefly review some of the key pieces of evidence that the three of us presented at the HPCSA hearing.

1. Epidemiological evidence

Modern studies show that there is no relationship between the amount of fat, including saturated fat, eaten in different countries and their respective rates of coronary heart disease. In contrast, the intake of polyunsaturated fat is directly related to CHD rates.

As I argued in the Centenary Debate,[22] modern data shows that total cardiovascular-disease mortality in a large number of European countries is an inverse function of total animal fat and protein intake, but is linearly related to energy intake from carbohydrates and alcohol, disproving the diet-heart hypothesis (see Figure 17.6 on page 344).[23]

Figure 17.5

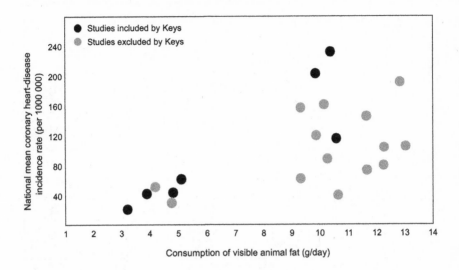

An analysis of 21 countries that Ancel Keys could have included in the Seven Countries Study shows they cluster into two groups: six with low rates of animal fat intake and the remaining 15 with higher rates of fat intake. By selecting four countries with low fat intakes, Keys ensured that he would achieve a significant relationship between fat intake and CHD death rates. Redrawn from P.D.P. Wood, 'A possible selection effect in medical science'[24]

Furthermore, those European countries with the greatest prevalence of raised blood cholesterol concentrations have the lowest rates of cardiovascular-disease mortality, disproving the lipid hypothesis. The prevalence of raised blood cholesterol concentrations is a linear function of (increasing) animal fat and protein intake; conversely, countries with the lowest prevalence of raised blood cholesterol concentrations have higher intakes of potatoes and cereals. Interestingly, the prevalence of high blood pressure in these countries is an inverse function of their prevalence of raised blood cholesterol concentrations.

P. Grasgruber *et al.* reported two other findings that are the converse of what the diet-heart hypothesis predicts:

- The prevalence of elevated blood pressures in these countries is an inverse function of total animal fat and protein intake, but is linearly related to energy intake from carbohydrates and alcohol.
- The prevalence of raised blood glucose concentrations in these countries is an inverse function of total animal fat and protein intake, but is linearly related to energy intake from carbohydrates and alcohol.

Figure 17.6

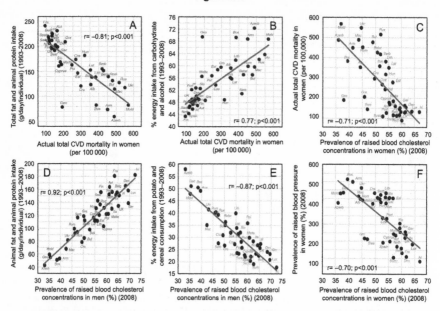

Total cardiovascular disease mortality in women in 42 European countries is an inverse function of mean daily consumption of total animal fat and protein (Panel A) and a linear function of carbohydrate and alcohol intake (Panel B). Cardiovascular disease mortality is an inverse function of raised blood cholesterol concentrations in women (Panel C), whereas prevalence of raised blood cholesterol concentrations in men is a linear function of total animal fat and protein intake (Panel D) and an inverse function of potato and cereal consumption (Panel E). The prevalence of raised blood pressure is an inverse function of raised blood cholesterol concentrations in women (Panel F). Redrawn from P. Grasgruber *et al*, 'Food consumption and the actual statistics of cardiovascular diseases: an epidemiological comparison of 42 European countries'[25]

Accordingly, the authors concluded: 'Irrespective of the possible limitations of the ecological study design, the undisputed finding of our paper is the fact that the highest CVD [cardiovascular disease] prevalence can be found in countries with the highest carbohydrate consumption whereas the lowest CVD prevalence is typical of countries with the highest intake of fat and protein.'[26] Thus: 'In the absence of any scientific evidence connecting saturated fat with CVDs, these findings show that current dietary recommendations regarding CVDs should be seriously reconsidered.'[27]

Additional data from some of these European countries shows a direct linear relationship between increasing heart-disease mortality rates and the intake of polyunsaturated fats – the 'vegetable' oils we are told to eat in place of saturated fats because they are supposedly more healthy (Chapter 7).[28]

Were Keys to repeat his study today, he would have to conclude (according to his flawed logic) that it is the consumption of 'vegetable' oils rich in omega-6 polyunsaturated fats (and perhaps other fats, the toxic effects of which have still to be identified) that causes arterial disease leading to heart attacks.

Figure 17.7

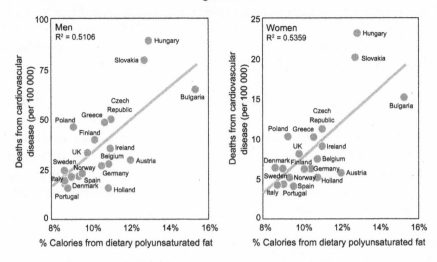

Linear relationship between polyunsaturated fat consumption and cardiovascular disease deaths in men and women in 19 European countries. Redrawn from Credit Suisse, 'Fat: The New Health Paradigm'[29]

In Chapter 7, I explained how Keys and his colleagues chose to bury the findings of the Minnesota Coronary Experiment, which found that substituting vegetable oils for saturated fats provided no health benefits, and may even have been harmful, especially for males over 65. The negative findings from that study and from Rossouw's WHI trial (Chapter 4) should have been sufficient to bury the diet-heart hypothesis. But this did not happen, because the authors of both studies, or their funders, did not see any value in accepting the null hypothesis.

2. It is not a high-fat diet that causes 'dangerous' cholesterol to rise
Ultimately, Keys acknowledged that cholesterol in the diet does not cause the blood cholesterol concentration to rise.[30] Interestingly, dietary cholesterol comes only from animal products, since plants do not contain cholesterol.

If dietary cholesterol does not cause blood cholesterol concentrations to rise, then logically, according to the diet-heart and lipid hypotheses, animal fats cannot cause heart disease (since cholesterol-containing animal fats do not cause blood cholesterol concentrations to rise). This obvious conclusion was first brought to our attention by Dr Zoë Harcombe.[31]

It is now clear that the dangerous atherogenic dyslipidaemia that produces arterial disease is caused by a high-carbohydrate diet that produces NAFLD. Heart attack is therefore a disease of carbohydrate, not fat, metabolism. Thus we need to understand the way in which carbohydrates, and not fats, alter blood 'cholesterol' (lipoprotein) values.*

3. *There is no evidence that blood cholesterol concentrations can predict the risk of future heart attack more effectively than measures of IR/pre-diabetes/T2DM*

The lipid hypothesis proposes that the key driver of arterial disease is an elevated blood cholesterol concentration. But evidence shows that the blood cholesterol concentration is such a poor predictor of heart-attack risk that it can, or should be, ignored. Rather, it is T2DM and other markers of IR and metabolic syndrome that are the better predictors.

Table 17.1 Predictors of cardiovascular disease risk

Predictor	Hazard ratio
T2DM	2.04
Smoking	1.79
Total cholesterol/HDL-C ratio	1.32
Systolic blood pressure (mmHg)	1.31
Apolipoprotein B:A-1 ratio	1.30
Apolipoprotein B (mmol/L)	1.24
Total cholesterol (mmol/L)	1.22
Triglyceride (mmol/L)	1.19
HDL-C (mmol/L)	0.83

Note that this is associational data. Independent scientists agree that only a hazard ratio of well over 2.0 might suggest a causal (not associational) relationship between two variables. Thus, in this table, the only variable that might be causally linked to heart-attack risk is T2DM. A hazard ratio of only 1.22 indicates that cholesterol can be exonerated of any role in the causation of heart attack. Data from E. di Angelantonio *et al*, 'Lipid-related markers and cardiovascular disease prediction'[32]

But perhaps the best evidence that cholesterol has little to do with heart disease comes from the very condition, familial hypercholesterolaemia, that cardiologists like to promote as definitive evidence that cholesterol drives the process of coronary atherosclerosis.

As I first suggested in Chapter 7, the evidence is the opposite; blood cholesterol

---

* Cholesterol is not water soluble, so it does not exist in the bloodstream as pure cholesterol. Rather, cholesterol exists in the blood in the form of water-soluble lipoproteins. Lipoproteins are specific particles containing fat in their centre surrounded by a single layer of phospholipid molecules (fats attached to a phosphorus-containing group), which make them water soluble. Specific lipoproteins were linked to heart disease by Dr John Gofman in the 1950s. But to simplify public understanding of the lipid hypothesis, the AHA and others decided that 'bad' cholesterol, not lipoproteins, determines risk of heart disease. This erroneous simplification became a pillar of the false diet-heart hypothesis and the subsequent damage it has caused to global health.

concentration is unable to predict who with FH will suffer from heart disease and who will not. The evidence shows that the longer people with FH survive, the more likely it is that they will have a normal life expectancy.[33] Even more perplexing for the cholesterol advocates is the recent finding that blood cholesterol concentration has essentially no predictive value for heart attack or stroke in the next 5–10 years in people with FH.[34] Rather, it is the usual suspects – age, previous history of atherosclerotic cardiovascular disease, obesity, diabetes, premature familial atherosclerotic CVD (all markers of IR) – that best predict risk of future heart attack in those with FH.

Table 17.2 Predictors of CVD risk in persons with FH

Variable		Hazard ratio	p values
Age	> 60 years	12.81	<0.001
History of ASCVD		6.64	<0.001
Body mass index	Obesity	6.12	<0.001
Age	30–59 years	5.88	<0.001
Body mass index	Overweight	4.69	<0.001
Diabetes mellitus		3.45	<0.001
Patient on ezetimibe		3.42	<0.001
Patient on maximum combined therapy		2.97	<0.001
Patient on maximum lipid-lowering therapy		2.88	<0.001
Male		2.76	<0.001
Premature familial ASCVD history		2.66	<0.001
Calculated pre-treatment LDL-C	> 160 mg/dl (4.5 mmol/L)	2.47	0.40
Patient on maximum statin dose		2.08	<0.001
Active smoking		1.77	0.004

ASCVD = atherosclerotic cardiovascular disease

Note that a hazard ratio of greater than 2.0 suggests an increasing probability that the risk predictor acts as a directly causal, rather than as an associational (but not causative), factor. Diabetes and obesity, both markers of IR, are therefore strongly implicated as directly causal factors for heart disease in these persons with FH. Note that p values <0.05 are not considered to be significant. A blood cholesterol concentration of >160mg/dl (4.5mmol/L) is the only variable on this table that is **not** a significant predictor of future cardiovascular disease. This dislodges a cornerstone of the lipid hypothesis

There are a number of unexpected observations on this table. First, that the predictors of future CVD in persons with FH are not greatly different from those in persons without the condition (Table 17.1), so that diabetes and obesity are again key risk factors.

Second, that the use of cholesterol-lowering statin drugs (ezetimibe; maximum combined therapy; maximum lipid-lowering therapy; maximum statin dose) are all significant predictors of future CVD risk in these patients. This probably does not mean that these drugs are the direct cause of future heart disease, but rather that those at greatest risk of future CVD are prescribed the most drugs. It might also mean that these drugs are rather less effective in preventing future heart disease in these patients than is usually acknowledged.

It's the fatty liver disease, stupid

We have known for some time that the added risks associated with obesity depend, in part, on where that extra fat is stored in the body. Fat that accumulates under the skin (subcutaneous fat) appears to be far less unhealthy than fat that accumulates within and between the organs in the abdomen – so-called visceral obesity. A group of hepatologists (liver specialists) have now gone one step further to show that the real killer in visceral obesity is the fat that accumulates within the liver causing NAFLD, a disease that is now also reaching epidemic proportions among people eating the 'displacing foods of modern commerce'.

By measuring the amount of fat in the livers of people with different metabolic conditions, including T2DM and NAFLD, Fernando Brill and his colleagues at the University of Florida have established that it is the presence of NAFLD, and not the overall level of body fatness, that predicts the presence of atherogenic dyslipidaemia.[35]

Their work therefore establishes that it is IR and NAFLD, and not obesity per se, that produces the abnormal metabolic state (atherogenic dyslipidaemia) that causes heart disease in those with IR and the related metabolic syndrome. The following are the metabolic features of atherogenic dyslipidaemia present in those with NAFLD and IR who eat high-carbohydrate (>25 grams per day) diets with high omega-6 to omega-3 ratios:

• Elevated blood HbA1c levels;
• Elevated fasting blood insulin levels;
• Elevated fasting blood glucose levels;
• Hyperinsulinaemia and hyperglycaemia (elevated blood glucose levels) in response to carbohydrate ingestion;
• Low blood HDL-cholesterol concentrations;
• High blood triglyceride concentrations;
• Elevated numbers of small dense LDL-particles;
• Elevated blood Apolipoprotein B concentrations; and
• Elevated blood gamma-glutamyl transferase (GGT) activity (indicating the presence of NAFLD).

But the absolutely key point is that it is dietary **carbohydrates**, especially fructose[36] present in sucrose, high-fructose corn syrup and fruit, allied to high intakes of unsaturated fats (oleate),[37] and not dietary saturated **fats**, that cause NAFLD. In part, this is because the major pathway by which fructose is cleared from the bloodstream is its conversion to liver fat (triglyceride). When the liver, skeletal muscles and adipose tissue are insulin resistant, a continuing high-carbohydrate diet causes liver fat to accumulate, worsening the IR. Thus, a vicious cycle results: as NAFLD develops, IR worsens, hyperinsulinaemia increases, atherogenic dyslipidaemia deteriorates, and the seeds for the chronic diseases of obesity, diabetes, heart disease and perhaps cancer and dementia are sown.

Importantly, caloric restriction, whether on a high- or low-carbohydrate diet, reduces liver fat in those with IR,[38] as can removing sugar, high-fructose corn syrup and refined carbohydrates from the diet.[39] Dietary carbohydrate restriction produces a significantly greater effect than caloric restriction.[40] Importantly, it is carbohydrate overfeeding that causes NAFLD, and this effect can be rapid, causing a more than tenfold greater increase in liver fat than in body weight within just three weeks.[41] In contrast, eating an LCHF diet reverses all the metabolic abnormalities of atherogenic dyslipidaemia,[42] presumably also by reversing NAFLD.

Thus, dietary carbohydrates, and not dietary fats, are the direct cause of this group of chronic diseases in people with IR. In contrast, a high-fat diet combined with carbohydrate restriction can reverse many of these conditions.[43]

Third, the one factor that does **not** predict future heart disease is an elevated blood cholesterol concentration. Remarkably, in both those with FH (Table 17.2) and without FH (Table 17.1), the least effective predictor of future risk is a raised blood 'cholesterol' concentration.

These findings in patients with FH effectively disprove the lipid hypothesis and the 'cholesterol-load' theory, which holds that the more cholesterol in the blood and the longer that cholesterol has had a chance to damage arteries, the greater is the individual's risk for future CVD. Rather, it is the conventional risk factors, specifically the presence of the markers of IR and perhaps abnormal blood clotting on a genetic basis,[44] that predict the development of arterial disease in those with FH.

So what is it about T2DM and IR that increases the risk for the development of disseminated obstructive arterial disease?

First, we have to suspect it is not blood cholesterol concentration, because these levels are 'elevated' in persons with T2DM whether or not they have or will develop CHD.[45] Ignored in that study are the much higher blood triglyceride concentrations (3.1 mmol/L) in people with T2DM who suffered heart attacks. This suggests that it is the presence of a fatty liver – the condition of NAFLD in people with IR who persevere in eating high-carbohydrate diets – that produces the atherogenic dyslipidaemia that causes the disseminated obstructive arterial disease that characterises T2DM.

4. There is no evidence that blood cholesterol concentration during life can predict the extent of coronary artery disease at death

If blood cholesterol concentration determines heart-attack risk, then autopsy studies should show a direct linear relationship between the extent of coronary artery disease at death and pre-morbid blood cholesterol concentration. But more than 19 studies, using many different methods, have failed to establish such a relationship. This has led W.R. Ware to conclude:

> The large number of null results for the association between serum LDL cholesterol levels and the prevalence or progression of both calcified and non-calcified plaque in the appropriate vascular bed and involving large numbers of men and women over a wide range of age, ethnic background, plaque burden and cholesterol levels cannot be easily dismissed. If the hypothesis is false, this has a significant impact on currently held views regarding risk factors and therapeutic interventions in the case of individuals who are asymptomatic, that is, issues associated with primary prevention. Also, if the hypothesis is false, then the use of changes in LDL as a surrogate marker for judging the importance of various risk factors for silent atherosclerosis and thus coronary artery disease can be called into question.[46]

The point is that your blood cholesterol concentration gives you absolutely no information about the state of your coronary arteries. However, your level of IR and the extent to which your daily carbohydrate intake has raised your HbA1c value will, in my opinion, prove to be excellent markers of how badly your arteries are likely to have been damaged.

For example, an HbA1c of 10 per cent in a person with uncontrolled T2DM increases the risk of having a limb amputation tenfold; the risk of any endpoint related to the disease fourfold; and the risk of having a heart attack or stroke twofold.[47] Measuring 'cholesterol' in patients with T2DM will have no such predictive value and is essentially useless.

Figure 17.8

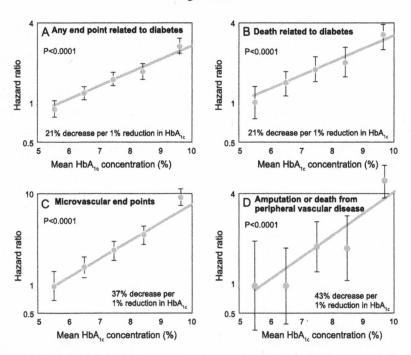

Hazard ratios for any endpoint related to diabetes (Panel A); for death related to diabetes (Panel B); for microvascular endpoints – kidney, heart, brain, eye, limb (Panel C); and for amputations or death from peripheral vascular disease (Panel D). Note that at HbA1c values greater than 8 per cent, the hazard ratios for all these outcomes is more than 2.0. Compare with predictive value for cholesterol and risk for developing heart disease (Table 16.2). Redrawn from I.M. Stratton *et al.*, 'Association of glycaemia with macrovascular and microvascular complications of type 2 diabetes'[48]

5. A low blood cholesterol concentration predicts a shorter life expectancy and increases risk for developing a range of diseases

If the body produces cholesterol solely to damage our coronary arteries and to kill us from heart disease, it follows that the lower the blood cholesterol concentration, the longer we will live.

But the evidence is clearly the opposite. As described in Chapter 7, low blood cholesterol concentrations are associated with a range of adverse health outcomes, including a shorter life expectancy and a greater risk for developing cancer and probably dementia. This is likely because cholesterol serves so many vital functions in the human body, such as:

- Maintaining the stiffness and stability of cell walls.
- Essential for the synthesis of neurotransmitters for propagation of nerve impulses through neurons.
- Essential for the production of enzymes and hormones, including aldosterone, cortisol, oestrogen, cortisone, progesterone, testosterone and ubiquinone.
- Essential for the synthesis of vitamin D3, which is responsible for proper bone calcification.
- Essential precursor of other molecules that are important for proper bodily functioning, including the production of bile.

By now it should be clear that all the evidence incriminates carbohydrates and IR as the key drivers of our current epidemics of ill health. Table 17.3 lists the blood parameters that really predict the extent to which one is insulin resistant, and hence one's real risk for developing the diseases linked to IR.

Table 17.3: Blood values, blood pressures and body mass indices indicating different levels of IR

Blood parameter	Insulin sensitive	Borderline	Insulin resistant/T2DM
HbA1c %	4.5	5.5	>6.0
Gamma-glutamyl transferase activity (U/L)	<45	>45	>100
Fasting insulin concentration (mIU/L)	<2.0	2.0–10.0	>10.0
Fasting glucose concentration (mmol/L)	<5.0	>5.5	>6.5
Fasting triglycerides (mmol/L)	0.5	1.0–1.5	>2.0
HDL-cholesterol concentration (mmol/L)	1.6	1.4	1.2
Fasting total cholesterol concentration (mmol/L)	Of no value in determining extent of insulin resistance. Minimal value for predicting risk of future heart attack.		
Fasting LDL-cholesterol concentration (mmol/L)	Of no value in determining extent of insulin resistance. Minimal value for predicting risk of future heart attack.		
Blood pressure (mm/Hg)	<120/80	140/90–150/95	>160/100
Body mass index (kg/m^2)	<24	24–28	>28

Reproduced from *The Banting Pocket Guide*, Cape Town: Penguin Books, 2017

We might never have known that it is carbohydrate, and not fat, that is the cause of our ill health were it not for the catastrophic change in our diet brought about by the introduction of the 1977 Dietary Guidelines for Americans. The idea that humans should increase their carbohydrate intake by eating more cereals and grains and less animal produce was not born from evidence that this would make us healthier. Nina Teicholz and Dr Zoë Harcombe made this clear in their testimony during the HPCSA hearing (Chapter 13). Instead, it followed the decision by President Richard Nixon in 1972 that in order to win re-election, he needed to reduce the cost of food and improve the wealth of US farmers.

To achieve this, he appointed Earl Butz as his secretary of agriculture. Butz's solution was to reward farmers in the Midwest so that they would produce wheat, maize and soy in 'industrial' amounts. As a result, US grain production increased dramatically to the point where, today, the US no longer has any reserve storage capacity for its grain surplus. Having industrialised the production of these grains, the next challenge faced by US politicians was how to sell this relatively cheap product not just to Americans, but also to the rest of the world. The solution was the 1977 US dietary guidelines, which demonised the high-fat foods that had allowed humans to become human, and romanticised the high-grain (poor people's) diet that, as I have shown, so damaged the health of the Egyptians and the poorest people on the Indian and African continents.

Removing fat from the diet also reduced the palatability of our foods. In a quest to return some flavour, food manufacturers discovered that by sweetening foods with sugar or high-fructose corn syrup, they could induce an addictive eating response.[49] As I wrote in *The Real Meal Revolution*: 'But one facet of processed foods is held sacrosanct by the industry. Any improvement to the nutritional profile of a product can in no way diminish its allure, and this has led to one of the industry's most devious moves: lowering one bad boy ingredient like fat while quietly adding more sugar to keep people hooked.'[50]

Over the next 35 years, the 1977 Dietary Guidelines for Americans produced a progressive and sustained increase in the addictive consumption of more and more carbohydrates.[51] This higher carbohydrate intake produced a 7–21 per cent increase in daily energy intake of men and women in the US, associated with large increases in the body mass indices of both genders.

Figure 17.9 on page 353 shows that following the introduction of the 1977 US dietary guidelines, the contribution of carbohydrate to the US daily energy intake increased from about 40 to 65 per cent. This increase was associated with the beginning of the obesity/diabetes tsunami that has since engulfed the world. I think there are two explanations for why this has happened.

The first is the addictive nature of sugar, which has hijacked the appestat controlling what we eat. The mechanism for this is fully described in *The Real Meal Revolution* and I will not repeat it here. The simple explanation is that

Figure 17.9

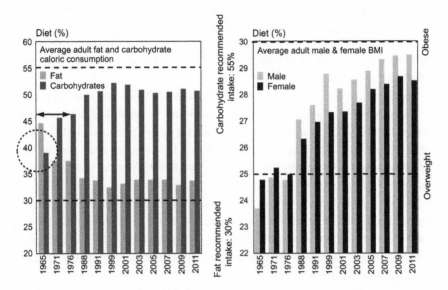

Left panel: changes in percentage calories from dietary fat and carbohydrates since adoption of the 1977 Dietary Guidelines for Americans. Note the dramatic changes between 1965 and 1999, and that in 1965 the percentage fat intake was 45% and carbohydrate intake 38% (circled). Right panel: there has been a progressive increase in the US average body mass index since the adoption of the guidelines. The logical assumption is that the increased carbohydrate consumption (left panel) caused the increase in body mass index (right panel). Redrawn from E. Cohen *et al.*, 'Statistical review of US macronutrient consumption data, 1965–2011'; L.S. Gross *et al.*, 'Increased consumption of refined carbohydrates and the epidemic of type 2 diabetes in the United States: An ecological assessment'[52]

carbohydrates make us hungry, whereas fats and proteins satiate. Chronic over-consumption of calories, especially carbohydrate calories, induces persistent hyperinsulinaemia that worsens IR, producing all the biological consequences of that condition.

The second factor has yet to be acknowledged by any biologist as far as I am aware. Here you will read it for the first time.

In Chapter 16, I described how the common ancestors of humans, chimpanzees and bonobos must have been hindgut fermenters. Although on occasion they ate fruit, which would have provided simple sugars (glucose and fructose) that travelled in the bloodstream directly to the liver in the portal vein, their main carbohydrate foods were in the form of cellulose.

Critically, microbial activity in their voluminous hindguts would have fermented the ingested carbohydrate (cellulose) anaerobically into volatile fatty acids, predominantly acetic, propionic and butyric acid. While superficially our hominin ancestors might have appeared to be eating high-carbohydrate diets, as a result of this microbial fermentation they were, in fact, eating diets high in fat, most of which was saturated. In fact, 60–70 per cent of the energy absorbed from the intestine in chimpanzees and gorillas is in the form of saturated fats. It is not an exaggeration to state that the large bowel of these great apes is an organ designed specifically to generate saturated fat.

The end result is that all mammals, carnivorous or herbivorous, subsist on high-fat diets. The sole exception is humans, who were advised to adopt a high-carbohydrate diet in 1977.

'Clearly from the standpoint of the host animal, VFAs [volatile fatty acids] are the important product of fermentation,' writes Richard Bowen of Colorado State University. 'These small lipids are used for many purposes, but the para-mount importance of VFAs to herbivores is that they are absorbed and serve the animal's major fuel for energy production',[53] providing 'greater than 70% of the ruminant's energy supply'.[54]

The first crucial point is that the ruminant's liver generates the glucose it requires from volatile fatty acids. As a result, ruminants are never exposed to high blood glucose concentrations following the ingestion of their high-carbohydrate (cellulose) diets, as now occurs in modern humans ingesting readily digested carbohydrates every few hours.

The second key point is that in their natural state, hindgut fermenters do not absorb large amounts of glucose directly into the portal vein and hence directly into the liver. Over the last two to four million years, our hominin ancestors reduced their reliance on dietary cellulose, replacing it with animal fat and protein, while the large bowel shortened (Figure 16.1). Until very recently, humans have had no long-term experience of the effects of dietary carbohydrates absorbed directly from the small bowel into the portal vein.

Crucially, we now know that if these increases happen repeatedly every few hours for decades on end, our IR worsens to the point at which insulin does not produce the desired outcome, however much is secreted. The result is T2DM. It is therefore IR, and not heart disease, that is our greatest medical threat. As a result of the promotion of the 1977 US dietary guidelines and the romantici-sation of the health benefits of the high-cereal diet, humans must now face – for the first time in the six million years of our evolutionary history – the frequent rapid delivery of glucose into the portal vein. For the first time, we must cope with repeated rapid rises in blood glucose and insulin concentrations each time we eat the 'displacing foods of modern commerce'.

IR is now certainly the most prevalent medical condition in the world, yet it is not taught or discussed in most medical schools.

An interesting part of Weston Price's work was that he did not find any populations existing on predominantly high-carbohydrate diets. Rather, in all the populations that he studied, fat and protein were the major contributors to daily caloric intake, as they were in our more ancient ancestors (*Homo erectus* and the Neanderthals), and in modern humans such as the Inuit, the Masai and modern foragers (Table 17.4). Only in the last 40 years since the introduction of the US dietary guidelines have carbohydrates begun to provide more than 40 per cent of our daily calories.

Table 17.4 Changes in dietary fat, protein and carbohydrate intakes in the course of human evolution

	Fat	Protein	Carbohydrate
Gorilla (ingested)	3	24	73
Gorilla (absorbed)	60		
Chimpanzee	3	21	76
Australopithecus africanus	?	?	?
Homo habilis	?	?	?
Homo erectus[55]	44	33	23
Neanderthals[56]	74-85	15-26	0
Homo sapiens – Masai	66	14	20
Homo sapiens – Inuit	48-70	14	16-38
Homo sapiens – modern foragers[57]	28-58	19-35	22-40
Homo sapiens[58]	33	14	53

Note that the proportion of energy derived from dietary fat has fallen, while that from carbohydrate has increased over the past few million years, but with the greatest change since 1977 (modern *Homo sapiens*)

Nevertheless, there are populations who are as healthy as those described by Price despite eating higher-carbohydrate diets. The 2300 inhabitants of the small island of Kitava off the east coast of New Guinea eat a diet based on tubers (cassava, yams, sweet potatoes and taro) and fruits (bananas, papaya, guavas, pineapple, mangoes and watermelon), supplemented with fish and coconuts. Despite their lifelong high-carbohydrate diet, Kitavans remain insulin sensitive for life,[59] and are therefore quite different from the Australian Aborigines, who are insulin resistant, apparently on a genetic basis.

The Kitavans are most likely an unusual population. This is important, because the majority of the world's population is more likely insulin resistant[60] (because they respond to an increased refined-carbohydrate intake by developing obesity and T2DM). Extrapolating the Kitavan experience or that of the Tsimané of Bolivia[61] to global populations may therefore lead to dietary advice that is the opposite of what is likely to be the healthiest.

Basically, insulin resistance, previously termed 'the thrifty genotype',[62] is a condition in which the insulin secreted normally in response to the carbohydrate, and to a lesser extent the protein, content of a meal fails to act appropriately on all the (insulin-receptive) bodily organs. The key abnormality is when the insulin fails to suppress glucose production by the liver (liver insulin resistance). In this case, following the ingestion of a carbohydrate meal, the liver continues to produce an excess of glucose. This causes blood glucose concentrations to remain elevated, stimulating further insulin secretion and producing hyperinsulinaemia (excessive levels of insulin circulating in the bloodstream).

The skeletal muscles and liver also have a reduced capacity to take up and store blood glucose (in the human form of starch – namely, glycogen). Instead, the excess glucose is converted to triglyceride for storage in the liver, producing NAFLD in the long term. The NAFLD in turn produces atherogenic dyslipidaemia, which leads to the disseminated obstructive arterial damage that is the characteristic feature of T2DM.

Once the fat cells in the adipose tissue become insulin resistant, they will fail to store fat appropriately, causing the continuous release of their contained fatty acids into the bloodstream; this fat will also end up in the visceral organs, including the liver and pancreas, worsening the IR.

But it is not the fat that causes the T2DM; rather the opposite. It is the high-carbohydrate diet in those with IR that sets up and perpetuates this vicious cycle.

Let us now look at how IR likely arose as a common human trait and why it is so damaging to our health in the presence of a high-carbohydrate diet.

1. It begins in the third trimester

Humans are the only land-based mammals whose babies are born with significant amounts of subcutaneous body fat. Since our nearest relatives, the chimpanzees and bonobos, do not produce fat babies, humans must have developed this adaptation in the past six million years. But to what possible advantage?

The answer is that the subcutaneous fat of the newborn provides the energy and the chemical building blocks for the rapid growth of the neonatal brain, as shown in Figure 16.3 on page 314. We know that this fat layer is laid down in normal pregnancy in the final trimester (12 weeks).

I suspect that the only way infants can lay down fat in this way is if they follow the same pattern as hibernating bears, which put on weight in the autumn before winter hibernation. They do this by developing (reversible) IR – becoming hyperinsulinaemic in the autumn and during the winter hibernation, but returning to normal insulin sensitivity during the spring and summer.[63] Recall in Chapter 16 I discussed the work of Professor Richard Johnson, who has investigated the role of sugar consumption in turning on the 'fat switch' to produce this metabolic change.

It is, therefore, not unreasonable to suggest that a heightened level of IR was programmed into human newborns sometime in the past six million years specifically to ensure that they became fat in the final 12 weeks of gestation; this fatness was then essential to generating the ketone bodies needed for the development of the large infant brain during the first two years after birth.

But we also know that infants born to mothers who develop gestational diabetes – a reversible form of T2DM that goes into remission immediately after the infant is born – are over-fat and at increased risk of developing obesity and T2DM. This indicates that infants exposed to continuously elevated maternal blood glucose concentrations become even more insulin resistant, and are pre-programmed to have higher levels of IR even before they are born.

So the infant in utero lives on a knife-edge: insufficient IR, and the infant will have inadequate body-fat stores to maximise its brain development during the first two years of life; too much, and the infant will likely develop obesity/T2DM, perhaps even in adolescence. But there is more.

Bears reverse their IR by fasting during their period of hibernation. But human infants, especially those born to mothers with gestational diabetes, will likely be weaned onto the same high-carbohydrate foods that caused their (insulin-resistant) mother's gestational diabetes in the first place. In this way, the environment converts a normal biological advantage, built into humans for the purpose of developing our large brains, into a trap for T2DM.

This interpretation has relevance to my HPCSA trial. By advocating weaning infants onto an LCHF diet, I was specifically trying to help mothers avoid this environmental diet trap.

My hypothesis is that, in order to produce the large brains that made us human, our evolution required that our babies develop (reversible) IR in the final 12 weeks before birth. When we lived in a low-carbohydrate environment this was fine, because infants would be weaned onto high-fat and moderate-carbohydrate foods similar in composition to breast milk. But with the introduction of modern convenience foods for infants by the Fremont Canning Company in Fremont, Michigan, in 1926 (to become Gerber in 1928), babies began to be weaned onto high-carbohydrate foods. Amy Bentley writes: 'By the postwar period, refined white rice cereal, introduced by Gerber in the 1940s, had become the iconic first food American families fed to their infants.'[64] As a result, the period of foetal and neonatal IR would have extended from the final 12 weeks of foetal life to beyond the neonatal period and, after the 1977 US dietary guidelines came into effect, into adolescence.

2. IR is the common condition that causes chronic diseases in those eating high-carb diets

Dr Gerald Reaven, now emeritus professor of medicine at Stanford University, has spent the past 60 years studying the condition that intellectually he now owns, insulin resistance. His academic interest was stirred early in his career, when he read that there are two forms of diabetes. The first, insulin-deficient T1DM, is caused when the pancreatic beta cells (which are destroyed in an auto-immune process perhaps related to wheat exposure causing leaky-gut syndrome) fail to produce insulin.[65] In the second, insulin-resistant T2DM, insulin must be secreted in abnormally high amounts, because the target cells on which the insulin normally acts are resistant to its action; hence the condition of IR or carbohydrate intolerance.

Reaven's great contribution has been to show that this persistent hyperinsulinaemia present in people with IR who eat high-carb diets (more than 50 grams per day), whether associated with T2DM or not, produces a collection of grave secondary consequences:[66]

- Weight gain
- Increased fat in the abdominal organs (visceral adiposity)
- High blood pressure
- Abnormal blood fat, glucose and insulin concentrations (atherogenic dyslipidaemia – Table 16.3 on page 314)
- Elevated blood uric-acid concentrations (gout)
- Impaired ability of arteries to dilate (endothelial dysfunction)
- Whole-body inflammation
- Dysfunction of the mitochondria (cellular organs that produce energy)
- Progressive increases in IR (insulin-induced IR)
- Impaired exercise performance

But Reaven's greatest (and bravest) intellectual contribution was to suggest that IR and hyperinsulinaemia are the necessary biological precursors for at least four, but perhaps for all six, of the most prevalent chronic medical conditions of our day[67] – the very six that will bankrupt our medical services within the next two decades, unless we understand the crucial importance of his work and act without delay. The six conditions most likely caused by high-carbohydrate diets in those with IR are:

1. Obesity
2. Arterial disease
   Local: Heart attack or stroke
   Disseminated: T2DM
3. High blood pressure
4. NAFLD
5. Cancer
6. Dementia (Alzheimer's disease, also known at type-3 diabetes)

Reaven's (Metabolic) Syndrome refers to the combination of obesity, diabetes, abnormal blood lipid levels and high blood pressure existing in the same individual. It is this singular combination that best predicts heart-attack risk.

The key finding from Reaven's work is that these conditions are not separate – **they are different expressions of the same underlying condition**. So patients should not be labelled as having high blood pressure or heart disease or diabetes or NAFLD. Instead, they should be diagnosed with the underlying condition – IR – with the understanding that the high blood pressure, obesity, diabetes, NAFLD, heart attack, stroke, perhaps even cancer or dementia, are simply markers, symptoms if you will, of the basic condition.

And that basic condition is IR, which, simply put, is the inability of the body to tolerate more than an absolute minimum amount of carbohydrates each day (without developing hyperinsulinaemia). We now know that for patients with more severe IR, a daily carbohydrate intake of 25–50 grams is the maximum that can be tolerated. But when Reaven began his work, this was not known.

To determine whether nutritional factors contribute to the development of metabolic syndrome, beginning in the 1980s, Reaven completed a number of RCTs of the effects of low-carbohydrate diets in patients with this condition. Without exception, his studies showed that removing carbohydrates from the diet uniformly improved all measures of health in those with IR and metabolic syndrome. This led him to the following conclusions:

> These results document that low-fat, high-carbohydrate diets, containing moderate amounts of sucrose, similar in composition to the recommendations of the American Diabetes Association, have deleterious metabolic effects when consumed by patients with NIDDM [non-insulin-dependent diabetes mellitus] for 15 days. Until it can be shown that these untoward effects are evanescent, and that long-term ingestion of similar diets will result in beneficial metabolic changes, it seems prudent to avoid the use of low-fat, high-carbohydrate diets containing moderate amounts of sucrose in patients with NIDDM.[68]

> The results of this study indicate that high-carbohydrate diets lead to several changes in carbohydrate and lipid metabolism in patients with NIDDM that could lead to an increased risk of coronary artery disease, and these effects persist for >6 [weeks]. Given these results, it seems reasonable to suggest that the routine recommendation of low-fat high-carbohydrate diets for patients with NIDDM be reconsidered.[69]

> In NIDDM patients, high-carbohydrate diets compared with high–monoun-saturated-fat diets caused persistent deterioration of glycemic control and accentuation of hyperinsulinemia, as well as increased plasma triglyceride and very-low-density lipoprotein cholesterol levels, which may not be desirable.[70]

So, besides establishing the fundamental role of IR in these chronic diseases, Reaven also discovered the optimum treatment: carbohydrate restriction. Yet he subsequently failed to emphasise the curative effects of low-carbohydrate diets that his studies had so clearly shown. Why is this?

I suspect that during his daily work at Stanford, Reaven was in close contact with some of the most influential cardiologists in the US and perhaps the world. They would not have taken kindly to their colleague's suggestion that, to prevent heart attacks, cardiologists should prescribe LCHF instead of the low-fat diet dictated, then as now, by the Dietary Guidelines for Americans, the AHA and the ADA. Had he chosen that route, Reaven's colleagues would have excommunicated him, his research funding would have dried up and his career would have been over, exactly as had happened to Dr John Yudkin for suggesting in the 1970s that sugar, not saturated fat, causes heart disease. So it seems to me that Reaven kept quiet, choosing rather to continue researching IR without paying much attention to how an LCHF diet might – simply, effectively and cheaply – prevent and reverse all the medical conditions caused by IR.

3. *One disease, one cause, many symptoms*

Reaven's problem was not unlike that faced by Darwin and Galileo, whose findings estranged them from religious orthodoxy. Reaven's unifying hypothesis of chronic disease not only offends his colleagues in cardiology; it strikes at the very heart (pun intended) of the pharmacological model practised in modern medicine.

If obesity, diabetes, heart disease, NAFLD, high blood pressure, and perhaps even cancer and dementia are, in fact, all symptoms of the same underlying condition – IR – then our current model of medical management must be wrong, requiring, as it does, specific but different pharmacological treatments for each separate condition, overseen by different hierarchies of medical specialists. And what if the cornerstone for the treatment of all these conditions is a low-carbohydrate diet, the very diet that has been vilified by my profession for the past 50 years? It must be an extremely frightening thought for many medical professionals. How do you come to terms with the possibility that, by following medical orthodoxy, you may have harmed many patients?

By producing a unifying theory for perhaps six chronic diseases, and by presenting the initial evidence that these conditions are initiated by high-carbohydrate diets in those with IR, Reaven has fundamentally changed our understanding of how these conditions develop, how they should be treated, and also how they might be prevented. Our challenge now is to incorporate this new understanding into our teaching and practise of medicine.

But time is short. We need to act expeditiously if we are to reverse the progressive slide to ill health and the ultimate bankruptcy of global medical services.

In Chapter 4, I explained why the current low-fat dietary advice does not prevent arterial disease, for example, of the coronary arteries supplying the heart. Instead, by causing atherogenic dyslipidaemia (as shown by Reaven's three studies and many others[71]), it is the direct cause of an unprecedented epidemic of arterial disease that threatens to overwhelm global medical services within the next 10 to 20 years.

In my HPCSA testimony, I presented one local study that clearly establishes the extent of the catastrophe facing South African medicine and why my profession is reluctant to acknowledge the existence of the IR that underpins it. T.E. Matsha and colleagues studied 1198 local volunteers from Bellville, Western Cape.[72] Importantly, the volunteers were all 'healthy' members of the community; they were not from a population being treated in hospital, for example.

Crucially, the researchers did not simply measure the volunteers' blood cholesterol concentrations according to the hopelessly incorrect theory that heart disease is the sole threat to the health of people living in the Western Cape. Rather, they measured a decent range of markers of IR and pre-diabetes (Table 17.5). The aim of the study was to determine whether these metabolic risk factors worsened with increasing levels of NAFLD, measured by the blood levels of the liver enzyme gamma-glutamyl transferase. It is known that blood GGT activity provides an excellent measure of the severity of IR and NAFLD.[73]

Table 17.5: Metabolic and other risk factors in 1 198 residents of a South African community grouped according to level of NAFLD (GGT) activity

Variables	Quarters of GGT			
	Q1	Q2	Q3	Q4
Number of subjects	292	272	318	316
Mean GGT (IU/L)	14	22	32	56
Mean age (years)	52.8	54.2	53.5	51.3
Mean systolic blood pressure (mmHg)	120	126	126	129
Mean diastolic blood pressure (mmHg)	73	76	76	79
Use of blood pressure–lowering agents (%)	32	40	42	42
Mean body mass index (kg/m^2)	28.6	29.5	31.1	30.3
Mean waist circumference (cm)	92.4	95.8	99.3	98.3
Current smoking (%)	33	42	41	46
Mean fasting blood [glucose] (mmol/L)	5.9	6.2	6.6	6.6
Median fasting blood [insulin] (uU/ml)	5.4	7.4	9.4	9.7
Mean HbA1c (%)	6.1	6.2	6.4	6.4
Mean blood [triglyceride] (mmol/L)	1.2	1.4	1.5	1.8
Mean blood [HDL cholesterol] (mmol/L)	1.3	1.3	1.2	1.3
Mean blood total [cholesterol] (mmol/L)	5.4	5.5	5.6	5.7
Median blood [C-reactive protein] (mg/L)	1.9	3.7	4.9	4.9
% with different features of the metabolic syndrome				
High waist circumference (%)	71	78	82	81
High blood pressure (%)	66	78	81	83
High fasting blood [glucose] (%)	34	49	51	56
High blood [triglyceride] (%)	15	27	31	39
Low blood [HDL cholesterol] (%)	43	47	56	51
Three components or more (%)	47	60	67	65

[ ] = concentration

Data from T.E. Matsha *et al.*, 'Gamma-glutamyl transferase, insulin resistance and cardiometabolic risk profile in a middle-aged African population'.[74] Note that Q1 were the 25 per cent of the study population with the lowest blood GGT activities; Q4 had the highest values and so the highest prevalence of NAFLD

The data clearly shows that the risk factors worsen across the table from left to right, indicating that increasing levels of NAFLD are associated with a worsening risk profile, as predicted by Reaven's model. The result is that the percentage in each group with Reaven's (Metabolic) Syndrome increases from 47 per cent in the group with the least NAFLD to 65 per cent in the group with the worst. But more frightening is the true incidence of diabetes in this group.

Even the 'healthiest' group (Q1) has elevated fasting glucose and insulin concentrations, as well as mean HbA1c concentrations of 6.1 per cent, indicating that essentially all in this group are already profoundly insulin resistant and will develop one or more of the serious consequences of IR in the next decade or so. Average HbA1c levels of 6.4 per cent and fasting blood glucose concentrations of 6.6 mmol/L in Q3 and Q4 indicate that the majority of people in these groups already have T2DM, although the authors fail to make this point in the table.

From the work of Reaven, Volek and their colleagues, and from my own study,[75] we know that the only chance these groups have of escaping the deadly complications of IR and T2DM is to drastically reduce their daily carbohydrate intake to below 50 grams per day. Those with T2DM should reduce to below 25 grams per day.

The problem is that because so many of these typical South Africans have blood cholesterol concentrations 'dangerously elevated' at more than 5.01 mmol/L, when they finally present themselves to conventionally trained physicians or cardiologists who believe that cholesterol causes heart disease and who do not understand IR, the majority will be prescribed a cholesterol-lowering statin drug and referred to a dietitian, who will prescribe the usual 'prudent, heart-healthy, low-fat diet in moderation'.

But statins will increase the risk for developing T2DM (Chapter 7), and the low-fat diet will expedite the development of T2DM and all its complications in the vast majority of these South Africans, whose IR is already so far advanced that their future development of T2DM is now an inevitability.

This is why I refused to run away from the HPCSA trial, no matter the cost to me, my wife and our family.

The future health of the South African nation depends almost entirely on health professionals finally getting to grips with the condition of IR. Once they do that and realise that the treatment is simple – the LCHF diet – the nation's health will be on the road to recovery, and the sacrifices my family and I have made in defending my position will have been more than justified.

Modern medicines don't work

If the arguments I have presented are correct, then the modern pharmacological model of disease management has to fail, because it ignores the cause of so much chronic disease – specifically, high-carbohydrate diets in those who are insulin resistant. Which raises the question: What is the evidence that treating the modern chronic diseases linked to IR with pharmacological drugs really makes any difference in the long term? I will detail the evidence only as it relates to those conditions linked to IR.

Obesity

Drugs for treating obesity are pretty ineffective – average weight loss in these trials is between three and six kilograms,[76] and the drugs come with many harmful side effects.[77] Whereas at least seven drugs have been passed for the treatment of obesity in the US, the European Union allows only one, orlistat.[78] The listed complications of using orlistat include decreased absorption of fat-soluble vitamins, steatorrhea (the presence of excess fat in faeces), oily spotting, flatulence with discharge, faecal urgency, oily evacuation, increased defecation and faecal incontinence.

When you see people losing 10–130 kilograms on the LCHF diet without any side effects, it is difficult to understand why medical practitioners continue to prescribe these drugs. There is an easier way.

Type-2 diabetes mellitus

In Chapter 7, I presented the evidence that more than 90 per cent of patients with T2DM can stop taking insulin if they follow the LCHF diet. Which raises the question: What is the effect of using insulin if you have T2DM? The answer: Not good.

Two recent studies show that progressive use of injected insulin is associated with increases in all-cause mortality, major cardiovascular events and, in one study, cancer rates.[79] Other large-scale observational studies from Canada and the UK show exactly the same outcomes. This fits with Reaven's model that insulin is the driver of much ill health.[80]

It is better to stop eating the carbohydrates that are driving the hyperinsulinaemia.

High blood pressure (hypertension)

According to a meta-analysis by M.R. Law, J.K. Morris and N.J. Wald, treatment of high blood pressure with medication reduces the relative (not absolute) risk for a subsequent heart attack by about 25 per cent, and for a stroke by about 33 per cent.[81] This effect requires that systolic blood pressure fall by 10 mmHg or diastolic blood pressure by 5 mmHg. In our Canadian intervention, studying the effects of the LCHF diet on metabolic syndrome, we achieved larger average reductions in systolic blood pressures (14 mmHg) with diet alone. Many of our subjects had also stopped taking their blood pressure–lowering medications during the trial.[82]

My point is that the LCHF diet might lower blood pressure more effectively than pharmacological treatments. In addition, the LCHF intervention includes many other benefits that can never be achieved by drugs, because the latter fail to address the primary cause: IR, hyperinsulinaemia and high-carbohydrate diets.

Furthermore, the authors of the aforementioned meta-analysis use *relative* not *absolute* risk reduction, and so, by default or design, dramatically inflate the apparent value of the drugs. For example, in this meta-analysis of 464 164 people, 22 115 (4.76 per cent) suffered heart attacks and 17 890 (3.85 per cent) strokes during the average of four years that the trials lasted. If the drugs reduced heart attack risk by 25 per cent and stroke risk by 33 per cent, the percentage of subjects suffering a heart attack would be 4.05 per cent and a stroke 2.54 per cent. Which means that the *absolute* risk reduction for a heart attack is 0.71 per cent (4.76 minus 4.05), and for stroke, 1.31 per cent (3.85 minus 2.54).

Which further means that to calculate the number needed to treat (NNT),* we divide the absolute risk reduction percentage into 100, giving NNTs for heart attack and stroke reduction of 141 and 76 respectively. Thus, to produce one beneficial outcome in one single patient, we must treat between 76 and 141 hypertensive patients with (expensive) medications for at least four years.

Interestingly, the NNTs for the 10 highest-grossing drugs in the US range between 3 and 24,[83] suggesting that the overwhelming majority of people in the US are not benefiting from the drugs they are prescribed.

Perhaps a dietary change might be more beneficial. And less expensive.

Coronary heart disease
The best possible absolute heart-attack risk reduction in people with established heart disease treated with cholesterol-lowering drugs (statins) is between 1 and 3 per cent, with little evidence that all-cause mortality is reduced or life is prolonged by much more than a few days (Chapter 3). This means that between 33 and 100 patients with heart disease must be treated for one person to benefit. Definitive evidence that people without heart disease benefit at all from the use of these drugs must still be provided.[84]

---

* The NNT provides a measure of the relative efficacy of different medical interventions. For example, if a specific intervention produces a 50 per cent absolute (not relative) risk reduction in a particular condition, the NNT for that intervention is 100/50, which equals 2. This means that the intervention will produce a benefit in every second patient. Most people I know will intentionally submit to an intervention that benefits every third or perhaps fourth patient. Compare this to the use of statins, which benefit one in between 50 and 140 treated patients. I conclude that if most patients were properly informed of the NNTs for statin drugs, they would probably not use them. The number needed to harm (NNH) is calculated in the same way, but for harmful outcomes.

Alzheimer's disease
There are no pharmacological drugs that make any difference to this disease. Some argue that promoting ketogenesis with a ketogenic LCHF diet may improve memory in patients with this condition. But because Alzheimer's is a form of diabetes (type-3 diabetes),[85] perhaps the best solution would be to prevent the condition in the first place by following the type of LCHF diet that has been shown to 'reverse' T2DM in a large number of people with advanced IR.[86]

Cancer
As discussed earlier in this chapter, cancer was essentially unheard of in populations eating their traditional diets. Even the mid-Victorian English did not suffer greatly from cancer (Figure 16.7 on page 324). That is why cancer is considered to be a disease of 'civilization'. Today, cancer is the second-leading cause of death among Americans, with one in four deaths in the US due to cancer. In 2013, 1 536 119 Americans received a new diagnosis of cancer and 584 872 died of the disease. The direct medical costs of cancer in the US are estimated at $74.8 billion.[87] Clearly, modern medicine does not yet have any answers for the prevention and treatment of cancer.

But perhaps the Inuit, the Plains Indians, the Masai, the Pathans and other 'manly, stalwart and resolute races of the north [of India]', the Australian Aborigines, the Nguni tribes of Southern Africa, the Swiss inhabitants of the Lötschental Valley, the New Zealand Maori and even the mid-Victorians, did.

Our fault is that perhaps we are just too proud to listen.

Closure

'Soon it became apparent, in interview after interview, that the story went far beyond the cold, empirical data, it tapped into base psychology, human limitations, economic incentives, and the deep-rooted, powerful forces of groupthink, forces that carry the inertia of the *Titanic*. Scientific progress doesn't glide from one exalted epiphany to the next, like the story of Isaac Newton getting hit on the head by an apple. It is a torch carried by human beings, it lurches, stumbles, wanders into dead ends, and then finds its way back out. It doesn't march in a straight line – it trips its way toward the truth. But the beautiful thing about science is no matter how bumpy the ride, eventually, because of the process itself, the truth is slowly, inevitably, mapped out.'

– **Travis Christofferson**, *Tripping Over the Truth*[1]

Advocate Joan Adams's comprehensive ruling achieved what Professor Tim Noakes and his lawyers had dedicated more than three years of their lives to accomplishing: complete vindication before a global audience. No longer did he have to endure the shame of being presumed guilty of nebulous charges by his peers. No longer could they consider him a mad, bad scientist and Public Health Enemy Number One.

Adams's ruling also confirmed that in a reasonable world, the HPCSA hearing would never have happened. In that world, universities are free of covert influences and are the supreme defenders of intellectual thought and scientific rigour. They do not throw their distinguished scientists to industry-led wolves for daring to challenge orthodoxy. But this is not a reasonable world, as we have demonstrated. Our book therefore reflects badly on all three of South Africa's top universities: Cape Town, Stellenbosch and Wits. UCT is arguably the most culpable, with Stellenbosch a close second and Wits not far behind. But that's only relatively speaking. North-West University does not acquit itself well, either.

We have also identified many imponderables weighing down the trial; so many, it's a wonder the HPCSA managed to get it off the ground.

One of those imponderables is whether the hearing would have happened at all were it not for the inordinately large, incestuous web of UCT academics that eventually spread to the other universities. And what can reasonably be perceived as coordinated smear campaigns against Noakes that began in the wake of his Damascene moment at the end of 2010.

Chief among those academics were cardiologists, lipidologists and dietitians from his scientific home, UCT's internationally renowned Faculty of Health Sciences. The faculty's nutrition department, headed by Professor Nelia Steyn, ably assisted by associate professor Marjanne Senekal, was a special hotbed of anti-Noakes and anti-LCHF sentiment.

In condoning and apparently colluding with what was effectively a scientific witch-hunt, UCT created the conditions for the smear campaigns to take root and spread nationally. UCT effectively declared open season on Noakes by condoning academic bullying from within its own ranks. It sent out a sinister signal to all its academics: it would exact a heavy price from even the most eminent scientists for the 'crime' of going against dogma. In colluding, all the other universities involved in this extraordinary saga sent the same signal.

The first sign of UCT's willingness to silence Noakes and suppress the science for LCHF was the cardiologists' letter to the press in September 2012. At the helm was Patrick Commerford, then cardiology professor and head of the cardiac clinic at UCT and Groote Schuur Hospital. Actually, an even earlier sign of UCT's innate antipathy towards boat-rocking scientists emanated from a far less scientific space: the personal blog of a lecturer in UCT's Faculty of Commerce, Jacques Rousseau.

Rousseau's first blog attacking Noakes appeared in 2012. At last count, he had devoted 30 posts to denigrating and demonising Noakes and LCHF, using religious and cultish terminology. He has compared Noakes to a 'faith healer' and called him a bad and dangerous scientist who 'sounds like a quack'. UCT's silence on such ad hominem attacks by one of its own lecturers was a prelude to what was to come.

Rousseau's obsession with Noakes can perhaps best be explained by who his father is: UCT graduate and epidemiology professor Jacques Rossouw, former head of the NIH Women's Health Initiative in the US. Rossouw is one of Noakes's most virulent and venomous critics. As we have shown in this book, the Rossouw family has made it their mission to malign Noakes at every turn.

A follow-up to the cardiologists' letter was also telling: the UCT Centenary Debate in December 2012, in which members of the Faculty of Health Sciences facilitated a debate between Noakes and Rossouw on the science behind diet and disease. What appeared to be a set-up from the start was not so much a debate as a kangaroo court. Rossouw was in Cape Town as a guest of his close friend Professor Krisela Steyn, a UCT Faculty of Health Sciences researcher and an implacable Noakes foe. In an interview with the *SAMJ* after the debate, Rossouw, Steyn and another UCT colleague, Professor Dinky Levitt, joined forces in coordinated attacks. Rossouw accused Noakes of going down a 'very dangerous path' and 'flouting the Hippocratic Oath'. Steyn called his theories on nutrition a 'public danger'. Levitt echoed by referring to Noakes as 'dangerous'.

That was followed by perhaps the most egregious attack on Noakes by his colleagues: the defamatory, inflammatory UCT professors' letter, published in the *Cape Times* in August 2014. Signatories included then faculty dean Professor Wim de Villiers, then department head Professor Bongani Mayosi, and Senekal.

Preceding that letter by just a few weeks was the publication of the Naudé review in *PLoS One*. As we've shown in this book, the HPCSA used the Naudé review to build its whole case against Noakes. The review became the oxygen for the ferocious prosecutorial fire that the HPCSA unleashed against him. Who requested the review is significant: the industry-fed Heart and Stroke Foundation of South Africa. The HSFSA is a mouthpiece of the food and drug industries that benefit from the conventional LFHC dietary guidelines. The HSFSA has yet to explain the rationale for requesting the review when there was already a robust Brazilian review on the same topic, which came to precisely the opposite conclusion. The Naudé review remains mired in accusations of scientific fraud, yet all the universities involved have blithely averted their eyes to claims of misconduct.

This raises the question of whether the hearing would have happened had the HSFSA not requested the review. It also raises another imponderable: Senekal's influence and the three 'hats' she wore in the war against Noakes (she was co-signatory of the UCT professors' letter, co-author of the Naudé review and consultant for the HPCSA during the hearing).

A prominent academic could have cut off the air supply to the HPCSA's case from the very start. One of the biggest imponderables is why Wits University professor Amaboo Dhai chose not to do so, as chair of the HPCSA's Fourth Preliminary Committee of Inquiry. The trial against Noakes might never have happened were it not for Dhai and her fellow committee members' 'highly irregular' conduct, as his lawyers diplomatically phrased it.

If Dhai were unbiased, she should have first sought the informed opinion of a paediatrician steeped in the science and practice of complementary feeding. If there was no such person of sufficient gravitas in South Africa, she should have looked further afield. Out of respect for Noakes as an internationally renowned scientist, one of few in the world with an A1 rating, she should have sought an opinion from an international expert.

One is Professor Nancy Krebs of the University of Colorado in Denver. Krebs is perhaps the world authority on this topic and has undertaken a series of RCTs of complementary feeding. Recall that RCTs are considered the 'gold standard' of scientific evidence. As Noakes presented in his evidence, Krebs has shown that the introduction of meat as an early complementary food for infant weaning has significant benefits. These include a reduction in childhood stunting,[2] increased linear growth without increased adiposity,[3] improved zinc[4] and iron status,[5] and what appears to be a superior gut microbiome.[6] Krebs also writes that infants should be weaned onto diets that contain 30–40 per cent fat. South Africa's dietary guidelines would consider this a high-fat diet. She continues:

> While median intakes of fat among US toddlers are within these guidelines, approximately one-quarter of toddlers consume diets below the recommended range of fat, while only 3% exceeded the recommended range. The traditional emphasis placed on cereal, fruits, and vegetables as first foods, all of which are low in fat, contributes to an overall sharp reduction in the percentage of energy from fats in older infants and may be associated with inadequate energy intake, especially in those who are breastfed.[7]

Instead of an expert of Krebs's stature, the HPCSA inexplicably turned first to a local registered dietitian, Marlene Ellmer. Unlike Krebs, Ellmer has yet to publish her first RCT of complementary feeding. In a summary of her evidence against Noakes, which Ellmer wisely ended up not giving, she claimed that there was no published evidence of the effects of a 'high-protein or a high-fat complementary diet' on infant growth and development. She also claimed that 'poor dietary intake' contributes to deteriorating child health in South Africa. Perhaps if Ellmer had acquainted herself with Krebs's work, including the study of the beneficial effects of increased meat consumption on infant stunting in Guatemala, Pakistan, Zambia and the Congo,[8] she might have shown the HPCSA where the real threat to infant health lies.

And if Dhai had done some basic homework, she might have consulted a recently published study showing that the early introduction of eggs as a complementary food significantly improved growth in infants in Ecuador. The authors concluded that: 'Generally accessible to vulnerable groups, eggs have the potential to contribute to global targets to reduce stunting.'[9] Despite the power of the grain industry, perhaps weaning onto eggs rather than maize could begin to address the problems of stunting among South African infants. Several of the prosecution's expert witnesses referred to the issue of childhood malnutrition in South Africa.

Instead, Dhai was on a different mission, as the contents of the now infamous file – the 'dodgy dossier' – revealed. She wanted the HPCSA to expedite the case against Noakes. She deemed him a threat to public health because of his 'high profile'. She therefore chose the opinion of the one person she could be fairly certain would support her view: North-West University nutrition professor Hester Vorster. Vorster was perhaps the South African academic with the most to gain from discrediting Noakes and burying the LCHF/Banting diet. As the author of the 2013 revision of the South African Food-based Dietary Guidelines, Vorster stands to lose the most from a move away from cereal- and grain-based high-carbohydrate diets to the LCHF lifestyle that Noakes advocates. Headlining the guidelines is her edict that we should all 'make starchy foods part of most meals'.[10] Besides her obvious conflict of interest, Vorster was demonstrably one of the least qualified South African academics to give an opinion on the complaint that her former student, dietitian Claire Julsing Strydom, made against Noakes.

Within the first five minutes of cross-examination, Advocate Dr Rocky Ramdass had blown Vorster's cover. He established that her undergraduate degree in home economics does not qualify her as a dietitian; that she has no other qualifications or training in dietetics; that she has never practised as a dietitian or treated a single patient; and, more importantly, that she has done no research on the LCHF diet. Vorster also has no expertise in ethics, knows little about social media and doesn't have a Twitter account. What Vorster does have is a long history of research funding from SASA and involvement with the Coca-Cola front company, the ILSI.

As US investigative journalist Russ Greene showed, Vorster was not the only one with this type of clear conflict of interest. Many, if not most, of the doctors, dietitians and academics involved in the HPCSA's case against Noakes have links with drug companies and/or the sugar industry in general, and the ILSI in particular.

Alternatively, the HPCSA could have just read the South African Food-based Dietary Guidelines. If they had done so, they would have read that: 'From six months of age, give your child meat, chicken, fish or egg every day, or as often as possible.'[11] That was essentially what Noakes recommended in his tweet to breastfeeding mother Pippa Leenstra. Both Vorster and her North-West University colleague, Professor Salome Kruger, should have seen that.

As we have shown in this book, the trial was never about infant feeding. The Naudé review clearly demonstrated that. It was also not about Noakes's conduct as a medical doctor on social media. After all, he hasn't practised clinical medicine for more than 15 years. Furthermore, the HPCSA doesn't have any guidelines for health professionals on social media. So how could the HPCSA go after Noakes for breaching non-existent guidelines?

Instead of relying on the acutely embarrassing testimony of Stellenbosch psychiatry professor Willie Pienaar, the HPCSA could have referred Noakes's tweet to Dr Brenda Kubheka of the University of the Witwatersrand's School of Public Health. In a recent editorial in the *SAMJ*, Kubheka clearly distinguishes between providing generic and patient-specific advice on Twitter: 'It is advisable that professionals share generic information online and avoid responding with direct medical advice to individuals.'[12] Which is exactly what Noakes did in responding to Leenstra's 'we' question.

In *Tim Noakes: The Quiet Maverick*, Daryl Ilbury considers the ethics of the tweet that started all the trouble. He concludes:

It's neither an offensive tweet by any stretch of the imagination, nor does it fall foul of any media law – it's not libellous and there's no encouragement of harm to others. People could disagree with him and had a voice to do so; that's the point of social media: it is a platform for public discussion ... Importantly, the question demanded a public, not a private response, which the person asking the question was free to accept or reject. And, as a medical doctor, Noakes didn't cross any ethical boundaries in replying on a public platform. He didn't publish any confidential patient information or dispense a diagnosis for a specific patient without seeing that patient; he simply provided generalised nutritional advice based on scientific evidence.[13]

Had the HPCSA followed this approach, they could have resolved Strydom's complaint in less than an hour. Instead, the HPCSA deliberately turned a single, innocuous tweet into a trial that lasted more than three years and cost millions of rands.

Which brings us to the most inexplicable imponderable: Leenstra's deafening silence. She was ostensibly the mother of a potential victim, yet the HPCSA did not call her to testify. Leenstra made it clear in media interviews that she thought the whole thing had become a circus. If the HPCSA had called her, she would have had to tell the truth: that she had no doctor–patient relationship with Noakes. In fact, if Leenstra's tweet was not a set-up from the start, as some suggest, she might have said that she didn't even know that Noakes was a doctor. His Twitter profile makes no mention of it, and his public profile is that of a scientist, not a doctor. Leenstra would have had to say that she hadn't tried to get a free consultation or medical advice out of Noakes; that all she did was ask Noakes for information and he gave it. End of story.

We speculated from the outset that this trial was a turf war between Noakes and dietitians. That leads to another major imponderable: Strydom's real motivation for going after him. It clearly wasn't his tweet, as evidence on the record at the hearing showed. Proof was found in an email chain that Noakes's instructing attorney, Adam Pike, uncovered in July 2017 after making a freedom-of-information request to ADSA under the Promotion of Access to Information Act.

Among other things, the emails show that Strydom and her successor as ADSA president, Maryke Gallagher, had Noakes, and not his tweet, firmly in their sights. In one email in June 2014, Strydom appeals emotively to the HPCSA about 'The Tim Noakes problem' and his 'bashing of the profession'. 'We need intervention from HPCSA as a matter of urgency,' she writes. Strydom also says that ADSA needs the HPCSA's 'much bigger clout'. In its replies, the HPCSA indicates that it will oblige.

Ironically, Strydom presents as proof of the 'bashing' a January 2014 media report that is highly critical of dietitians. However, Noakes is not the one doing the bashing. The article, by Gary Watson, is also highly supportive of Noakes, which clearly infuriated Strydom.[14]

This would account for emails in which Strydom encourages another ADSA executive to lodge a complaint against Noakes with the HPCSA in July 2014. Catherine Pereira's grounds were even more frivolous than Strydom's: outrage at Noakes opining that he didn't know of any dietitian who tells people in poor communities not to drink Coca-Cola or eat potato crisps. In reality, Strydom had no proof that Noakes had ever said anything remotely antagonistic towards any dietitian personally, because he hadn't ever done so.

The emails Pike uncovered show that it was the publication of *The Real Meal Revolution* in 2013 that really caused an uproar among some dietitians. The book had stimulated a public uprising against the advice that dietitians regularly dished up. The public was demanding proof of their claims that the Banting diet was dangerous. All they could come up with was what Watson exposed: nothing at all, although he put it in stronger language. Watson's article appears to have been the tipping point that set Strydom and Gallagher on their quest to muzzle Noakes: the public wouldn't accept their explanations for why Banting wasn't brilliant. Instead of thinking of a properly scientific answer, they tried to shoot the messenger of *The Real Meal Revolution*. They thought that if they cut off Noakes's scientific head, they would stop the revolt.

ADSA clearly had Noakes in its sights for years. It took the freedom-of-information request in mid-2017 by Noakes's lawyers for ADSA to give up an email chain. In one email, Strydom begged the HPCSA to expedite the case against Noakes. She appeared to assume, oddly though correctly enough, that the HPCSA would automatically do her and Gallagher's bidding.

What also stands out as an imponderable is the ethics of the connection between Strydom and the HPCSA's Dietetics and Nutrition Board member: North-West University nutrition professor Edelweiss Wentzel-Viljoen. In an email on 4 June 2015, Wentzel-Viljoen apologises to Strydom for not being able to disclose the HPCSA's 'plan' for Noakes. The fact that there was a 'plan' suggests the HPCSA's bias towards a guilty verdict from the outset. She says that the HPCSA's legal department told her she was not allowed to tell Strydom about the 'plan'. One could reasonably have assumed that as a Dietetics and Nutrition Board member, Wentzel-Viljoen would have been cognisant of her responsibility to act without prejudice towards a fellow health professional.

Yet another imponderable is why the HPCSA chose so speedily and enthusiastically to enter the turf war on the dietitians' side. After all, HPCSA hearings are supposed to be dispassionate inquiries into the truth of a matter.

In an email on 11 July 2015, Gallagher makes similar emotional appeals to the HPCSA's registrar, Dr Buyiswa Mjamba-Matshoba, for assistance against Noakes. She states that ADSA used its 'limited budget' to appoint a firm of specialist attorneys on a 'watching brief' over the HPCSA proceedings. Quite why ADSA needed lawyers to watch over them is anyone's guess, since Strydom and Gallagher were not facing charges.

But Gallagher doesn't stop there. She says that ADSA's attorneys had 'to date assisted [HPCSA prosecuting counsel Advocate Meshack Mapholisa] with preparation for the hearing'. In reply, Mjamba-Matshoba sees nothing unusual or inappropriate in ADSA's lawyers assisting the HPCSA to build a case against Noakes. If proof were needed that the HPCSA had colluded with ADSA from the outset, Gallagher provided it in her emailed letter.

Gallagher's comments in that email are a prelude to later dissembling and semantic gymnastics in claims that ADSA had never lodged a complaint and had no vendetta against Noakes. Gallagher has tried claiming that ADSA only 'sought guidance' from the HPCSA on the conduct of health professionals on social media. The emails show that to be untrue. Furthermore, the HPCSA has no guidelines for health professionals on social media. If Gallagher had indeed asked the HPCSA for guidelines, she would have learnt as much.

Both Strydom and Gallagher also show inordinate anxiety over whether the HPCSA was throwing sufficient resources behind its efforts to succeed against Noakes. They make clear their desire for a guilty verdict.

The emails therefore also show how remarkably apposite were comments made by Advocate Michael van der Nest for Noakes in closing arguments. He described Strydom as a 'disgruntled dietitian' who was angry because the public seemed to be listening to Noakes and not to her. He also said that the tweet was just a pretext for the HPCSA and ADSA to go after Noakes.

Strydom and Gallagher can look like the prime movers behind Noakes's trial, as both are food-industry consultants. However, they could not have succeeded without a little help from strategically placed friends within the HPCSA, such as Wentzel-Viljoen. She tried to get onto the HPCSA's Professional Conduct Committee to hear the charge against Noakes, and saw no conflict of interest in her well-documented opposition to Noakes and LCHF. She was happy to be a fox guarding the hen house. She only recused herself after Noakes's lawyers forced her to do so.

This leads to another imponderable: would the hearing have happened without so many 'cuddly dietitians in the cosy embrace of industry fat cats'? British health writer Jerome Burne used that phrase to describe the antics of dietitians in his own country.[15] He could just as easily have been talking about South Africa.

In this book, Noakes and I have named many dietitians, doctors and assorted academics who contributed, directly or indirectly, to the HPCSA's prosecution of him. The list is not exhaustive, but it is long. So long, it may be tempting to think that it's not possible for so many doctors, dietitians and academics to be out of step. We have shown that it's both possible and probable.

Of course, Noakes and I are not insinuating that all those who helped the HPCSA are mad, bad people, on the payroll or in the thrall of food and drug companies. Many are decent enough, even as they may be ignorant, fearful and suffering prolonged bouts of cognitive dissonance. As Noakes has proved, it takes courage to change your mind when you've believed and taught wrongly for decades.

We have also shown the intricate web of industry-led ties that bind the dietitians, doctors and academics who have tried to bully Noakes into silence. All have careers, reputations, livelihoods, funding, sponsors and/or businesses to protect. Noakes and LCHF threaten them all. For proof, you only have to look at the knee-jerk responses of ADSA dietitians and HPCSA witnesses to the bestselling *The Real Meal Revolution*, of which Noakes is a co-author. Vorster, Kruger and another HPCSA expert witness, Dr Muhammad Ali Dhansay, attacked his chapter on the extensive science for LCHF, claiming that the evidence he presented was 'not peer reviewed'. Yet much of the evidence is from peer-reviewed journals. More bizarrely, all freely admitted that they hadn't even read it. They seemed to take the book's commercial success as a personal affront.

That pointed to another imponderable: would the hearing have happened if Noakes had not contributed a chapter to *The Real Meal Revolution*?

But perhaps the biggest imponderable of all may lie in yet another incestuous web: ADSA's leadership profile. ADSA's executive committees throughout this case have comprised a coterie of mostly privileged white females from similar middle-class cultural and conservative backgrounds, a closed shop of mostly friends, or friends of friends. Many appear to be undeclared vegetarians or vegans, or at least strongly pushing planet-based agendas, without any evidence and with significant industry ties of one sort or another. What if the leadership had been more open, less overtly conflicted and more reflective of the diversity of South Africa's population and scientific views on diet and nutrition? What if they were not all so irrationally fat- and red-meat-phobic?

After the UCT professors' letter, Noakes took the view that moves were afoot to isolate him from his colleagues and destroy his scientific reputation. He had two choices: he could defend himself, or he could terminate his registration as a medical practitioner with the HPCSA. This would have been without consequence, because he hasn't practised as a medical doctor for more than 15 years and has no plans to do so again. But the public might have interpreted this as evidence of guilt. So it was never really an option. Noakes had no choice but to defend himself to the best of his ability.

When Noakes asked me to co-author this book, I accepted in a heartbeat. As a journalist with a hard-news background, I knew it would be a dream opportunity. I would get to delve into and document the murky world of medicine, nutrition science and academia in South Africa. I knew it would be another step on a remarkable journey. It would be a chance to expose the many doctors, dietitians and academics in the thrall, if not the pay, of food and drug industries. I would also get to reveal the many health professionals who put patients before profits, and the price they pay for having the courage to do so.

Noakes possesses many qualities that enticed me to travel with him on this journey: not just his formidable intellect, but also his honesty and integrity. To the uninitiated, Noakes can at times seem almost brutally honest. But as the Jewish proverb goes: 'When con men meet a legitimately honest man, they are so bewildered that they consider him a greater con man than themselves.'

On this journey, I witnessed first-hand the nightmare that Noakes endured. I saw the pillar that enabled him to handle the ordeal with the strength, courage and dignity that he did: his family – wife Marilyn, son Travis and daughter Candice. Noakes describes Marilyn's support as 'absolutely critical'. He says that the actions of those intent on 'breaking' him followed the classic CIA modus operandi: first isolate the individual from his colleagues, and then from his spouse. 'They might have been able to do the former; they were never going to achieve the latter,' he says. 'I and my family have emerged changed but stronger from the experience.'

Noakes has had many 'angels' helping him on his journey, among them his expert witnesses, Dr Zoë Harcombe, Nina Teicholz and Dr Caryn Zinn. Despite the best efforts of the HPCSA's expensive team of external lawyers, Tim's Angels stood firm. Their evidence was the angelic and scientific equivalent of landmines, which they exploded in the faces of the HPCSA's witnesses.

Perhaps the real turning point in Noakes's fortune was earlier, when his hyper-energetic instructing attorney, Adam Pike, took charge, and advocates Dr Rocky Ramdass and Mike van der Nest SC offered their support *pro Deo*. I call them 'Tim's Avenging Angels'. From that moment on, there was only ever going to be one outcome – the one that Advocate Joan Adams delivered on 21 April 2017.

Noakes says of his legal team: 'Rocky, Mike and Adam are three of the most honourable, upstanding and outstanding people I have ever had the privilege to meet.' To him, Ramdass is 'Brother' Rocky, a devout Hindu who epitomises the Vedic definition of a man of God: 'Softer than the flower, where kindness is concerned; stronger than the thunder, where principles are at stake.' To the HPCSA, Noakes says that his entire legal team was 'stronger than the thunder'. To him and Marilyn, 'they were softer than the flower'.

Then, of course, there are the many LCHF scientists and doctors and many millions of Banters who continue to speak up for Noakes worldwide.

Noakes's lawyers are very much 'old-school' in their approach to law and in their dedication to fighting injustice. They saw the HPCSA's prosecution of Noakes as stifling legitimate scientific debate and eroding his constitutional right to freedom of speech. All looked forward to a vigorous scientific debate in the hearing. All were to be bitterly disappointed. They saw the case as veering between farce and Greek tragedy. As an arguably 'old-fashioned' lawyer, Van der Nest had demanded to see the science to build the case for his client. Noakes gave it to him in spades. Yet when it came to Noakes's cross-examination, as Van der Nest argued, the HPCSA simply ignored vast swathes of the scientific material. He saw the ultimate irony in the HPCSA's argument contending that the scientific material was irrelevant because it related to adults. The reality appeared to be, he said, that the HPCSA simply could not answer Noakes's scientific evidence.

Van der Nest is respected and revered as one of South Africa's top senior counsel, a person of formidable intellect, integrity and courage. He has seen the effects of prosecutions by bodies such as the HPCSA and the negative effects on the lives of those prosecuted, even when they've won their cases down the line. He knows that there is almost always a negative impact on the accused's life. He knows that, despite the obvious, some will want to believe that Noakes was found not guilty on legal technicalities. Van der Nest also knows that reputation is never fully restored in cases like this. Ramdass is a physician and vegetarian, who at the age of nearly 50 had the courage to change careers and start out as a junior advocate. He brought to the table his encyclopaedic medical knowledge, legal talent and a rare ability to make people listen to him and find themselves wanting to agree with him. Pike, along with his prodigious intelligence, has an acting background and thus naturally tends to see the theatrical side of litigation. However, while he sees the drama, he also sees the extensive damage.

As Van der Nest argued, statutory bodies such as the HPCSA have a duty to take care and never to prosecute for the wrong reasons. After all, anyone is free to agree or disagree with Noakes, but it is completely inappropriate for the HPCSA to prosecute him for his scientific views and to side with those who disagree with him. As we have shown in this book, the HPCSA showed an utter dereliction of duty.

And while Noakes won a decisive victory in Adams's ruling, ADSA, the HPCSA and others have made it clear that their war with him continues. As our journey progressed, I frequently ended my emails to him with the following: *A luta continua, vitória é certa.*[*] It resonated with him.

Does he have any regrets? Of course. Only a fool has no regrets, and Noakes is clearly no fool. For more than three years – that Noakes has described as his 'descent into darkness' – the trial dominated his and his family's life. Perhaps the worst part, he says, was the failure of his university to do anything to support him.

---

[*] 'The struggle continues, victory is certain'. This was the rallying cry of the FRELIMO movement during Mozambique's war for independence. The phrase is Portuguese and was used by FRELIMO leader Samora Machel to cultivate popular support against the Portuguese colonial presence.

Instead, it betrayed him. 'It has estranged me from an organisation to which I have dedicated my working life,' Noakes told me.

The unrecognised hero, the most powerful avenging angel who lifted him out of the darkness, is unquestionably Noakes's wife of 45 years, Marilyn Anne. It is only fitting that she should have the last word in this book.

On 2 July 2017, Noakes's 68th birthday, Marilyn gave him a card showing a magical blue malachite kingfisher rising effortlessly from the water. Inside, she had written the following:

Did you know that the Kingfisher is a symbol of Halcyon Days? According to the legend, during the 10 days around the winter solstice, the Kingfisher laid her eggs in a nest floating on the Aegean Sea. The bird, it is said, charmed the waves and the eggs were hatched on a tranquil sea beneath cloudless skies. These are the Halcyon Days; they signify peace and happiness.

I am so proud of how you weathered the storm of that most vindictive and harrowing HPCSA Hearing/Trial. The only blessing was the splendid performance of your defence team and those caring friends who came to support you. Getting to know these emotionally intelligent people was humbling and special.

When you were at last given the space to present your evidence to support the LCHF argument you did it with such integrity and eloquence. Well done! It is no wonder that Advocate Joan Adams found you Not Guilty!

Hold your head up high and don't allow 'them' to rob you of your enthusiasm, optimism and wonderful engaging smile.

I wish you Happy Halcyon Days for ever more ...

Abbreviations and Acronyms

ADA	American Diabetes Association
ADSA	Association for Dietetics in South Africa
AHA	American Heart Association
AHPRA	Australian Health Practitioner Regulation Agency
AND	Academy of Nutrition and Dietetics
AUT	Auckland University of Technology
BMJ	*British Medical Journal*
CDE	Centre for Diabetes and Endocrinology
CHD	coronary heart disease
CICO	calories in, calories out
CNE	Continuing Nutrition Education
CNF	Cochrane Nutrition Field
CORIS	Coronary Risk Factor Intervention Study
CPD	Continuing Professional Development
CVD	cardiovascular disease
EAHE	exercise-associated hyponatraemic encephalopathy
ESSM	Exercise Science and Sports Medicine
FH	familial hypercholestrolaemia
GGT	gamma-glutamyl transferase
GLiMMER	Global Lifestyle Medicine Mobilizing to Effect Reform
HbA1c	glycated haemoglobin
HDL	high-density lipoprotein
HELP	Healthy Eating & Lifestyle Program
HFCS	high-fructose corn syrup
HPCSA	Health Professions Council of South Africa
HSFSA	Heart and Stroke Foundation of South Africa
ILSI	International Life Sciences Institute
IR	insulin resistance
JAMA	*Journal of the American Medical Association*
LCHF	low carbohydrate, high fat
LDL	low-density lipoprotein
LFHC	low fat, high carbohydrate

mmol/L	millimoles per litre
NAFLD	non-alcoholic fatty liver disease
NCD	non-communicable diseases
NCGS	non-coeliac gluten sensitivity
NIH	National Institutes of Health
NRF	National Research Foundation
NSRD	Nutritional Solutions Registered Dietitians
NSSA	Nutrition Society of South Africa
PAD	peripheral artery disease
PAIA	Promotion of Access to Information Act
PAJA	Promotion of Administrative Justice Act
PoPI	Protection of Personal Information Act
RCT	randomised controlled trial
SAHA	South African Heart Association
SAJCN	*South African Journal of Clinical Nutrition*
SAMA	South African Medical Association
SAMJ	*South African Medical Journal*
SAMRC	South African Medical Research Council
SASA	South African Sugar Association
SSISA	Sports Science Institute of South Africa
T1DM	type-1 diabetes mellitus
T2DM	type-2 diabetes mellitus
THUSA	Transition and Health during Urbanisation of South Africans
UCT	University of Cape Town
USDA	United States Department of Agriculture
WHIRCDMT	Women's Health Initiative Randomized Controlled Dietary Modification Trial
WHO	World Health Organization
Wits	University of the Witwatersrand

Select Bibliography

Atkins, Robert. *Dr Atkins' New Diet Revolution.* London: Vermilion 2002

Banting, William. *Letter on Corpulence, Addressed to the Public.* London: Harrison, 1864

Cleave, Thomas L. *The Saccharine Disease: Conditions caused by the taking of refined carbohydrates, such as sugar and white flour.* Bristol: John Wright & Sons Ltd, 1974

————, and D. George. *Diabetes, Coronary Thrombosis and the Saccharine Disease.* Bristol: John Wright & Sons Ltd, 1966

Colpo, Anthony. *The Great Cholesterol Con: Why everything you've been told about cholesterol, diet, and heart disease is wrong!* Self-published: Lulu, 2006

Creed, Sally-Ann, David Grier, Jonno Proudfoot and Tim Noakes. *The Real Meal Revolution.* Cape Town: Quivertree, 2013

Davis, William. *Wheat Belly: Lose the Wheat, Lose the Weight, and Find Your Path Back to Health.* New York: Rodale, 2011

De Lorgeril, Michel. *Cholesterol and Statins: Sham Science and Bad Medicine.* Kindle edition, 2014

Dreger, Alice. *Galileo's Middle Finger: Heretics, Activists, and One Scholar's Search for Justice.* New York: Penguin Press, 2015

Eades, Michael R. and Mary Dan Eades. *Protein Power.* New York: Bantam Books, 1996

Ebstein, Wilhelm. *Corpulence and Its Treatment on Physiological Principles.* London: H. Grevel, 1884

————. *The Regimen to be Adopted in Cases of Gout.* London: J. & A. Churchill, 1885

Eenfeldt, Andreas. *Low Carb, High Fat Food Revolution: Advice and Recipes to Improve Your Health and Reduce Your Weight.* New York: Skyhorse Publishing, 2014

Forslund, Monique. *Low-carb Living for Families.* Cape Town: Struik Lifestyle, 2013

Fung, Jason. *The Obesity Code: Unlocking the Secrets of Weight Loss.* Vancouver/ Berkeley: Greystone Books, 2016

Gøtzsche, Peter. *Deadly Medicines and Organised Crime: How Big Pharma has Corrupted Healthcare.* Florida: CRC Press, 2013

Harari, Yuval Noah. *Sapiens: A Brief History of Humankind.* London: Harvill Secker, 2014

Harcombe, Zoë. *The Obesity Epidemic: What Caused It? How Can We Stop It?*
Cwmbran, Wales: Columbus Publishing, 2010

Ilbury, Daryl. *Tim Noakes: The Quiet Maverick*. Cape Town: Penguin Books, 2017

Le Fanu, James. *The Rise and Fall of Modern Medicine*. London: Abacus, 2000

Lustig, Robert. *Fat Chance: Beating the Odds Against Sugar, Processed Food, Obesity
and Disease*. New York: Hudson Street Press, 2013

McCarrison, Robert. *Nutrition and Health*. London: The McCarrison Society, 1982

Morgan, William. *Diabetes Mellitus: Its History, Chemistry, Anatomy, Pathology,
Physiology, and Treatment*. London: The Homeopathic Publishing Company,
1877

Noakes, Tim. *Lore of Running*. Champaign, IL: Human Kinetics, 2003

———. *Waterlogged: The Serious Problem of Overhydration in Endurance Sports*.
Champaign, IL: Human Kinetics, 2012

——— and Michael Vlismas. *Challenging Beliefs: Memoirs of a Career*. Cape Town:
Zebra Press, 2012

———, Bernadine Douglas and Bridgette Allan. *The Banting Pocket Guide*, Cape
Town: Penguin Books, 2017

———, Jonno Proudfoot and Bridget Surtees. *Raising Superheroes*. Cape Town:
Burnett Media, 2015

Oppenheimer, Rebecca W. *Diabetic Cookery: Recipes and Menus*. London:
Forgotten Books, 2017

Osler, William. *The Principles and Practice of Medicine*. New York: D. Appleton and
Company, 1978

Perlmutter, David. *Grain Brain: The Surprising Truth About Wheat, Carbs, and
Sugar – Your Brain's Silent Killers*. New York: Little, Brown and Company, 2013

Poland, Marguerite, David Hammond-Tooke and Leigh Voight. *The Abundant
Herds: A Celebration of the Nguni Cattle of the Zulu People*. Cape Town:
Fernwood Press, 2006

Price, Weston. *Nutrition and Physical Degeneration*. Oxford: Benediction Classics,
2010

Roberts, Barbara. *The Truth About Statins: Risks and Alternatives to Cholesterol-
lowering Drugs*. New York: Pocket Books, 2012

Sandler, Benjamin P. *How to Prevent Heart Attacks*. Milwaukee: Lee Foundation for
Nutritional Research, 1958

Schofield, Grant, Caryn Zinn and Craig Rodger. *What The Fat? Fat's IN, Sugar's
OUT*. Auckland: The Real Food Publishing Company, 2015

Taubes, Gary. *Good Calories, Bad Calories*. New York: Anchor Books, 2007

———. *The Case Against Sugar*. New York: Alfred A. Knopf, 2016

———. *Why We Get Fat and What To Do About It*. New York: Alfred A. Knopf,
2011

Teicholz, Nina. *The Big Fat Surprise: Why Butter, Meat and Cheese Belong in a
Healthy Diet*. New York: Simon & Schuster, 2014

Thomson, Karen. *Sugar Free: 8 Weeks to Freedom from Sugar and Carb Addiction.* Cape Town: Sunbird Publishers, 2015

Voegtlin, Walter L. *The Stone Age Diet: Based on In-depth Studies of Human Ecology and the Diet of Man.* New York: Vantage Press, 1975

Volek, Jeff and Stephen Phinney. *The Art and Science of Low Carbohydrate Living.* Florida: Beyond Obesity LLC, 2011

———. *The Art and Science of Low Carbohydrate Performance.* Florida: Beyond Obesity LLC, 2012

Westman, Eric, Stephen Phinney and Jeff Volek. *The New Atkins for a New You.* New York: Fireside, 2010

Yellowlees, Walter. *A Doctor in the Wilderness.* Perthshire: Dr W.W. Yellowlees, 2001

Yudkin, John. *Pure, White and Deadly: How Sugar is Killing Us and What We Can Do to Stop It.* London: Penguin Books, 1972

Notes

Preface: Tim Noakes

1. R.A. Irving, T.D. Noakes, R. Buck *et al.*, 'Evaluation of renal function and fluid homeostasis during recovery from exercise-induced hyponatremia', *Journal of Applied Physiology* 70(1), 1991: 342–48.
2. T.D. Noakes, *Waterlogged: The Serious Problem of Overhydration in Endurance Sports* (Champaign, IL: Human Kinetics, 2012).
3. D. Ilbury, *Quiet Maverick: Tim Noakes Chews the Fat* (Johannesburg: Mampoer Shorts, 2015), 23.
4. T.D. Noakes, 'Tainted glory: Doping and athletic performance', *New England Journal of Medicine* 351(9), 2004: 847–49.
5. USADA, 'Statement from USADA CEO Travis T. Tygart regarding the U.S. Postal Service Pro Cycling Team doping conspiracy', 10 October 2012.
6. D. Walsh, *The Program: Seven Deadly Sins – My Pursuit of Lance Armstrong* (London: Simon & Schuster, 2012), 444.
7. Ibid., 413.
8. Ibid., 449.
9. L.G. Pugh, *Achieving the Impossible: A Fearless Leader. A Fragile Earth* (London: Simon & Schuster, 2010).
10. G. Claassen, *Kwakke, Kwinte & Kwale* (Cape Town: XLibris Publishing, 2014).
11. T.D. Noakes, 'Low-carbohydrate and high-fat intake can manage obesity and associated conditions: Occasional survey', *SAMJ* 103(11), 2013: 826–30.
12. P.C. Gøtzsche, *Deadly Medicines and Organised Crime: How Big Pharma Has Corrupted Healthcare* (Florida: CRC Press, 2013).

Preface: Marika Sboros

1. M. Jones, 'Noakes goes too far - doctors', *IOL*, 14 September 2012, available at http://www.iol.co.za/lifestyle/noakes-goes-too-far---doctors-1383310 (last accessed 31 July 2017).
2. K. Child, 'Tim Noakes diet is "criminal" says doctor', *Times*, 4 August 2014.
3. R. Smith, 'Are some diets "mass murder"?', *BMJ* 2014;349:g7654.
4. C.E Naudé, A. Schoonees, M. Senekal *et al.*, 'Low carbohydrate versus isoenergetic balanced diets for reducing weight and cardiovascular risk: A systematic review and meta-analysis', *PLoS One* 9(7), 2014: e100652.

Introduction

1. Russ Greene, 'Big Food vs. Tim Noakes: The final crusade', *The Russells*, 5 January 2017, available at https://therussells.crossfit.com/2017/01/05/big-food-vs-tim-noakes-the-final-crusade/ (last accessed 31 July 2017).

PART I: THE LOW-CARB REVOLUTION
Chapter 1: The Low-carb Summit

1. C. Choi, 'Study details sugar industry attempt to shape science', *Observer-Reporter US and World*, 12 September 2016, available at http://www.observer-reporter.com/20160912/study_details_sugar_industry_attempt_to_shape_science (last accessed 22 September 2017).
2. A. O'Connor, 'Coca-Cola funds scientists who shift blame for obesity away from bad diets', *New York Times*, 9 August 2015, available at https://www.google.com/search?client=safari&rls=en&q=Coca-Cola+Funds+Scientists+Who+Shift+Blame+for+Obesity+Away+From+Bad+DietsBY+ANAHAD+O%E2%80%99CONNOR++AUGUST+9,+2015&ie=UTF-8&oe=UTF-8 (last accessed 22 September 2017).
3. I. Shai, D. Schwarzfuchs, Y. Henkin *et al.*, 'Weight loss with a low-carbohydrate, Mediterranean, or low-fat diet', *New England Journal of Medicine* 359(3), 2008: 229–41.
4. M.L. Dansinger, J.A. Gleason, J.L. Griffith *et al.*, 'Comparison of the Atkins, Ornish, Weight Watchers, and Zone diets for weight loss and heart disease risk reduction: A randomized trial', *JAMA* 293(1), 2005: 43–53.
5. Z. Harcombe, 'An examination of the randomised controlled trial and epidemiological evidence for the introduction of dietary fat recommendations in 1977 and 1983: A systematic review and meta-analysis', PhD thesis, University of the West of Scotland, March 2016.
6. Z. Harcombe, J.S. Baker, S.M. Cooper *et al.*, 'Evidence from randomised controlled trials did not support the introduction of dietary fat guidelines in 1977 and 1983: A systematic review and meta-analysis', *Open Heart* 2(1), 2015: e000196.
7. A. Malhotra, J.J. DiNicolantonio and S. Capewell, 'It is time to stop counting calories, and time instead to promote dietary changes that substantially and rapidly reduce cardiovascular morbidity and mortality', *Open Heart* 2(1), 2015: e000273.
8. A. Malhotra, 'Saturated fat is not the major issue', *BMJ* 2013;347:f6340.
9. O. Warburg, 'The prime cause and prevention of cancer', Lindau Lecture, 30 June 1966, available at http://www.healingcancernaturally.com/warburgcancer-cause-prevention.html (last accessed 31 July 2017).
10. J. Rousseau, 'Lessons in bad science – Tim Noakes and the *SAMJ*', *Synapses*, 24 October 2013, available at http://synapses.co.za/lessons-bad-science-tim-noakes-samj/comment-page-1/ (last accessed 31 July 2017).
11. J. Rousseau, 'More lessons in bad science (and reasoning) from Noakes', *Synapses*, 27 October 2013, available at http://synapses.co.za/lessons-bad-science-reasoning-noakes/ (last accessed 31 July 2017).
12. S. Rousseau, 'The celebrity quick-fix: When good food meets bad science', *Food, Culture & Society* 18(2), 2015: 265–87.
13. J. Rousseau, 'Roundup – 2015 LCHF summit', *Synapses*, 22 February 2015, available at http://synapses.co.za/2015-lchf-summit/ (last accessed 31 July 2017).

14. S. Hawking, *Black Holes and Baby Universes and Other Essays* (London: Bantam Press, 1993), 36.

Chapter 2: The Most Important Experiment of My Life

1. W. Yellowlees, *A Doctor in the Wilderness* (Perthshire: Dr W.W. Yellowlees, 2001), 14.
2. Ibid.
3. Ibid.
4. Ibid., 17.
5. Ibid., 195.
6. Ibid., 15.
7. Ibid., 15–16.
8. Ibid., 195.
9. S.D. Phinney, B.R. Bistrian, W.J. Evans *et al.*, 'The human metabolic response to chronic ketosis without caloric restriction: Preservation of submaximal exercise capability with reduced carbohydrate oxidation', *Metabolism* 32(8), 1983: 769–76.
10. E.V. Lambert, D.P. Speechly, S.C. Dennis *et al.*, 'Enhanced endurance in trained cyclists during moderate intensity exercise following 2 weeks adaptation to a high fat diet', *European Journal of Applied Physiology and Occupational Physiology* 69(4), 1994: 287–93; J.H. Goedecke, C. Christie, G. Wilson *et al.*, 'Metabolic adaptations to a high-fat diet in endurance cyclists', *Metabolism* 48(12), 1999: 1509–17; E.V. Lambert, J.H. Goedecke, C. Zyle *et al.*, 'High-fat diet versus habitual diet prior to carbohydrate loading: Effects of exercise metabolism and cycling performance', *International Journal of Sport Nutrition and Exercise Metabolism* 11(2), 2001: 209–25; L. Havemann, S.J. West, J.H. Goedecke *et al.*, 'Fat adaptation followed by carbohydrate loading compromises high-intensity sprint performance', *Journal of Applied Physiology* 100(1), 2006: 194–202.
11. A.L. Carey, H.M. Staudacher, N.K. Cummings *et al.*, 'Effects of fat adaptation and carbohydrate restoration on prolonged endurance exercise', *Journal of Applied Physiology (Bethesda, Md: 1985)* 91(1), 2001: 115–22; N.K. Stepto, A.L. Carey, H.M. Staudacher *et al.*, 'Effect of short-term fat adaptation on high-intensity training. *Medicine & Science in Sports & Exercise* 34(3), 2002: 449–55.
12. E.C. Westman, S.D. Phinney and J.S. Volek, *The New Atkins for a New You* (New York: Fireside, 2010), xi.
13. J. Yudkin, E. Evans and M.G. Smith, 'The low-carbohydrate diet in the treatment of chronic dyspepsia', *Proceedings of the Nutrition Society* 31(1), 1972: 12A.
14. S.D. Pointer, J. Rickstew, J.C. Slaughter *et al.*, 'Dietary carbohydrate intake, insulin resistance and gastro-oesophageal reflux disease: A pilot study in European- and African-American obese women', *Alimentary Pharmacology & Therapeutics* 44(9), 2016: 976–88. Austin GL, Thiny MT, Westman EC, et al. 'A very low-carbohydrate diet improves gastroephageal reflux and its symptoms'. *Digestive Diseases and Sciences* 2006; 53(8): 1307–1312.
15. C. Catassi, J.C. Bai, B. Bonaz *et al.*, 'Non-celiac gluten sensitivity: The new frontier of gluten related disorders', *Nutrients* 5(10), 2013: 3839–53.
16. G. Taubes, 'What if it's all been a big fat lie?', *New York Times Magazine*, 7 July 2002, available at http://www.nytimes.com/2002/07/07/magazine/what-if-it-s-all-been-a-big-fat-lie.html (last accessed 31 July 2017).

17. See N. Teicholz, *The Big Fat Surprise: Why Butter, Meat and Cheese Belong in a Healthy Diet* (New York: Simon & Schuster, 2014); Z. Harcombe, 'An examination of the randomised controlled trial and epidemiological evidence for the introduction of dietary fat recommendations in 1977 and 1983: A systematic review and meta-analysis', PhD thesis, University of the West of Scotland, March 2016.

Chapter 3: The Backlash Begins

1. J. Achenbach, 'Why do many reasonable people doubt science?', *National Geographic*, March 2015.
2. M. Jones, 'Noakes goes too far – doctors', *IOL*, 14 September 2012, available at http://www.iol.co.za/lifestyle/noakes-goes-too-far---doctors-1383310 (last accessed 31 July 2017).
3. P.C. Gøtzsche, *Deadly Medicines and Organised Crime: How Big Pharma Has Corrupted Healthcare* (Florida: CRC Press, 2013).
4. G. Orwell, *Nineteen Eighty-Four* (London: The Folio Society, 2001).
5. J.D. Abramson, H.G. Rosenberg, N. Jewell *et al.*, 'Should people at low risk of cardiovascular disease take a statin?', *BMJ* 2013;347:f6123.
6. Ibid.
7. D. Newman, 'Statins given for 5 years for heart disease prevention (with known heart disease)', *The NNT*, 2 November 2013, available at http://www.thennt.com/nnt/statins-for-heart-disease-prevention-with-known-heart-disease/ (last accessed 31 July 2017).
8. Abramson, Rosenberg, Jewell *et al.*, 'Should people at low risk of cardiovascular disease take a statin?'; Newman, 'Statin drugs given for 5 years for heart disease prevention without known heart disease'; D. Diamond and U. Ravnskov, 'How statistical deception created the appearance that statins are safe and effective in primary and secondary prevention of cardiovascular disease', *Expert Review of Clinincal Pharmacology* 8(2), 2015: 201–10; M. de Lorgeril and M. Rabaeus, 'Beyond confusion and controversy: Can we evaluate the real efficacy and safety of cholesterol-lowering with statins?', *Journal of Controversies in Biomedical Research* 1(1), 2015: 67–92; M. Rabaeus, P.V. Nguyen and M. de Lorgeril, 'Recent flaws in evidence-based medicine: Statin effects in primary prevention and consequences of suspending the treatment', *Journal of Controversies in Biomedical Research* 3(1), 2017: 1–10; R. DuBroff, 'Cholesterol paradox. A correlate does not a surrogate make', *Evidence-Based Medicine* 22(1), 2016: 15–19.
9. M.L. Kristensen, P.M. Christensen and J. Hallas, 'The effect of statins on average survival in randomised trials, an analysis of end point postponement', *BMJ Open* 5(9), 2015: e007118.
10. Newman, 'Statins given for 5 years for heart disease prevention (with known heart disease)'; A.L. Culver, I.S. Ockene, R. Balasubramanian *et al.*, 'Statin use and risk of diabetes mellitus in postmenopausal women in the Women's Health Initiative', *Archives of Internal Medicine* 172(2), 2012: 144–52.
11. X. Huang, A. Alonso, X. Guo *et al.*, 'Statins, plasma cholesterol, and risk of Parkinson's disease: A prospective study', *Movement Disorders* 30(4), 2015: 552–9.
12. Abramson, Rosenberg, Jewell *et al.*, 'Should people at low risk of cardiovascular disease take a statin?'; R.F. Redberg and M.H. Katz, 'Healthy men should not take

statins', *JAMA* 307(14), 2012: 1491–2; R.F. Redberg and M.H. Katz, 'Statins for primary prevention: The debate is intense, but the data are weak', *JAMA* 316(19), 2016: 1979–81; A. Malhotra, J. Abramson, M. de Lorgeril *et al.*, 'More clarity needed on the true benefits and risks of statins', *Prescriber*, Dec 2016: 15–17.

13. J.P. Ioannidis, 'More than a billion people taking statins?: Potential implications of the new cardiovascular guidelines', *JAMA* 311(5), 2014: 463–4.

14. DuBroff, 'Cholesterol paradox. A correlate does not a surrogate make'.

15. Ibid.

16. B. Lown, 'A maverick's lonely path in cardiology (Essay 28)', *Dr Bernard Lown's Blog*, 10 March 2012, available at https://bernardlown.wordpress.com/2012/03/10/mavericks-lonely-path-in-cardiology/ (last accessed 31 July 2017); P.J. Podrid, T.B. Graboys and B. Lown, 'Prognosis of medically treated patients with coronary-artery disease with profound ST-segment depression during exercise testing', *The New England Journal of Medicine* 305(19), 1981: 1111–6; T.B. Graboys, A. Headley, B. Lown *et al.*, 'Results of a second-opinion program for coronary artery bypass graft surgery', *JAMA* 258(12), 1987: 1611–4; S. Jabbour, Y. Young-Xu, T.B. Graboys *et al.*, 'Long-term outcomes of optimized medical management of outpatients with stable coronary artery disease', *American Journal of Cardiology* 93(3), 2004: 294–9; T.B. Graboys and B. Lown, 'Good outcomes in coronary artery disease without invasive procedures', *Archives of Internal Medicine* 166(12), 2006: 1325, author reply 26.

17. S.C. Knipp, N. Matatko, H. Wilhelm *et al.*, 'Cognitive outcomes three years after coronary artery bypass surgery: Relation to diffusion-weighted magnetic resonance imaging', *The Annals of Thoracic Surgery* 85(3), 2008: 872–9.

18. D.G. Katritsis and J.P. Ioannidis, 'Percutaneous coronary intervention versus conservative therapy in nonacute coronary artery disease: A meta-analysis', *Circulation* 111(22), 2005: 2906–12. See also A. Malhotra, 'Too much angioplasty. Stenting offers no prognostic benefit over drugs in stable coronary disease', *BMJ* 2013;347:f5741; A. Malhotra, 'The whole truth about coronary stents. The elephant in the room', *JAMA* 174(8), 2014: 1367–8.

19. Podrid, Graboys and Lown, 'Prognosis of medically treated patients with coronary-artery disease with profound ST-segment depression during exercise testing'.

20. A. Malhotra, R. Redberg and P. Meier, 'Saturated fat does not clog the arteries: Coronary heart disease is a chronic inflammatory condition, the risk of which can be effectively reduced from healthy lifestyle interventions', *British Journal of Sports Medicine* 51(15), 2017: 1111–2.

21. Lown, 'A maverick's lonely path in cardiology (Essay 28)'.

22. J.A. Ambrose, M.A. Tannenbaum, D. Alexopoulos *et al.*, 'Angiographic progression of coronary artery disease and the development of myocardial infarction', *Journal of the American College of Cardiology* 12(1), 1988: 56–62; W.C. Little, M. Constantinescu, R.J. Applegate *et al.*, 'Can coronary angiography predict the site of a subsequent myocardial infarction in patients with mild-to-moderate coronary artery disease?', *Circulation* 78(5 Pt 1), 1988: 1157–66.

23. Graboys and Lown, 'Good outcomes in coronary artery disease without invasive procedures'.

24. Lown, 'A maverick's lonely path in cardiology (Essay 28)'.

25. T.D. Noakes and J. Windt, 'Evidence that supports the prescription of low-carbohydrate high-fat diets: A narrative review', *British Journal of Sports Medicine* 51(2), 2017: 133–9.

26. M. Stilwell, 'Is Tim Noakes the Malema of medicine?', *Mail & Guardian*, 21 September 2012, available at https://mg.co.za/article/2012-09-21-00-is-tim-noakes-the-malema-of-medicine (last accessed 31 July 2017).

27. Ambrose, Tannenbaum, Alexopoulos *et al.*, 'Angiographic progression of coronary artery disease and the development of myocardial infarction'; Little, Constantinescu, Applegate *et al.*, 'Can coronary angiography predict the site of a subsequent myocardial infarction in patients with mild-to-moderate coronary artery disease?'.

28. K. Sliwa, J.G. Lyons, M.J. Carrington *et al.*, 'Different lipid profiles according to ethnicity in the Heart of Soweto study cohort of de novo presentations of heart disease', *Cardiovascular Journal of Africa* 23(7), 2012: 389–95.

29. A. Sachdeva, C.P. Cannon, P.C. Deedwania *et al.*, 'Lipid levels in patients hospitalized with coronary artery disease: An analysis of 136,905 hospitalizations in Get With The Guidelines', *American Heart Journal* 157(1), 2009: 111–7; M.D. Miedema, R.F. Garberich, L.J. Schnaidt *et al.*, 'Statin eligibility and outpatient care prior to ST-segment elevation myocardial infarction', *Journal of the American Heart Association* 6(4), 2017: e005333.

30. B.H. Roberts, *The Truth About Statins: Risks and Alternatives to Cholesterol-lowering Drugs* (New York: Pocket Books, 2012), 97–8.

31. A.L. Stock and J. Yudkin, 'Nutrient intake of subjects on low carbohydrate diet used in treatment of obesity', *American Journal of Clinical Nutrition* 23(7), 1970: 948–52.

32. See endnote 8.

33. A.P. DeFilippis, R. Young, C.J. Carrubba *et al.*, 'An analysis of calibration and discrimination among multiple cardiovascular risk scores in a modern multiethnic cohort', *Annals of Internal Medicine* 162(4), 2015: 266–75.

34. Ibid.

Chapter 4: The Centenary Debate

1. A. Dreger, *Galileo's Middle Finger: Heretics, Activists, and One Scholar's Search for Justice* (New York: Penguin Press, 2015), 262.

2. B.V. Howard, L. van Horn, J. Hsia *et al.*, 'Low-fat dietary pattern and risk of cardiovascular disease: The Women's Health Initiative Randomized Controlled Dietary Modification Trial', *JAMA* 295(6), 2006: 655–66.

3. J.M. Shikany, K.L Margolis, M. Pettinger *et al.*, 'Effects of a low-fat dietary intervention on glucose, insulin, and insulin resistance in the Women's Health Initiative (WHI) Dietary Modification trial', *American Journal of Clinical Nutrition* 94(1), 2011: 75–85.

4. J.E. Rossouw, J.P. du Plessis, A.J. Benade *et al.*, 'Coronary risk factor screening in three rural communities: The CORIS baseline study', *SAMJ* 64(12), 1983: 430–6.

5. K. Steyn, M. Steyn, A.S. Swanepoel *et al.*, 'Twelve-year results of the Coronary Risk Factor Study (CORIS)', *International Journal of Epidemiology* 26(5), 1997: 964–71.

6. Ibid.

7. C.E. Naudé, A. Schoonees, M. Senekal *et al.*, 'Low carbohydrate versus isoenergetic balanced diets for reducing weight and cardiovascular risk: A systematic review and meta-analysis', *PLoS One* 9(7), 2014: e100652.

8. The lecture was subsequently published. See T.D. Noakes, 'The 2012 University of Cape Town Faculty of Health Sciences Centenary Debate', *SAJCN* 28(1), 2016: 19–33.

9. J.A. Cutler, J.D. Neaton, S.B. Hulley *et al.*, 'Coronary heart disease and all-causes mortality in the Multiple Risk Factor Intervention Trial: Subgroup findings and comparisons with other trials', *Preventive Medicine* 14(3), 1985: 293–311; X. Pi-Sunyer, 'The Look AHEAD trial: A review and discussion of its outcomes', *Current Nutrition Reports* 3(4), 2014: 387–91.

10. T.D. Noakes, 'The Women's Health Initiative Randomized Controlled Dietary Modification Trial: An inconvenient finding and the diet-heart hypothesis', *SAMJ* 103(11), 2013: 824–5.

11. J.E. Rossouw and B.V. Howard, 'Noakes misses the point', *SAMJ* 103(12), 2013: 882.

12. T.D. Noakes, 'WHIDMT: Rossouw and Howard blatantly miss the point', *SAMJ* 104(4), 2014: 261–2.

13. J.E. Rossouw, 'The diet-heart hypothesis, obesity and diabetes', *SAJCN* 28(1), 2015: 38–43.

14. B. Unal, J.A. Critchley and S. Capewell, 'Explaining the decline in coronary heart disease mortality in England and Wales between 1981 and 2000', *Circulation* 109(9), 2004: 1101–7.

15. A. Sekikawa, Y. Miyamoto, K. Miura *et al.*, 'Continuous decline in mortality from coronary heart disease in Japan despite a continuous and marked rise in total cholesterol: Japanese experience after the Seven Countries Study', *International Journal of Epidemiology* 44(5), 2015: 1614–24.

16. M. Murata, 'Secular trends in growth and changes in eating patterns of Japanese children', *American Journal of Clinical Nutrition* 72(5 Suppl), 2000: 1379s–83s.

17. N. Nago, S. Ishikawa, T. Goto *et al.*, 'Low cholesterol is associated with mortality from stroke, heart disease, and cancer: The Jichi Medical School Cohort Study', *Journal of Epidemiology* 21(1), 2011: 67–74.

18. P. Cheng, J. Wang, W. Shao *et al.*, 'Can dietary saturated fat be beneficial in prevention of stroke risk? A meta-analysis', *Neurological Sciences: Official Journal of the Italian Neurological Society and of the Italian Society of Clinical Neurophysiology* 37(7), 2016: 1089–98.

19. E. Vartiainen, P. Puska, J. Tuomilehto *et al.*, 'Changes in risk factors explain changes in mortality from ischaemic heart disease in Finland', *BMJ* 309, 1994: 23–7.

20. J. McCormick and P. Skrabanek, 'Coronary heart disease is not preventable by population interventions', *The Lancet* 2(8615), 1988: 839–41.

21. Ibid.

22. P.V. Luoma, S. Nayha, K. Sikkila *et al.*, 'High serum alpha-tocopherol, albumin, selenium and cholesterol and low mortality from coronary heart disease in northern Finland', *Journal of Internal Medicine* 237, 1995: 49–54.

23. S. Nayham, 'Low mortality from ischaemic heart disease in the Sami district of Finland', *Social Science & Medicine* 44(1), 1997: 129.

24. C. Stout, J. Morrow, E.N. Brandt *et al.*, 'Unusually low incidence of death from myocardial infarction: Study of an Italian American community in Pennsylvania',

JAMA 188(10), 1964: 845–9; S. Wolf, R.C. Herrenkohl, J. Lasker *et al.*, 'Roseto, Pennsylvania 25 years later: Highlights of a medical and sociological survey', *Transactions of the American Clinical Climatological Association* 100, 1989: 57–67; B. Egolf, J. Lasker, S. Wolf et al., 'The Roseto effect: A 50-year comparison of mortality rates', *American Journal of Public Health* 82, 1992: 1089–92.

25. Wolf, Herrenkohl, Lasker *et al.*, 'Roseto, Pennsylvania 25 years later: Highlights of a medical and sociological survey', 58.

26. S. Wolf, 'Mortality from myocardial infarction in Roseto', *JAMA* 195, 1966: 142.

27. Wolf, Herrenkohl, Lasker *et al.*, 'Roseto, Pennsylvania 25 years later: Highlights of a medical and sociological survey', 67.

28. Ibid., 66.

29. Egolf, Lasker, Wolf *et al.*, 'The Roseto effect: A 50-year comparison of mortality rates', 1092.

30. Ibid.

31. D. Yam, A. Eliraz and E.M. Berry, 'Diet and disease – the Israeli paradox: Possible dangers of a high omega-6 polyunsaturated fatty acid diet', *Israel Journal of Medical Sciences* 32(11), 1996: 1134–43.

32. D.S. Ludwig, 'Lifespan weighed down by diet', *JAMA* 315(21), 2016: 2269–70.

33. M. de Lorgeril, S. Renaud, P. Salen *et al.*, 'Mediterranean alpha-linolenic acid-rich diet in secondary prevention of coronary heart disease', *The Lancet* 343, 1994: 1454–9; M. de Lorgeril, P. Salen, J-L. Martin *et al.*, 'Mediterranean diet, traditional risk factors, and the rate of cardiovascular complications after myocardial infarction: Final report of the Lyon Diet Heart Study', *Circulation* 99, 1999: 779–85.

34. K. Okada, M. Gohbara, S. Kataoka *et al.*, 'Association between blood glucose variability and coronary plaque instability in patients with acute coronary syndromes', *Cardiovascular Diabetology* 14, 2015: 111–23.

35. Rossouw, 'The diet-heart hypothesis, obesity and diabetes', 43.

36. C. Ford, S. Chang, M.Z. Vitolins *et al.*, 'Evaluation of diet pattern and weight gain in postmenopausal women enrolled in the Women's Health Initiative Observational Study', *British Journal of Nutrition* 117, 2017; 1189–97

37. Ibid., 1196.

38. D. Williams, 'Innovative disagreement', *Leader.co.za*, 27 February 2013, available at http://www.leader.co.za/article.aspx?s=23&f=1&a=4279 (last accessed 1 August 2017).

39. C. Bateman, 'Inconvenient truth or public health threat?', *SAMJ* 103(2), 2013: 69–71.

40. American Diabetes Association, 'Statistics about Diabetes', available at http://www.diabetes.org/diabetes-basics/statistics/ (last accessed 1 August 2017).

41. J.R. Kraft, *Diabetes Epidemic & You* (La Vergne: Trafford Publishing, 2008).

42. C. Crofts, 'Understanding and diagnosing hyperinsulinaemia', PhD thesis, Auckland University of Technology, 2015, available at http://aut.researchgateway.ac.nz/bitstream/handle/10292/9906/CroftsC.pdf?sequence=3 (last accessed 1 August 2017); C. Crofts, G. Schofield, C. Zinn *et al.*, 'Identifying hyperinsulinaemia in the absence of impaired glucose tolerance: An examination of the Kraft database', *Diabetes Research and Clinical Practice* 118(8), 2016: 50–7.

43. National Institute of Diabetes and Digestive and Kidney Diseases, 'Overweight and Obesity Statistics', available at https://www.niddk.nih.gov/health-information/health-statistics/overweight-obesity (last accessed 1 August 2017).

44. J.M. Lee, W.H. Herman, M.J. Okumura *et al.*, 'Prevalence and determinants of insulin resistance among US adolescents: A population-based study', *Diabetes Care* 29, 2006: 2427–32. K.A. Erion and B.E. Corkey, 'Hyperinsulinemia: A cause of obesity?', *Current Obesity Reports* 6(2), 2017: 178–86; M.P. Czech, 'Insulin action and resistance in obesity and type 2 diabetes', *Nature Medicine* 23, 2017: 804–14.

45. R. DuBroff, 'Cholesterol paradox. A correlate does not a surrogate make', *Evidence-Based Medicine* 22(1), 2016: 15.

46. A. Mente, M. O'Donnell, S. Rangarajan *et al.*, 'Associations of urinary sodium excretion with cardiovascular events in individuals with and without hypertension: A pooled analysis of data from four studies', *The Lancet* 388(10043), 2016: 465–75.

47. K. Stolarz-Skrzypek, T. Kuznetsova, L. Thijs *et al.*, 'European project on genes in hypertension (EPOGH) investigators: Fatal and nonfatal outcomes, incidence of hypertension, and blood pressure changes in relation to urinary sodium excretion', *JAMA* 305, 2011: 1777–85; M.J. O'Donnell, S. Yusuf, A. Mente *et al.*, 'Urinary sodium and potassium excretion and risk of cardiovascular events', *JAMA* 306, 2011: 2229–38; M. O'Donnell, A. Mente, S. Rangarajan *et al.*, 'Urinary sodium and potassium excretion, mortality, and cardiovascular events', *New England Journal of Medicine* 371, 2014: 612–23; N. Graudal, G. Jürgens, B. Baslund and M.H. Alderman, 'Compared with usual sodium intake, low and excessive-sodium diets are associated with increased mortality: A meta-analysis', *American Journal of Hypertension* 27, 2014: 1129–37; M.M. Joosten, R.T. Gansevoort, K.J. Mukamal *et al.*, 'PREVEND Study Group: Sodium excretion and risk of developing coronary heart disease', *Circulation* 129, 2014: 1121–8. M.L. Thomas, J. Moran, C. Forsblom, *et al.* 'The association between dieting sodium intake, ESRD, and all-cause mortality in patients with type 1 diabetes'. *Diabetes Care* 34(4); 2011: 861–866

48. E. O'Brien, 'Salt: Too much or too little?', *The Lancet* 388(10043), 2016: 439–40.

49. K. Kitada, S. Daub, Y. Zhang *et al.*, 'High salt intake reprioritizes osmolyte and energy metabolism for body fluid conservation', *Journal of Clinical Investigation* 127(5), 2017: 1944–59.

50. M-S. Zhou, A. Wang and H. Yu, 'Link between insulin resistance and hypertension: What is the evidence from evolutionary biology?', *Diabetology and Metabolic Syndrome* 6, 2014: 12; G. Schofield, G. Henderson and C. Crofts, 'Beyond salt: Where next for hypertension epidemiology', *The Lancet* 388, 2016: 2110. G.M. Reaven, 'Insulin resistance/compensatory hyperinsulinemia, essential hypertension, and cardiovascular disease', Journal of Clinical Endocrinology and Metabolism 88(6), 2003: 2399–403.

51. J.J. DiNicolantonio and S.C. Lucan, 'The wrong white crystals: Not salt but sugar as aetiological in hypertension and cardiometabolic disease', *Open Heart* 1, 2014: e000167; J.J. DiNicolantonio, *The Salt Fix: Why the Experts Got It All Wrong – and How Eating More Might Save Your Life* (New York: Harmony Books, 2017).

52. J. Webster, C. Clickmore, K. Charlton *et al.*, 'South Africa's salt reduction strategy: Are we on track, and what lies ahead', *SAMJ* 107(1), 2017: 20–1.

53. 'Experts warn against Noakes diet', *Health24*, 31 July 2014, available at http://www.health24.com/Medical/Heart/Foods-diet-and-your-heart/Experts-warn-against-Noakes-diet-20130212 (last accessed 1 August 2017).

54. B.M. Mayosi and T. Forrester, 'Commentary: "Serum-cholesterol, diet, and coronary heart-disease in Africans and Asians in Uganda" by AG Shaper and KW Jones', *International Journal of Epidemiology* 41(5), 2012: 1233–5.

55. P.D.P. Wood, 'A possible selection effect in medical science', *The Statistician* 30(2), 1981: 131–5.

56. I.D. Frantz Jr, E.A. Dawson, P.L. Ashman *et al.*, 'Test of effect of lipid lowering by diet on cardiovascular risk. The Minnesota Coronary Survey', *Arteriosclerosis* 9(1), 1989: 129–35.

57. C.E. Ramsden, D. Zamora, S. Majchrzak-Hong *et al.*, 'Re-evaluation of the traditional diet-heart hypothesis: Analysis of recovered data from Minnesota Coronary Experiment (1968–73)', *BMJ* 2016;353:i1246.

58. A. O'Connor, 'A decades-old study, rediscovered, challenges advice on saturated fat', *New York Times*, 13 April 2016, available at https://well.blogs.nytimes.com/2016/04/13/a-decades-old-study-rediscovered-challenges-advice-on-saturated-fat/?_r=0 (last accessed 1 August 2017); P. Whoriskey, 'This study 40 years ago could have reshaped the American diet. But it was never fully published', *Washington Post*, 12 April 2016, available at https://www.washingtonpost.com/news/wonk/wp/2016/04/12/this-study-40-years-ago-could-have-reshaped-the-american-diet-but-it-was-never-fully-published/?utm_term=.ad8097d6bd8b (last accessed 1 August 2017).

59. O'Connor, 'A decades-old study, rediscovered, challenges advice on saturated fat'.

60. Whoriskey, 'This study 40 years ago could have reshaped the American diet. But it was never fully published'.

61. Ramsden, Zamora, Majchrzak-Hong *et al.*, 'Re-evaluation of the traditional diet-heart hypothesis: Analysis of recovered data from Minnesota Coronary Experiment (1968–73)'.

62. Whoriskey, 'This study 40 years ago could have reshaped the American diet. But it was never fully published'.

63. M. Planck, *Scientific Autobiography, and Other Papers* (New York: Philosophical Library, 1949), 33–4.

64. Dreger, *Galileo's Middle Finger*, 137.

65. Ibid., 262.

66. Ibid., 137.

67. Ibid.

68. Ibid., 262.

Chapter 5: The UCT Professors' Letter

1. D. Spence, 'What happened to the doctor–patient relationship?', *BMJ* 2012;344:e4349.

2. T.D. Noakes, 'Low-carbohydrate and high-fat intake can manage obesity and associated conditions: Occasional survey', *SAMJ* 103(11), 2013: 826–30.

3. B. Ndenze, 'SA's ticking time bomb', *Cape Times*, 19 August 2014.

4. Curriculum Vitae (abridged): Wim de Villiers, available at http://www.sun.ac.za/english/management/wim-de-villiers/Documents/Abridged%20Curriculum%20Vitae%20%28CV%29%20Prof%20Wim%20de%20Villiers%20%28Nov%202014%29.pdf (last accessed 1 August 2017).

5. C. Ancelotti, *Quiet Leadership: Winning Hearts, Minds and Matches* (Kindle edition: Penguin Books, 2016).

6. L. Opie, 'Noakes diet carries risks', *Sunday Times*, 27 July 2014.

7. University of Stellenbosch, 'Profile sketch – Prof Wim de Villiers', available at http://www.sun.ac.za/english/management/wim-de-villiers/Documents/Wim%20de%20Villiers%20profile%20on%20letterhead.pdf (last accessed 1 August 2017).

8. F. Howells and L. Ronnie, 'Academic bullying: Shadows across the Ivory Tower', *Aggression and Violent Behavior*, manuscript submitted, 2017.

9. J. Hoepner, 'With us or against us: Using the wind turbine syndrome case study to examine implications of contested enquiry on individual researchers', PhD thesis, Australian National University, 2015.

10. HPCSA, 'General ethical guidelines for the health care professions', Booklet 1, Pretoria, May 2008, available at http://www.hpcsa.co.za/downloads/conduct_ethics/rules/generic_ethical_rules/booklet_1_guidelines_good_prac.pdf (last accessed 1 August 2017).

11. HPCSA, 'Ethical and professional rules of the Health Professions Council of South Africa as promulgated in Government Gazette R717/2006', Booklet 2, Pretoria, May 2008, www.hpcsa.co.za/Uploads/editor/UserFiles/downloads/conduct_ethics/rules/generic_ethical_rules/booklet_2_generic_ethical_rules_with_anexures.pdf (last accessed 1 August 2017).

12. University of Cape Town, 'Declaration for Health Science Graduands', available at http://www.uct.ac.za/usr/calendar/faculties_EBE_Healthsciences_science.pdf (last accessed 1 August 2017).

13. W. Osler, *The Principles and Practice of Medicine* (New York: D. Appleton and Company, 1978).

14. S. Mark, S. du Toit, T.D. Noakes *et al.*, 'A successful lifestyle intervention model replicated in diverse clinical settings', *SAMJ* 106(8), 2016: 763–6.

15. I. Shai, D. Schwarzfuchs, Y. Henkin *et al.*, 'Weight loss with a low-carbohydrate, Mediterranean, or low-fat diet', *New England Journal of Medicine* 359(3), 2008: 229–41; H. Guldbrand, B. Dizdar, B. Bunjaku *et al.*, 'In type 2 diabetes, randomisation to advice to follow a low-carbohydrate diet transiently improves glycaemic control compared with advice to follow a low-fat diet producing a similar weight loss', *Diabetologia* 55(8), 2012: 2118–27; G.D. Foster, H.R. Wyatt, J.O. Hill *et al.*, 'Weight and metabolic outcomes after 2 years on a low-carbohydrate versus low-fat diet: A randomized trial', *Annals of Internal Medicine* 153(3), 2010: 147–57; N. Iqbal, M.L. Vetter, R.H. Moore *et al.*, 'Effects of a low-intensity intervention that prescribed a low-carbohydrate vs. a low-fat diet in obese, diabetic participants', *Obesity (Silver Spring, Md)* 18(9), 2010: 1733–8.

16. C.D. Gardner, A. Kiazand, S. Alhassan *et al.*, 'Comparison of the Atkins, Zone, Ornish, and LEARN diets for change in weight and related risk factors among overweight premenopausal women: The A to Z Weight Loss Study: A randomized trial', *JAMA* 297(9), 2007: 969–77; G.D. Brinkworth, M. Noakes, J.D. Buckley *et al.*, 'Long-term effects of a very-low-carbohydrate weight loss diet compared with an isocaloric low-fat diet after 12 mo.', *American Journal of Clinical Nutrition* 90(1), 2009: 23–32; L.A. Bazzano, T. Hu, K. Reynolds *et al.*, 'Effects of low-carbohydrate and low-fat diets: A randomized trial', *Annals of Internal Medicine* 161(5), 2014: 309–18; N.J. Davis, N. Tomuta, C. Schechter *et al.*, 'Comparative study of the effects of a 1-year dietary intervention of a low-carbohydrate diet versus a low-fat diet on

weight and glycemic control in type 2 diabetes', *Diabetes Care* 32(7), 2009: 1147–52; M.L. Dansinger, J.A. Gleason, J.L. Griffith *et al.*, 'Comparison of the Atkins, Ornish, Weight Watchers, and Zone diets for weight loss and heart disease risk reduction: A randomized trial. *JAMA* 293(1), 2005: 43–53; M. Flechtner-Mors, B.O. Boehm, R. Wittmann *et al.*, 'Enhanced weight loss with protein-enriched meal replacements in subjects with the metabolic syndrome', *Diabetes/Metabolism Research and Reviews* 26(5), 2010: 393–405; S.S. Lim, M. Noakes, J.B. Keogh *et al.*, 'Long-term effects of a low carbohydrate, low fat or high unsaturated fat diet compared to a no-intervention control', *Nutrition, Metabolism and Cardiovascular Diseases* 20(8), 2010: 599–607.

17. Mark, Du Toit, Noakes *et al.*, 'A successful lifestyle intervention model replicated in diverse clinical settings'.

18. A. Malhotra, T. Noakes and S. Phinney, 'It is time to bust the myth of physical inactivity and obesity: You cannot outrun a bad diet', *British Journal of Sports Medicine* 49(15), 2015: 967–8.

19. J.H. Koeslag, T.D. Noakes and A.W. Sloan, 'Post-exercise ketosis', *Journal of Physiology* 301, 1980: 79–90.

20. T. Noakes, J.S. Volek and S.D. Phinney, 'Low-carbohydrate diets for athletes: What evidence?', *British Journal of Sports Medicine* 48(14), 2014: 1077–8.

21. Mark, Du Toit, Noakes *et al.*, 'A successful lifestyle intervention model replicated in diverse clinical settings'.

22. C.C. Webster, T.D. Noakes, S.K. Chacko *et al.*, 'Gluconeogenesis during endurance exercise in cyclists habituated to a long-term low carbohydrate high-fat diet', *Journal of Physiology* 594(15), 2016: 4389–405.

23. F. Villette, 'Noakes diet unproven – UCT scientists', *Cape Times*, 25 August 2014.

24. Bazzano, T. Hu, K. Reynolds *et al.*, 'Effects of low-carbohydrate and low-fat diets: A randomized trial'.

25. 'New study supports Noakes's low-carb, high-fat diet', *Cape Times*, 4 September 2014.

26. R. Smith, 'Are some diets "mass murder"?' *BMJ* 2014;349:g7654.

27. S. Spencer, 'Fat and heart disease: Challenging the dogma', *The Lancet* 390, 2017: 731.

Chapter 6: The Naudé Review

1. C.E. Naudé, A. Schoonees, M. Senekal *et al.*, 'Low carbohydrate versus isoenergetic balanced diets for reducing weight and cardiovascular risk: A systematic review and meta-analysis', *PLoS One* 9(7), 2014: e100652.

2. C. Bateman, 'Inconvenient truth or public health threat?', *SAMJ* 103(2), 2013: 69–71.

3. N.B. Bueno, I.S. de Melo, S.L. de Oliveira *et al.*, 'Very-low-carbohydrate ketogenic diet v. low-fat diet for long-term weight loss: A meta-analysis of randomised controlled trials', *British Journal of Nutrition* 110(7), 2013: 1178–87.

4. W. Stassen, 'Noakes's popular low-carb diet is not healthier, better for weight loss – study', *Cape Times*, 10 July 2014, available at http://www.iol.co.za/capetimes/news/noakess-low-carb-diet-not-healthier-1717305 (last accessed 2 August 2017).

5. A. Keys, J. Brozek, A. Henschel *et al.*, 'Psychological effects – interpretation and synthesis', in *The Biology of Human Starvation Volume II* (Minneapolis: University of Minnesota Press, 1950), 905–18.

6. G. Taubes, 'Diet advice that ignores hunger', *New York Times*, 29 August 2015,

available at https://www.nytimes.com/2015/08/30/opinion/diet-advice-that-ignores-hunger.html (last accessed 2 August 2017).

7.   Keys, Brozek, Henschel *et al.*, 'Psychological effects – interpretation and synthesis', 911.

8.   Ibid., 912.

9.   A.L. Stock and J. Yudkin, 'Nutrient intake of subjects on low carbohydrate diet used in treatment of obesity', *American Journal of Clinical Nutrition* 23(7), 1970: 948–52.

10.   R.C. Atkins, *Dr Atkins New Diet Revolution* (London: Vermilion, 2002).

11.   E.C. Westman, S.D. Phinney and J.S. Volek, *The New Atkins for a New You* (New York: Fireside, 2010).

12.   'New research shows Noakes diet no more than dangerous fad', *SA Breaking News*, 10 July 2014, available at http://www.sabreakingnews.co.za/2014/07/10/new-research-shows-noakes-diet-no-more-than-dangerous-fad/ (last accessed 2 August 2017).

13.   Z. Harcombe, 'An examination of the randomised controlled trial and epidemiological evidence for the introduction of dietary fat recommendations in 1977 and 1983: A systematic review and meta-analysis', PhD thesis, University of the West of Scotland, March 2016; Z. Harcombe, J.S. Baker, S.M. Cooper *et al.*, 'Evidence from randomised controlled trials did not support the introduction of dietary fat guidelines in 1977 and 1983: A systematic review and meta-analysis', *Open Heart* 2(1), 2015: e000196; Z. Harcombe, J.S. Baker and B. Davies, 'Evidence from prospective cohort studies did not support the introduction of dietary fat guidelines in 1977 and 1983: A systematic review', *British Journal of Sports Medicine*, 29 June 2016, doi: 10.1136/bjsports-2016-096409; Z. Harcombe, J.S. Baker, J.J. DiNicolantonio *et al.*, 'Evidence from randomised controlled trials does not support current dietary fat guidelines: A systematic review and meta-analysis', *Open Heart* 3(2), 2016: e000409; Z. Harcombe, 'Dietary fat guidelines have no evidence base: Where next for public health nutritional advice?', *British Journal of Sports Medicine* 51, 2017: 769–74.

14.   Z. Harcombe and T.D. Noakes, 'The universities of Stellenbosch/Cape Town low-carbohydrate diet review: Mistake or mischief?', *SAMJ* 106(12), 2016: 1179–82.

15.   (1) N.D. Luscombe, P.M. Clifton, M. Noakes *et al.*, 'Effect of a high-protein, energy-restricted diet on weight loss and energy expenditure after weight stabilization in hyperinsulinemic subjects', *International Journal of Obesity and Related Metabolic Disorders: Journal of the International Association for the Study of Obesity* 27(5), 2003: 582–90; (2) E. Farnsworth, N.D. Luscombe, M. Noakes *et al.*, 'Effect of a high-protein, energy-restricted diet on body composition, glycemic control, and lipid concentrations in overweight and obese hyperinsulinemic men and women', *American Journal of Clinical Nutrition* 78(1), 2003: 31–9; (3) J.B. Keogh, G.D Brinkworth, M. Noakes *et al.*, 'Effects of weight loss from a very-low-carbohydrate diet on endothelial function and markers of cardiovascular disease risk in subjects with abdominal obesity', *American Journal of Clinical Nutrition* 87(3), 2008: 567–76; (4) F.M. Sacks, G.A. Bray, V.J. Carey *et al.*, 'Comparison of weight-loss diets with different compositions of fat, protein, and carbohydrates', *New England Journal of Medicine* 360(9), 2009: 859–73; (5) D.A. de Luis, M.G. Sagrado, R. Conde *et al.*, 'The effects of two different hypocaloric diets on glucagon-like peptide 1 in obese adults, relation with insulin response after weight loss', *Journal of Diabetes and Its Complications* 23(4), 2009: 239–43; (6) D.A. de Luis, R. Aller,

O. Izaola *et al.*, 'Evaluation of weight loss and adipocytokines levels after two hypocaloric diets with different macronutrient distribution in obese subjects with rs9939609 gene variant', *Diabetes/Metabolism Research and Reviews* 28(8), 2012: 663–8; (7) S. Frisch, A. Zittermann, H.K. Berthold *et al.*, 'A randomized controlled trial on the efficacy of carbohydrate-reduced or fat-reduced diets in patients attending a telemedically guided weight loss program', *Cardiovascular Diabetology* 8, 2009: 36; (8) D.K. Layman, E.M. Evans, D. Erickson *et al.*, 'A moderate-protein diet produces sustained weight loss and long-term changes in body composition and blood lipids in obese adults', *Journal of Nutrition* 139(3), 2009: 514–21; (9) S.S. Lim, M. Noakes, J.B. Keogh *et al.*, 'Long-term effects of a low carbohydrate, low fat or high unsaturated fat diet compared to a no-intervention control', *Nutrition, Metabolism and Cardiovascular Diseases* 20(8), 2010: 599–607; (10) T.P. Wycherley, G.D. Brinkworth, P.M. Clifton *et al.*, 'Comparison of the effects of 52 weeks weight loss with either a high-protein or high-carbohydrate diet on body composition and cardiometabolic risk factors in overweight and obese males', *Nutrition & Diabetes* 2, 2012: e40; (11) R.M. Krauss, P.J. Blanche, R.S. Rawlings *et al.*, 'Separate effects of reduced carbohydrate intake and weight loss on atherogenic dyslipidemia', *American Journal of Clinical Nutrition* 83(5), 2006: 1025–31; (12) T.O. Klemsdal, I. Holme, H. Nerland *et al.*, 'Effects of a low glycemic load diet versus a low-fat diet in subjects with and without the metabolic syndrome', *Nutrition, Metabolism and Cardiovascular Diseases* 20(3), 2010: 195–201; (13) Y.W. Aude, A.S. Agatston, F. Lopez-Jimenez *et al.*, 'The national cholesterol education program diet vs a diet lower in carbohydrates and higher in protein and monounsaturated fat: A randomized trial', *Archives of Internal Medicine* 164(19), 2004: 2141–6; (14) D.A. Lasker, E.M. Evans and D.K. Layman, 'Moderate carbohydrate, moderate protein weight loss diet reduces cardiovascular disease risk compared to high carbohydrate, low protein diet in obese adults: A randomized clinical trial', *Nutrition & Metabolism* (Lond.) 5, 2008: 30.

16. Harcombe and Noakes, 'The universities of Stellenbosch/Cape Town low-carbohydrate diet review: Mistake or mischief?'.

17. L. Isaacs, 'Noakes disputes diet study', *Cape Times*, 20 December 2016.

18. Z. Harcombe and T.D. Noakes, 'Response to study: Mistake or mischief?', *Cape Times*, 23 December 2016.

19. I. Coetzee, 'Noakes hits back at researchers', *News24*, 10 January 2017, available at http://www.news24.com/SouthAfrica/News/noakes-hits-back-at-researchers-20170110 (last accessed 2 August 2017).

20. C.E. Naudé, A. Schoonees, M. Senekal *et al.*, 'Reliable systematic review of low-carbohydrate diets shows similar weight-loss effects compared with balanced diets and no cardiovascular risk benefits: Response to methodological criticisms', *SAMJ* 107(3), 2017: 170.

21. Z. Harcombe and T.D. Noakes, 'Naudé *et al.* avoid answering the essential question: Mistake or mischief?', *SAMJ* 107(5), 2017: 360–1.

22. FMHS Marketing and Communications, 'SU researcher is co-director of new Cochrane Nutrition Field', 23 August 2016, available at http://www.sun.ac.za/english/Lists/news/DispForm.aspx?ID=4189 (last accessed 2 August 2017).

23. C. Naudé, 'Would an increase in vegetables and fruit intake help to reduce the

burden of nutrition-related disease in South Africa? An umbrella review of the evidence', *SAJCN* 26(3), 2013: 104–14.

24. Ibid.

25. M.E. Stuijvenberg, S.E. Schoeman, S.J. Lombard *et al.*, 'Serum retinol in 1–6-year-old children from a low socio-economic South African community with a high intake of liver: Implications for blanket vitamin A supplementation', *Public Health Nutrition* 15(4), 2012: 716–24.

26. FMHS Marketing and Communications, 'Dean honoured for his contribution to evidence-based healthcare, November 2016, available at http://www0.sun.ac.za/vivus/vivus-4-november-2016/excellence/dean-honoured-for-his-contribution-to-evidence-based-healthcare.html (last accessed 2 August 2017).

27. J.P.A. Ioannidis, 'The mass production of redundant, misleading, and conflicted systematic reviews and meta-analyses', *Milbank Quarterly* 94(3), 2016: 485–514.

28. E. Archer, G. Pavela and C.J. Lavie, 'The inadmissibility of what we eat in America and NHANES Dietary Data in Nutrition and Obesity Research and the scientific formulation of National Dietary Guidelines', *Mayo Clinic Proceedings* 90(7), 2015: 911–26.

Chapter 7: Responses of Official Bodies

1. L. Tolstoy, *The Kingdom of God Is Within You* (Mineola, NY: Dover Publications, 2006).

2. S. Landau, M. Daniels, V. Mufamadi *et al.*, 'Position statement on the role of low-carbohydrate diets for people with diabetes', 29 March 2012, available at http://bit.ly/2lGrlep (last accessed 2 August 2017).

3. R. Catsicas, *The Complete Nutritional Solution to Diabetes* (Cape Town: Random House Struik, 2009); D. Daniels, V. Mufamadi, G. Eksteen *et al.*, *Cooking From the Heart* 3 (Cape Times: Trident Press Printing, 2015).

4. R.D. Feinman, W.K. Pogozelski, A. Astrup *et al.*, 'Dietary carbohydrate restriction as the first approach in diabetes management: Critical review and evidence base', *Nutrition* 31(1), 2015: 1–13; O. Hamdy, 'Nutrition revolution – The end of the high carbohydrates era for diabetes: Prevention and management', *US Endocrinology* 10(2), 2014: 103–4; O. Snorgaard, G.M. Poulsen, H.K. Andersen *et al.*, 'Systematic review and meta-analysis of dietary carbohydrate restriction in patients with type 2 diabetes', *BMJ* 2017;5:e000354; L.R. Saslow, A.E. Mason, S. Kim *et al.*, 'An online intervention comparing a very low-carbohydrate ketogenic diet and lifestyle recommendations versus a plate method diet in overweight individuals with type 2 diabetes: A randomized controlled trial', *Journal of Medical Internet Research* 19(2), 2017: e36; A.L. McKenzie, S.J. Hallberg, B.C.C. Creighton *et al.*, 'A novel intervention including individualized nutritional recommendations reduces hemoglobin A1c level, medication use, and weight in type 2 diabetes', *JMIR Diabetes* 2(1), 2017: e5; M.R. McKenzie and S. Illingworth, 'Should a low carbohydrate diet be recommended for diabetes management?', *Proceedings of the Nutrition Society* 76(OCEI), 2017: E19.

5. Institute of Medicine, 'Dietary Reference Intakes for Energy, Carbohydrate, Fiber, Fat, Fatty Acids, Cholesterol, Protein and Amino Acids' (Washington, DC: National Academies Press, 2005), 275.

6. L. Cordain, S.B. Eaton, A. Sebastian *et al.*, 'Origins and evolution of the Western

diet: Health implications for the 21st century', *American Journal of Clinical Nutrition* 81(2), 2005: 341–54.

7. CDC, 'Trends in intake of energy and macronutrients – United States, 1971–2000', MMWR 53(4), 2004: 80–2, available at https://www.cdc.gov/mmwr/preview/mmwrhtml/mm5304a3.htm (last accessed 2 August 2017).

8. Collaboration NRF, 'Worldwide trends in diabetes since 1980: A pooled analysis of 751 population-based studies with 4.4 million participants', *The Lancet* 387(10027), 2016: 1513–30. R.T. Erasmus, D.J. Soita, M.S. Hassan *et al.*, 'High prevalence of diabetes mellitus and metabolic syndrome in a South African coloured population: Baseline data of a study in Bellville, Cape Town', *SAMJ* 102(11), 2012: 841–4. T.E. Matsha, M. Macharia, Y.Y. Yako *et al.*, 'Gamma-glutamyltransferase, insulin resistance and cardiometabolic risk profile in a middle-aged African population', *European Journal of Preventive Cardiology* 21(12), 2012: 1541–8. T.R. Hird, F.J. Pirie, T.M. Esterhuizen *et al.*, 'Burden of diabetes and first evidence for the utility of HbA1c for diagnosis and detection of diabetes in urban black South Africans: The Durban diabetes study', *PLoS One* 11(8), 2016: e0161966. doi: 10.1371/journal.pone.0161966. N. Peer, C. Lombard, K. Steyn *et al.*, 'High prevalence of metabolic syndrome in the black population of Cape Town: The Cardiovascular Risk in Black South Africans (CRIBSA) study', *European Journal of Preventive Cardiology* 22(8), 2015: 1036–42.

9. G. Collier and K. O'Dea, 'The effect of coingestion of fat on the glucose, insulin, and gastric inhibitory polypeptide responses to carbohydrate and protein', *American Journal of Clinical Nutrition* 37(6), 1983: 941–4.

10. J.M. Falko, S.E. Crockett, S. Cataland *et al.*, 'Gastric inhibitory polypeptide (GIP) stimulated by fat ingestion in man', *Journal of Clinical Endocrinology & Metabolism* 41(2), 1975: 260–5.

11. F.Q. Nuttall, A.D. Mooradian, M.C. Gannon *et al.*, 'Effect of protein ingestion on the glucose and insulin response to a standardized oral glucose load', *Diabetes Care* 7(5), 1984: 465–70.

12. M. Bliss, *The Discovery of Insulin* (Chicago: The University of Chicago Press, 1984).

13. W. Morgan, *Diabetes Mellitus: Its History, Chemistry, Anatomy, Pathology, Physiology And Treatment* (London: The Homeopathic Publishing Company, 1877), 156.

14. K.F. Petersen, S. Dufour, D.B. Savage *et al.*, 'The role of skeletal muscle insulin resistance in the pathogenesis of the metabolic syndrome', *Proceedings of the National Academy of Sciences* 104(31), 2007: 12587–94.

15. Ibid., 12.

16. Ibid., 159.

17. Ibid., 162–3.

18. I. Seegen, 'The treatment of diabetes mellitus'. *Boston Medical and Surgical Journal* 73(12), 1890: 265–7.

19. F.M. Allen, E. Stillman and R. Fitz, *Total Dietary Regulation in the Treatment of Diabetes* 11th ed. (New York: The Rockerfeller Institute for Medical Research, 1919), 90.

20. E.P. Joslin, *The Treatment of Diabetes Mellitus* (Utah: Repressed Publishing, 2012), 254.

21. E.P. Joslin, *A Diabetic Manual for the Mutual Use of Doctor and Patient* (Philadelphia: Lea & Febiger, 1919), 9.

22. L.H. Newburgh and P.L. Marsh, 'The use of a high fat diet in the treatment of diabetes mellitus', *Archives of Internal Medicine* 26(6), 1920: 647–62; L.H. Newburgh and P.L. Marsh, 'Further observations on the use of a high fat diet in the treatment of diabetes mellitus', *Archives of Internal Medicine* 31(4), 1923: 455–90; L.H. Newburgh and D.S. Waller, 'Studies of diabetes mellitus: Evidence that the disability is concerned solely with the metabolism of glucose. The mode of action of insulin', *Journal of Clinical Investigation* 11(5), 1932: 995–1002.

23. E.C. Westman, W.S. Yancy Jr and M. Humphreys, 'Dietary treatment of diabetes mellitus in the pre-insulin era (1914–1922)', *Perspectives in Biology and Medicine* 49(1), 2006: 77–83.

24. Joslin, *A Diabetic Manual for the Mutual Use of Doctor and Patient*, 62.

25. E. Cersosimo, C. Triplitt, L.J. Mandarino *et al.*, 'Pathogenesis of type 2 diabetes mellitus', in L.J. de Groot, P. Beck-Peccoz, G. Chrousos *et al.* (eds), *Endotext* (South Dartmouth, MA: MDText.com, Inc., 2000).

26. R. Rodriguez-Gutierrez and V.M. Montori, 'Glycemic control of patients with type 2 diabetes mellitus: Our evolving faith in the face of evidence', *Circulation: Cardiovascular Quality and Outcomes* 9, 2016: 504–512.

27. S. Erpeldinger, M.B. Rehman, C. Berkhout *et al.*, 'Efficacy and safety of insulin in type 2 diabetes: Meta-analysis of randomized controlled trials', *BMC Endocrine Disorders* 16, 2016: 39.

28. X. Pi-Sunyer, 'The Look AHEAD trial: A review and discussion of its outcomes', *Current Nutrition Reports* 3(4), 2014: 387–91.

29. K. Child, 'Experts refute Noakes's diabetes diet claims', *Times*, 4 April 2012.

30. Hamdy, 'Nutrition revolution – The end of the high carbohydrates era for diabetes: Prevention and management'.

31. R. Taylor, 'Banting Memorial Lecture 2012: Reversing the twin cycles of type 2 diabetes', *Diabetic Medicine: A Journal of the British Diabetic Association* 30(3), 2013: 267–75.

32. J.R. Poortmans and O. Dellalieux, 'Do regular high protein diets have potential health risks on kidney function in athletes?', *International Journal of Sports Nutrition and Exercise Metabolism* 10(1), 1999: 28–38.

33. A. Tirosh, R. Golan, I. Harman-Boehm *et al.*, 'Renal function following three distinct weight loss dietary strategies during 2 years of randomized controlled trial', *Diabetes Care* 36(8), 2013: 2225–32.

34. C.E. Berryman, S. Agarwal, H.R. Lieberman *et al.*, 'Diets higher in animal and plant protein are associated with lower adiposity and do not impair renal function in US adults', *American Journal of Clinical Nutrition* 104(3), 2016: 743–9.

35. J.V. Nielsen, P. Westerlund and P. Bygren, 'A low-carbohydrate diet may prevent end-stage renal failure in type 2 diabetes: A case report', *Nutrition & Metabolism* 3, 2006: 23.

36. A.J. Hahr and M.E. Molitch, 'Management of diabetes mellitus in patients with chronic kidney disease', *Clinical Diabetes and Endocrinology* 1, 2015: 2.

37. C.C. Webster, T.D. Noakes, S.K. Chacko *et al.*, 'Gluconeogenesis during endurance exercise in cyclists habituated to a long-term low carbohydrate high-fat diet', *Journal of Physiology* 594(15), 2016: 4389–405.

38. F. Bril and K. Cusi, 'Nonalcoholic fatty liver disease: The new complication of type

2 diabetes mellitus', *Endocrinology and Metabolism Clinics of North America* 45(4), 2016: 765–81.

39. F. Bril, J.J. Sninsky, A.M. Baca *et al.*, 'Hepatic steatosis and insulin resistance, but not steatohepatitis, promote atherogenic dyslipidemia in NAFLD', *Journal of Clinical Endocrinology & Metabolism* 101(2), 2016: 644–52; R. Lomonaco, F. Bril, P. Portillo-Sanchez *et al.*, 'Metabolic impact of nonalcoholic steatohepatitis in obese patients with type 2 diabetes', *Diabetes Care* 39(4), 2016: 632–8.

40. M.B. Rothberg, 'Coronary artery disease as clogged pipes: A misconceptual model', *Circulation: Cardiovascular Quality and Outcomes* 6, 2013: 129–32; A. Malhotra, R.F. Redberg and P. Meier, 'Saturated fat does not clog the arteries: Coronary heart disease is a chronic inflammatory condition, the risk of which can be effectively reduced from healthy lifestyle interventions', *British Journal of Sports Medicine* 51(15), 2017: 1111–2.

41. HPSCA statement on low-carb diet, 'Balance – not carb restriction – is key to good health', 29 October 2012, available at http://myrunnersworld.co.za/low-carb-high-protein-diet-warning/ (last accessed 2 August 2017).

42. C. Becker, 'Government vs Tim Noakes', chrislbecker.com, 9 October 2012, available at http://chrislbecker.com/2012/10/09/government-vs-tim-noakes/ (last accessed 2 August 2017).

43. V. Mungal-Singh, 'Heart Foundation's open letter to Tim Noakes', *Health 24*, updated 27 September 2016, available at http://bit.ly/X4ekuD (last accessed 2 August 2017).

44. HSFSA, 'Getting to the heart of the heart mark', available at http://www.heartfounda tion.co.za/heart-mark (last accessed 16 August 2017).

45. M.G. Enig, R.J. Munn and M. Keeney, 'Dietary fat and cancer trends: A critique', *Federation Proceedings* 37(9), 1978: 2215–20; M.G. Enig, S. Atal, M. Keeney *et al.*, 'Isomeric trans fatty acids in the U.S. diet', *Journal of the American College of Nutrition* 9(5), 1990: 471–86; M.G. Enig, *Know Your Fats: The Complete Primer for Understanding the Nutrition of Fats, Oils, and Cholesterol* (Bethesda, MA: Bethesda Press, 2000); M. Enig and S. Fallon, *Eat Fat Lose Fat* (London: Plume Printing, 2006). W.C. Willett, M.J. Stampfer, J.E. Manson, *et al.* 'Intake of trans fatty acids and risk of coronary heart disease among woman'. *The Lancet* 341, 1993: 581–585.

46. Enig and Fallon, *Eat Fat Lose Fat*, 38.

47. C.E. Ramsden, D. Zamora, B. Leelarthaepin *et al.*, 'Use of dietary linoleic acid for secondary prevention of coronary heart disease and death: Evaluation of recovered data from the Sydney Diet Heart Study and updated meta-analysis', *BMJ* 2013;346:e8707.

48. C.E. Ramsden, D. Zamora, S. Majchrzak-Hong *et al.*, 'Re-evaluation of the traditional diet-heart hypothesis: Analysis of recovered data from Minnesota Coronary Experiment (1968–73)', *BMJ* 2016;353:i1246.

49. G.A. Rose, W.B. Thomson and R.T. Williams, 'Corn oil in treatment of ischaemic heart disease', *BMJ* 1(5449), 1965: 1531–3.

50. T.E. Standberg, V.V. Salomaa, V.A. Naukkarinen *et al.*, 'Long-term mortality after 5-year multifactorial primary prevention of cardiovascular diseases in middle-aged men', *JAMA* 266(9), 1991: 1226–9; T.E. Standberg, V.V. Salomaa, V.A. Naukkarinen *et al.*, 'Cardiovascular morbidity and multifactorial primary prevention: Fifteen

year follow-up of the Helsinki Businessmen Study', *Nutrition, Metabolism and Cardiovascular Diseases* 5, 1995: 7–15; T.E. Standberg, V.V. Salomaa, H.T. Vanhanen et al., 'Mortality in participants and non-participants of a multifactorial prevention study of cardiovascular diseases: A 28 year follow up of the Helsinki Businessmen Study', *British Heart Journal* 74, 1995: 449–54.

51. D. Mozaffarian, R. Micha and S. Wallace, 'Effects on coronary heart disease of increasing polyunsaturated fat in place of saturated fat: A systematic review and meta-analysis of randomized controlled trials', *PLoS Medicine* 7(3), 2010: e1000252.

52. D. Mozaffarian, E.B. Rimm and D.M. Herrington, 'Dietary fats, carbohydrate, and progression of coronary atherosclerosis in postmenopausal women', *American Journal of Clinical Nutrition* 80(5), 2004: 1175–84.

53. U. Ravnskov, J.J. DiNicolantonio, Z. Harcombe et al., 'The questionable benefits of exchanging saturated fat with polyunsaturated fat', *Mayo Clinic Proceedings* 89(4), 2014: 451–3; J.J. DiNicolantonio, 'The cardiometabolic consequences of replacing saturated fats with carbohydrates or omega-6 polyunsaturated fats: Do the dietary guidelines have it wrong?', *Open Heart* 1, 2014: 1–4.

54. B.A. Hannon, S.V. Thompson, R. An et al., 'Clinical outcomes of dietary replacement of saturated fatty acids with unsaturated fat sources in adults with overweight and obesity: A systematic review and meta-analysis of randomized control trials', *Annals of Nutrition and Metabolism* 71, 2017: 107–17.

55. B.E. Phillipson, D.W Rothrock, W.E. Connor et al., 'Reduction of plasma lipids, lipoproteins, and apoproteins by dietary fish oils in patients with hypertriglyceridemia', *New England Journal of Medicine* 312, 1985: 1210–6.

56. M-L. Silaste, M. Rantala and G. Alfthan, 'Changes in dietary fat intake alter plasma levels of oxidized low-density lipoprotein and lipoprotein(a)', *Arteriosclerosis Thrombosis Vascular Biology* 24, 2004: 498–503.

57. L.F. Chang, S.R. Vethakkan, K. Nesaretnam et al., 'Adverse effects on insulin secretion of replacing saturated fat with refined carbohydrate but not with monounsaturated fat: A randomized controlled trial in centrally obese subjects', *Journal of Clinical Lipidology* 10, 2016: 1431–41.

58. K-T. Teng, L.F. Chang, S.R. Vethakkan et al., 'Effects of exchanging carbohydrate or monounsaturated fat with saturated fat on inflammatory and thrombogenic responses in subjects with abdominal obesity: A randomized controlled trial', *Clinical Nutrition* 36, (2017): 1250–8.

59. S. Hamley, 'The effect of replacing saturated fat with mostly n-6 polyunsaturated fats on coronary heart disease: A meta-analysis of randomised controlled trials', *Nutrition Journal* 16, 2017: 30.

60. Taubes G. Vegetable oils, (Francis) Bacon, Bing Crosby, and the American Heart Association. http://garytaubes.com/vegetable-oils-francis-bacon-bing-crosby-and-the-american-heart-association/. (last accessed 28 July 2017).

61. 'Why you should never cook with sunflower oil', *Health24*, 4 October 2016, available at http://www.health24.com/Medical/Heart/News/why-you-should-never-cook-with-sunflower-oil-20151215 (last accessed 2 August 2017). See also R.M. Doctor, 'Scientists recommend cooking with lard, butter: Frying with vegetable oil releases toxic, cancer-causing chemicals', *Tech Times*, 9 November 2015, available at http://bit.ly/2mSC2tj (last accessed 2 August 2017).

62. M.L. Pearce and S. Dayton, 'Incidence of cancer in men on a diet high in polyunsaturated fat', *The Lancet* 1(7697), 1971: 464–7.

63. D. Yam, A. Eliraz and E.M. Berry, 'Diet and disease – the Israeli paradox: Possible dangers of a high omega-6 polyunsaturated fatty acid diet', *Israel Journal of Medical Sciences* 32(11), 1996: 1134–43.

64. R. Mousley, 'Molokai: Chalupsky makes it number 12!', Surfski.info, 21 May 2012, available at http://www.surfski.info/races/aus-nz/story/1406/molokai-chalupsky-makes-it-number-12.html (last accessed 2 August 2017).

65. 'The highs and lows of a low-carb-high-fat (LCHF) diet', HSFSA, 2016, available at http://www.heartfoundation.co.za/topical-articles/highs-and-lows-low-carb-high-fat-lchf-diet (last accessed 2 August 2017).

66. M.M. Shams-White, M. Chung, M. Du, *et al.* 'Dietary protein and bone health: a systematic review and meta-analyysis from the National osteoporosis Foundation.' *American Journal of Clinical Nutrition* 105, 2017: 1528–1543.

67. S. Mark, S. du Toit, T.D. Noakes *et al.*, 'A successful lifestyle intervention model replicated in diverse clinical settings', *SAMJ* 106(8), 2016: 763–6.

68. SAHA, 'Diet for prevention of cardiovascular disease', available at https://www.saheart.org/files/banting.pdf (last accessed 22 August 2017).

69. See the Heart Mark product list: http://www.heartfoundation.co.za/products.

70. J.S. Volek, S.D. Phinney, C.E. Forsythe *et al.*, 'Carbohydrate restriction has a more favorable impact on the metabolic syndrome than a low fat diet', *Lipids* 44(4), 2009: 297–309.

71. S. Mark, S. du Toit, T.D. Noakes *et al.*, 'A successful lifestyle intervention model replicated in diverse clinical settings', *SAMJ* 106(8), 2016: 763–6.

72. G. Taubes, *Good Calories, Bad Calories* (New York: Anchor Books, 2007), 34.

73. J.P. Ioannidis, 'Why most published research findings are false', *PLoS Medicine* 2(8), 2005: e124; J.P. Ioannidis, 'Evidence-based medicine has been hijacked: A report to David Sackett', *Journal of Clinical Epidemiology* 73, 2016: 82–6; J.P. Ioannidis, 'Acknowledging and overcoming nonreproducibility in basic and preclinical research', *JAMA* 317(10), 2017: 1019. J.P. Ioannidis, M.E. Stuart, S. Brownlee *et al.* 'How to survive the medical misinformation mess.' *European Journal of Clinical Investigation* 2017 Sept 7. doi 10.1111/eci. 12834 [Epub ahead of print].

74. J.P. Ioannidis, 'We need more randomized trials in nutrition-preferably large, long-term, and with negative results', *American Journal of Clinical Nutrition* 103(6), 2016: 1385–6.

75. J.P. Ioannidis, 'Implausible results in human nutrition research', *BMJ* 2013;347:f6698.

76. A.W. Brown, J.P. Ioannidis, M.B. Cope *et al.*, 'Unscientific beliefs about scientific topics in nutrition', *Advances in Nutrition (Bethesda, Md)* 5(5), 2014: 563–5.

77. Ibid.

78. J.P. Ioannidis, 'The mass production of redundant, misleading, and conflicted systematic reviews and meta-analyses', *Milbank Quarterly* 94(3), 2016: 485–514.

79. J. le Fanu, *The Rise and Fall of Modern Medicine* (London: Abacus, 2013), 398–9.

80. E. Klug, 'South African dyslipidaemia guideline consensus statement', *SAMJ* 102(3 Pt 2), 2012: 178–87.

81. L.H. Opie and A.J. Dalby, 'Cardiovascular prevention: Lifestyle and statins – competitors or companions?', *SAMJ* 104(3), 2014: 168–73.

82. P.C. Gøtzsche, *Deadly Medicines and Organised Crime: How Big Pharma has Corrupted Healthcare* (Florida: CRC Press, 2013), 26–32.

83. Ibid., 61.

84. K. Child, 'Tim Noakes diet is "criminal" says doctor', *Times*, 4 August 2014.

85. F.B. Kraemer and H.N. Ginsberg, 'Gerald M. Reaven, MD: Demonstration of the central role of insulin resistance in type 2 diabetes and cardiovascular disease', *Diabetes Care* 37(5), 2014: 1178–81.

86. G. Reaven, 'Insulin resistance and coronary heart disease in nondiabetic individuals', *Arteriosclerosis, Thrombosis, and Vascular Biology* 32(8), 2012: 1754–9.

87. A. Fasano, 'Leaky gut and autoimmune diseases', *Clinical Reviews in Allergy & Immunology* 42(1), 2012: 71–8.

88. Discovery Holdings press release, 'The Big Fat Debate lives up to its billing at the Discovery Vitality Summit', 1 August 2014, available at http://bit.ly/2mBFEgx (last accessed 2 August 2017).

89. W. Stassen, 'Noakes diet particularly dangerous for Afrikaans population', *Health-E News*, 11 August 2014, available at https://www.health-e.org.za/2014/08/11/noakes-diet-particularly-dangerous-afrikaans-population/ (last accessed 2 August 2017).

90. Credit Suisse Research Institute, 'Fat: The New Health Paradigm', September 2015: 6, available at http://publications.credit-suisse.com/tasks/render/file/index.cfm?fileid=9163B920-CAEF-91FB-EE5769786A03D76E (last accessed 2 August 2017).

91. Z. Harcombe, 'Familial hypercholesterolemia', ZoeHarcombe.com, 7 November 2016, available at http://www.zoeharcombe.com/2016/11/familial-hypercholesterolemia-fh/ (last accessed 2 August 2017).

92. Scientific Steering Committee on behalf of the Simon Broome Register Group, 'Risk of fatal coronary heart disease in familial hypercholesterolaemia', *BMJ* 303(6807), 1991: 893–6.

93. H.A. Neil, M.M. Hawkins, P.N. Durrington *et al.*, 'Non-coronary heart disease mortality and risk of fatal cancer in patients with treated heterozygous familial hypercholesterolaemia: A prospective registry study', *Atherosclerosis* 179(2), 2005: 293–7.

94. E.J. Sijbrands, R.G. Westendorp, J.C. Defesche *et al.*, 'Mortality over two centuries in large pedigree with familial hypercholesterolaemia: family tree mortality study', *BMJ* 322(7293), 2001: 1019–23.

95. R.R. Williams, S.J. Hasstedt, D.E. Wilson *et al.*, 'Evidence that men with familial hypercholesterolemia can avoid early coronary death: An analysis of 77 gene carriers in four Utah pedigrees', *JAMA* 255(2), 1986: 219–24.

96. W.R. Harlan Jr, J.B. Graham and E.H. Estes, 'Familial hypercholesterolemia: A genetic and metabolic study', *Medicine* 45(2), 1966: 77–110.

97. L. Pérez de Isla, R. Alonso, N. Mata *et al.*, 'Predicting cardiovascular events in familial hypercholesterolemia: The SAFEHEART Registry', *Circulation* 135(22), 2017: 2133–44.

98. M. Sebestjen, B. Zegura, B. Guzic-Salobir *et al.*, 'Fibrinolytic parameters and insulin resistance in young survivors of myocardial infarction with heterozygous familial hypercholesterolemia', *Wiener klinische Wochenschrift* 113(3–4), 2001: 113–8.

99. M. Paquette, M. Chong, S. Theriault *et al.*, 'Polygenic risk score predicts prevalence of cardiovascular disease in patients with familial hypercholesterolemia', *Journal of Clinical Lipidology* 11, 2017: 725–32.

100. J. Versmissen, D.M. Oosterveer, M. Yazdanpanah *et al.*, 'Efficacy of statins in familial hypercholesterolaemia: A long term cohort study', *BMJ* 2008;337:a2423; F.J. Raal, G.J. Pilcher, V.R. Panz *et al.*, 'Reduction in mortality in subjects with homozygous familial hypercholesterolemia associated with advances in lipid-lowering therapy', *Circulation* 124(20), 2011: 2202–7.

101. J.S. Hill, M.R. Hayden, J. Frohlich *et al.*, 'Genetic and environmental factors affecting the incidence of coronary artery disease in heterozygous familial hypercholesterolemia', *Arteriosclerosis and Thrombosis: A Journal of Vascular Biology* 11(2), 1991: 290–7; T.A. Miettinen and H. Gylling, 'Mortality and cholesterol metabolism in familial hypercholesterolemia: Long-term follow-up of 96 patients', *Arteriosclerosis (Dallas, Tex)* 8(2), 1988: 163–7; A.C. Jansen, E.S. van Aalst-Cohen, M.W. Tanck *et al.*, 'The contribution of classical risk factors to cardiovascular disease in familial hypercholesterolaemia: Data in 2400 patients', *Journal of Internal Medicine* 256(6), 2004: 482–90; I. Skoumas, C. Masoura, C. Pitsavos *et al.*, 'Evidence that non-lipid cardiovascular risk factors are associated with high prevalence of coronary artery disease in patients with heterozygous familial hypercholesterolemia or familial combined hyperlipidemia', *International Journal of Cardiology* 121(2), 2007: 178–83; Pérez de Isla, Alonso, Mata *et al.*, 'Predicting cardiovascular events in familial hypercholesterolemia: The SAFEHEART Registry'.

102. A. Postiglione, A. Nappi, A. Brunetti *et al.*, 'Relative protection from cerebral atherosclerosis of young patients with homozygous familial hypercholesterolemia', *Atherosclerosis* 90(1), 1991: 23–30.

103. D.D. Sugrue, I. Trayner, G.R. Thompson *et al.*, 'Coronary artery disease and haemostatic variables in heterozygous familial hypercholesterolaemia', *British Heart Journal* 53(3), 1985: 265–8; A.C. Jansen, E.S. van Aalst-Cohen, M.W. Tanck *et al.*, 'Genetic determinants of cardiovascular disease risk in familial hypercholesterolemia', *Arteriosclerosis, Thrombosis, and Vascular Biology* 25(7), 2005: 1475–81; Sebestjen, Zegura, Guzic-Salobir *et al.*, 'Fibrinolytic parameters and insulin resistance in young survivors of myocardial infarction with heterozygous familial hypercholesterolemia'; Skoumas, Masoura, Pitsavos *et al.*, 'Evidence that non-lipid cardiovascular risk factors are associated with high prevalence of coronary artery disease in patients with heterozygous familial hypercholesterolemia or familial combined hyperlipidemia'.

104. M. Kendrick, 'Should women be offered cholesterol lowering drugs to prevent cardiovascular disease? No', *BMJ* 334(7601), 2007: 983; B.H. Roberts, *The Truth About Statins* (New York: Pocket Books, 2012).

105. L.H. Opie, 'Exercise-induced myalgia may limit the cardiovascular benefits of statins', *Cardiovascular Drugs and Therapy* 27(6), 2013: 569–72; P. de Souich, G. Roederer and R. Dufour, 'Myotoxicity of statins: Mechanism of action', *Pharmacology & Therapeutics* 175, 2017: 1–16; J. Hippisley-Cox, 'Unintended effects of statins in men and women in England and Wales: Population based cohort study using the QResearch database', *BMJ* 2010;340:c2197.

106. D. Gaist, U. Jeppesen, M. Andersen *et al.*, 'Statins and risk of polyneuropathy: A case-control study', *Neurology* 58(9), 2002: 1333–7.

107. R. Cai, Y. Yuan, J. Sun *et al.*, 'Statins worsen glycemic control of T2DM in target

LDL-c level and LDL-c reduction dependent manners: A meta-analysis', *Expert Opinion in Pharmacotherapy* 17(14), 2016.

108. D. Preiss, S.R. Seshasai, P. Welsh *et al.*, 'Risk of incident diabetes with intensive-dose compared with moderate-dose statin therapy: A meta-analysis', *JAMA* 305(24), 2011: 2556–64; S.G. Chrysant, 'New onset diabetes mellitus induced by statins: Current evidence', *Postgraduate Medicine* 129(4), 2017: 430–5.

109. Hippisley-Cox, 'Unintended effects of statins in men and women in England and Wales: population based cohort study using the QResearch database'.

110. N.A. Melville, 'Statin use linked to increased Parkinson's risk', *Medscape*, 26 October 2016. G. Liu, N.W. Sterling, L. Kong, *et al.* 'Statins may facilitate Parkinson's disease: Insight gained from a large, national claims database'. *Movement Disorders* 32(6), 2017: 913–917.

111. A.A. Alsheikh-Ali, P.V. Maddukuri, H. Han *et al.*, 'Effect of the magnitude of lipid lowering on risk of elevated liver enzymes, rhabdomyolysis, and cancer: Insights from large randomized statin trials', *Journal of the American College of Cardiology* 50(5), 2007: 409–18.

112. M.W. Moyer, 'It's not dementia, it's your heart medication: Cholesterol drugs and memory', *Scientific American*, 1 September 2010, available at https://www.scientific american.com/article/its-not-dementia-its-your-heart-medication/ (last accessed 3 August 2017).

113. D. Graveline and P.J. Rosch, 'Why reported statin side effects are just the tip of a *Titanic* iceberg', in Rosch (ed.), *Fat and Cholesterol Don't Cause Heart Attacks: And Statins are Not The Solution* (Cwmbran: Columbus Publishing Ltd, 2016).

114. H. Okuyama, P.H. Langsjoen, T. Hamazaki *et al.*, 'Statins stimulate atherosclerosis and heart failure: Pharmacological mechanisms', *Expert Review of Clinical Pharmacology* 8(2), 2015.

115. Roberts, *The Truth About Statins*, 16–17; K.K. Ray, S.R. Seshasai, S. Erqou *et al.*, 'Statins and all-cause mortality in high-risk primary prevention: A meta-analysis of 11 randomized controlled trials involving 65,229 participants', *Archives of Internal Medicine* 170(12), 2010: 1024–31.

116. Y. Ma, G.M. Persuitte, C. Andrews *et al.*, 'Impact of incident diabetes on atherosclerotic cardiovascular disease according to statin use history among postmenopausal women', *European Journal of Epidemiology* 31(8), 2016: 747–61.

117. Gøtzsche, *Deadly Medicines and Organised Crime: How Big Pharma has Corrupted Healthcare*, 129.

118. U. Ravnskov, D.M. Diamond, R. Hama *et al.*, 'Lack of an association or an inverse association between low-density-lipoprotein cholesterol and mortality in the elderly: A systematic review', *BMJ Open* 6(6), 2016: e010401.

119. R. Mamtani, J.D. Lewis, F.I. Scott *et al.*, 'Disentangling the association between statins, cholesterol, and colorectal cancer: A nested case-control study', *PLoS Medicine* 13(4), 2016: e1002007.

120. R.S. Newson, J.F. Felix, J. Heeringa *et al.*, 'Association between serum cholesterol and noncardiovascular mortality in older age', *Journal of the American Geriatrics Society* 59(10), 2011: 1779–85.

121. Y. Takata, T. Ansai, I. Soh *et al.*, 'Serum total cholesterol concentration and 10-year mortality in an 85-year-old population', *Clinical Interventions in Aging* 9, 2014:

293–300; A.W. Weverling-Rijnsburger, G.J. Blauw, A.M. Lagaay *et al.*, 'Total cholesterol and risk of mortality in the oldest old', *The Lancet* 350(9085), 1997: 1119–23; P. Tuikkala, S. Hartikainen, M.J. Korhonen *et al.*, 'Serum total cholesterol levels and all-cause mortality in a home-dwelling elderly population: A six-year follow-up', *Scandinavian Journal of Primary Health Care* 28(2), 2010: 121–7.

122. T.B. Horwich, M.A. Hamilton, R. Maclellan *et al.*, 'Low serum total cholesterol is associated with a marked increase in mortality in advanced heart failure', *Journal of Cardiac Failure* 8(4), 2002: 216–24.

123. C. Iribarren, D.R. Jacobs Jr, S. Sidney *et al.*, 'Cohort study of serum total cholesterol and in-hospital incidence of infectious diseases', *Epidemiology and Infection* 121(2), 1998: 335–47.

124. A.J. Claxton, D.R. Jacobs Jr, C. Iribarren *et al.*, 'Association between serum total cholesterol and HIV infection in a high-risk cohort of young men', *Journal of Acquired Immune Deficiency Syndromes and Human Retrovirology* 17(1), 1998: 51–7.

125. J.D. Neaton and D.N. Wentworth, 'Low serum cholesterol and risk of death from AIDS', *AIDS (London, England)* 11(7), 1997: 929–30.

126. G. Zuliani, M. Cavalieri, M. Galvani *et al.*, 'Relationship between low levels of high-density lipoprotein cholesterol and dementia in the elderly: The InChianti study', *The Journals of Gerontology Series A, Biological Sciences and Medical Sciences* 65(5), 2010: 559–64; X. Huang, H. Chen, W.C. Miller *et al.* 'Lower low-density lipoprotein cholesterol levels are associated with Parkinson's disease'. *Movement Disorders* 22(3), 2007: 377–381; L.M.L. de Lau, P.J. Koudstaal, A. Hofman, *et al.* 'Serum cholesterol levels and the risk of Parkinson's Disease'. *American Journal of Epidemiology* 164(10), 2006: 998–1002.

127. L.F. Ellison and H.I. Morrison, 'Low serum cholesterol concentration and risk of suicide', *Epidemiology* 12(2), 2001: 168–72.

128. R.M. Mufti, R. Balon and C.L. Arfken, 'Low cholesterol and violence', *Psychiatric Services (Washington, DC)* 49(2), 1998: 221–4.

129. Mark, Du Toit, Noakes *et al.*, 'A successful lifestyle intervention model replicated in diverse clinical settings'.

130. E.J. Sijbrands, R.G. Westendorp, J.C. Defesche *et al.*, 'Mortality over two centuries in large pedigree with familial hypercholesterolaemia: Family tree mortality study', *BMJ* 322(7293), 2001: 1019–23; Pérez de Isla, Alonso, Mata *et al.*, 'Predicting cardiovascular events in familial hypercholesterolemia: The SAFEHEART Registry'.

Chapter 8: The Banting for Babies Tweet

1. Watch Sharyl Attkisson's TEDx Talk, 'Astroturf and manipulation of media messages', for an explanation of astroturfers. Available at https://www.youtube.com/watch?v=-bYAQ-ZZtEU (last accessed 2 August 2017). S. Attkisson. *The Smear. How shady political operatives and fake news control what you see, what you think and how you vote.* New York: Harper Collins, 2017.

2. T.D. Noakes, 'Low-carbohydrate and high-fat intake can manage obesity and associated conditions: Occasional survey', *SAMJ* 103(11), 2013: 826–30.

3. 'Prof Tim Noakes: Clarifying the controversy', *Nutritional Solutions*, 31 January 2014, available at http://www.nutritionalsolutions.co.za/prof-tim-noakes-clarifying-the-controversy/ (last accessed 2 August 2017).

4. M. Ellmer, 'The nutritional management of adult burn wound patients in South Africa', master's thesis, University of Stellenbosch, 2007.

5. M. Bishay, J. Pichler, V. Horn *et al.*, 'Intestinal failure-associated liver disease in surgical infants requiring long-term parenteral nutrition', *Journal of Pediatric Surgery* 47(2), 2012: 359–62.

6. 'Conversations with Prof Tim Noakes', *Nutritional Solutions*, 6 February 2014, available at http://www.nutritionalsolutions.co.za/conversations-with-prof-tim-noakes/ (last accessed 2 August 2017).

7. N. Teicholz, 'The scientific report guiding the US dietary guidelines: Is it scientific?', *BMJ* 2015;351:h4962; '*BMJ* won't retract controversial dietary guidelines article; issues lengthy correction', *Retraction Watch*, 2 December 2016.

8. Z. Harcombe, 'An examination of the randomised controlled trial and epidemiological evidence for the introduction of dietary fat recommendations in 1977 and 1983: A systematic review and meta-analysis', PhD thesis, University of the West of Scotland, March 2016.

9. A.L. McKenzie, S.J. Hallberg, B.C. Creighton *et al.*, 'A novel intervention including individualized nutritional recommendations reduces hemoglobin A1c level, medication use, and weight in type 2 diabetes', *JMIR Diabetes* 2(1), 2017: e5.

10. Credit Suisse Research Institute, 'Fat: The New Health Paradigm', September 2015: 21, available at http://publications.credit-suisse.com/tasks/render/file/index.cfm?fileid=9163B920-CAEF-91FB-EE5769786A03D76E (last accessed 2 August 2017).

11. M. Ellmer, 'Is the LCHF diet suitable and safe for infants?', *Nutritional Solutions*, 4 March 2014, http://www.nutritionalsolutions.co.za/is-the-lchf-diet-suitable-and-safe-for-infants/ (last accessed 2 August 2017).

12. A.C. Estampador and P.W. Franks, 'Genetic and epigenetic catalysts in early-life programming of adult cardiometabolic disorders', *Diabetes, Metabolic Syndrome and Obesity* 7, 2014: 575–86.

13. M. Ellmer, 'LCHF diets continued: Are they safe for pregnant and/or breastfeeding mothers?', *Nutritional Solutions*, 5 March 2014, available at http://www.nutritional solutions.co.za/lchf-diets-continued-are-they-safe-for-pregnant-andor-breastfeeding-mothers/ (last accessed 2 August 2017).

14. Health Professions Act 56 of 1974, 'Regulations Defining the Scope of the Profession of Dietetics', available at http://www.hpcsa.co.za/Uploads/editor/UserFiles/downloads/legislations/regulations/dn/regulations/regulations_gnr891_91.pdf (last accessed 2 August 2017).

15. T.D. Noakes, J. Proudfoot and B. Surtees, *Raising Superheroes* (Cape Town: Burnett Media, 2015).

16. J. Chang and L. Salahi, 'Rice cereal controversy: Does it make kids fat?', *abcNews*, 31 January 2011, available at http://abcnews.go.com/Health/w_ParentingResource/baby-diet-white-rice-cereal-pediatrician-dr-alan-greene-focuses/story?id=12801589 (last accessed 2 August 2017).

17. L. Jansen van Rensburg, 'Noakes se verhoor? "Ek voel 'n veer!"', *Netwerk24*, 28 November 2015, available at http://www.netwerk24.com/Nuus/Gesondheid/noakes-se-verhoor-ek-voel-n-veer-20151128 (last accessed 2 August 2017).

18. 'Yale doc loses 2 HuffPo blog posts after secretly promoting his novel', *Retraction Watch*, 20 November 2015, available at http://retractionwatch.com/2015/11/20/yale-

doc-loses-2-huffpo-blog-posts-after-secretly-pushing-his-novel/ (last accessed 2 August 2017).

19. R. Greene, 'David Katz: Junk food's slyest defender', *The Russells*, 26 September 2016, available at https://therussells.crossfit.com/2016/09/26/david-katz-junk-foods-slyest-defender/ (last accessed 2 August 2017).

20. C. Labos, 'Don't be fooled by big fat surprises, fat is still bad for you', *CBC News*, 2 March 2015, available at http://www.cbc.ca/news/health/don-t-be-fooled-by-big-fat-surprises-fat-is-still-bad-for-you-1.2965140 (last accessed 2 August 2017).

21. C. Julsing Strydom, 'Interview with Sylvia Escott Stump – Claire Julsing-Strydom', *SAJCN* 27(2), 2014: 82–4.

22. Academy of Nutrition and Dietetics press release, 'In wake of New York soda ban proposal, Academy of Nutrition and Dietetics encourages education, moderation', *newswise*, 31 May 2012, available at http://www.newswise.com/articles/in-wake-of-new-york-soda-ban-proposal-academy-of-nutrition-and-dietetics-encourages-education-moderation (last accessed 2 August 2017).

23. F. Gomes, 'Words for our sponsors', *World Nutrition* 4(8), 2013, available at http://bit.ly/2ndzhmG (last accessed 2 August 2017).

24. G. Schofield, C. Zinn, N. Harris *et al.*, 'Response to draft dietary guidelines submitted to the Ministry of Health', *AUT University*, April 2014.

PART II: NUTRITION ON TRIAL
Chapter 9: The Hearing: June 2015

1. M. Phillips, 'Absolute objectivity the ideal: Perspectivism the reality', *Kleio* 28(1), 1996: 32–42.

2. R.F. Taflinger, 'The myth of objectivity in journalism: A commentary', Washington State University, May 1996, available at http://public.wsu.edu/~taflinge/mythobj.html (last accessed 3 August 2017).

3. A. Novak, 'Capital sentencing discretion in Southern Africa: A human rights perspective on the doctrine of extenuating circumstances in death penalty cases; African Human Rights Law Journal (Chapter 2 Vol 1)', *African Human Rights Law Journal* 2, 2014, available at http://www.saflii.org/za/journals/AHRLJ/2014/2.html (last accessed 3 August 2017).

4. N.P. Steyn, N.G. Myburgh and J.H. Nel, 'Evidence to support a food-based dietary guideline on sugar consumption in South Africa', *Bulletin of the World Health Organization* 81(8), 2003: 599–608, available at http://www.scielosp.org/scielo.php?script=sci_arttext&pid=S0042-96862003000800010 (last accessed 3 August 2017).

5. N. Steyn and N. Temple, 'Evidence to support a food-based dietary guideline on sugar consumption in South Africa', *BMC Public Health*, 2012, available at http://bmcpublichealth.biomedcentral.com/articles/10.1186/1471-2458-12-502 (last accessed 3 August 2017).

6. R. Greene, 'Big Food vs. Tim Noakes: The final crusade', *The Russells*, 5 January 2017, available at https://therussells.crossfit.com/2017/01/05/big-food-vs-tim-noakes-the-final-crusade/ (last accessed 3 August 2017).

7. 'Report of South African ministerial task team (MTT) to investigate allegations of administrative irregularities, mismanagement and poor governance at the Health Professions Council of South Africa (HPCSA): A case of multi-system failure',

18 October 2015, available at http://section27.org.za/wp-content/uploads/2016/05/Report-of-the-Ministerial-Task-Team-to-Investigate-Allegations-at-the-HPCSA.pdf (last accessed 3 August 2017).

8. www.saspen.com/upcoming-events/nutrition-in-non-communicable-diseases-prevention-roadshow.

Chapter 10: The Second Session: November 2015

1. H.H. Vorster et al., 'The nutrition and health transition in the North West Province of South Africa: A review of the THUSA (Transition and Health during Urbanisation of South Africans) study', Public Health Nutrition 8(5), 2005: 480–90.

2. R. Greene, 'Big Food vs. Tim Noakes: The final crusade', The Russells, 5 January 2017, available at https://therussells.crossfit.com/2017/01/05/big-food-vs-tim-noakes-the-final-crusade/ (last accessed 3 August 2017).

3. J.A. Wessels in Coopers (South Africa) (Pty) Ltd v Deutsche Gesellschaft Für Schädlingsbekämpfung mbH 1976 (3) SA 352 (A).

Chapter 11: The Start of the Third Session: February 2016

1. University of the Witwatersrand, 'Staff profile: Professor Ames Dhai', available at https://www.wits.ac.za/staff/academic-a-z-listing/d/amesdhaiwitsacza/ (last accessed 3 August 2017).

2. The Big Fat Debate, available at http://www.humannutrition.uct.ac.za/nutrition/thebigfatdebate (last accessed 3 August 2017).

3. N. Steyn et al., 'Assessment of the dietary intake of schoolchildren in South Africa: 15 years after the first national study', Nutrients 8(509), 2016, available at www.mdpi.com/2072-6643/8/8/509/pdf (last accessed 3 August 2017).

4. C.E. Naudé, A. Schoonees, M. Senekal et al., 'Low carbohydrate versus isoenergetic balanced diets for reducing weight and cardiovascular risk: A systematic review and meta-analysis', PLoS One 9(7), 2014: e100652.

5. Z. Harcombe and T.D. Noakes, 'The universities of Stellenbosch/Cape Town low-carbohydrate diet review: Mistake or mischief?', SAMJ 106(12), 2016: 1179–82.

6. 'Food-based Dietary Guidelines for South Africa 2013 No 3 (Suppl)', SAJCN, available at http://sajcn.co.za/index.php/SAJCN/issue/view/67 (last accessed 3 August 2017).

7. H.H. Vorster, et al., 'An introduction to the revised food-based dietary guidelines for South Africa', SAJCN 26(3)(Supplement), 2013: S5–S12.

8. N. Steyn and R. Ochse, '"Enjoy a variety of foods": As a food-based 2 dietary guideline for South Africa', SAJCN 26(3)(Supplement), 2013: S13–S17.

9. H.H. Voster, '"Make starchy foods part of most meals": A food-based dietary guideline for South Africa', SAJCN 26(3)(Supplement), 2013: S28–S35.

10. C. Smuts and P. Wolmarans, 'The importance of the quality or type of fat in the diet: A food-based dietary guideline for South Africa', SAJCN 26, 2013: s87–s99.

11. S. Pagot and B. Appelhans, 'A call for an end to the diet debates', JAMA 310(7), 2013: 687–8.

12. Department of Justice and Constitutional Development, 'Promotion of Administrative Justice Act, 2000 (Act 3 of 2000)', available at http://www.justice.gov.za/paja/about/terms.htm (last accessed 3 August 2017).

13. Department of Justice and Constitutional Development, 'Promotion of Administrative Justice Act, 2000 (Act 3 of 2000)', available at http://www.justice.gov.za/paja/about/action.htm (last accessed 3 August 2017).

14. K. Horsley, 'Trials and tribunals: Administrative justice after PAJA and *New Clicks* with particular reference to the financial services industry', Public Law dissertation, UCT, 15 February 2006, available at http://www.publiclaw.uct.ac.za/usr/public_law/LLMPapers/horsley.pdf (last accessed 3 August 2017).

15. L. Jansen van Rensburg, 'Noakes se verhoor? "Ek voel 'n veer!"', *Netwerk24*, 28 November 2015.

Chapter 12: Finally, Noakes Speaks

1. A. Dreger, *Galileo's Middle Finger: Heretics, Activists, and One Scholar's Search for Justice* (New York: Penguin Press, 2015), 11.

2. Ibid., 262.

3. H. Lategan, *Healthy and Tasty: Diabetes* (Pretoria: LAPA Publishers, 2014).

4. J.A. Hawley, S.C. Dennis, B.J. Laidler, A.N. Bosch, T.D. Noakes and F. Brouns, 'High rates of exogenous carbohydrate oxidation from starch ingested during prolonged exercise', *Journal of Applied Physiology* 71(5), 1991: 1801–6.

5. C.E. Naudé, A. Schoonees, M. Senekal *et al.*, 'Low carbohydrate versus isoenergetic balanced diets for reducing weight and cardiovascular risk: A systematic review and meta-analysis', *PLoS One* 9(7), 2014: e100652.

6. Z. Harcombe and T.D. Noakes, 'The universities of Stellenbosch/Cape Town low-carbohydrate diet review: Mistake or mischief?', *SAMJ* 106(12), 2016: 1179–82.

7. L. Isaacs, 'LCHF diet "actually works"', *Cape Times*, 20 December 2016.

8. C.E. Naudé *et al.*, 'Reliable systematic review of low-carbohydrate diets shows similar weight-loss effects compared with balanced diets and no cardiovascular risk benefits: Response to methodological criticisms', *SAMJ* 107(3), 2017: 170.

9. N.B. Bueno *et al.*, 'Very-low-carbohydrate ketogenic diet v. low-fat diet for long-term weight loss: A meta-analysis of randomised controlled trials', *British Journal of Nutrition*, 110(7), 2013: 1178–87.

10. L.M. Burke *et al.*, 'Carbohydrate loading failed to improve 100-km cycling performance in a placebo-controlled trial', *Journal of Applied Physiology (1985)* 88(4), 2000: 1284–90.

11. S.C. Cunnane and M.A. Crawford, 'Survival of the fattest: Fat babies were the key to evolution of the large human brain', *Comparative Biochemistry and Physiology Part A* 136, 2003: 17–26.

12. I. Leslie, 'The sugar conspiracy', *The Guardian*, 7 April 2016, available at https://www.theguardian.com/society/2016/apr/07/the-sugar-conspiracy-robert-lustig-john-yudkin (last accessed 4 August 2017).

13. D.A. Graber, *Just the Facts 101: Mass Media and American Politics*, 9th ed., Cram101 Textbook Reviews and Content Technologies, 2017, available at https://books.google.co.uk/books?id=IWfYAwAAQBAJ&pg=PT41&lpg=PT41&dq=Astroturfing+nutrition&source=bl&ots=oHLBjn6wG-&sig=ct8uPfWgO5yYRaZphK6wElUdZQE&hl=en&sa=X&ved=oahUKEwjQxIKj-a3UAhWHDsAKHS1BBhcQ6AEISjAI#v=onepage&q=Astroturfing%20nutrition&f=false (last accessed 4 August 2017).

14. J. Walters, 'Nutrition experts alarmed by nonprofit downplaying role of junk food

in obesity', *The Guardian*, 11 August 2015, available at https://www.theguardian.com/society/2015/aug/11/obesity-junk-food-exercise-global-energy-balance-network-coca-cola (last accessed 4 August 2017).

15. Leslie, 'The sugar conspiracy'.

16. M. Skotnicki, '"The dog that didn't bark": What we can learn from Sir Arthur Conan Doyle about using the absence of expected facts', *Briefly Writing*, 25 July 2012, available at https://brieflywriting.com/2012/07/25/the-dog-that-didnt-bark-what-we-can-learn-from-sir-arthur-conan-doyle-about-using-the-absence-of-expected-facts/ (last accessed 4 August 2017).

17. L. Jansen van Rensburg, 'Noakes se verhoor? "Ek voel 'n veer!"', *Netwerk24*, 28 November 2015.

18. ADSA, 'Raising Superheroes - book review', *Nutrition Confidence*, 22 September 2015, available at https://nutritionconfidence.wordpress.com/2015/09/22/raising-superheroes-book-review/ (last accessed 4 August 2017).

Chapter 13: The Angels

1. Z. Harcombe, J.S. Baker, S.M. Cooper *et al.*, 'Evidence from randomised controlled trials did not support the introduction of dietary fat guidelines in 1977 and 1983: A systematic review and meta-analysis', *Open Heart* 2, 2015: e000196.

2. Z. Harcombe, J.S. Baker and B. Davies, 'Evidence from prospective cohort studies does not support current dietary fat guidelines: A systematic review and meta-analysis', *British Journal of Sports Medicine*, Published online first: 03 October 2016; doi: 10.1136/bjsports-2016-096550.

3. C. Crofts *et al.*, 'Hyperinsulinemia: Best management practice', *Diabesity* 2(1), 2016: 1–11.

4. Harcombe, J.S. Baker, S.M. Cooper *et al.*, 'Evidence from randomised controlled trials did not support the introduction of dietary fat guidelines in 1977 and 1983: A systematic review and meta-analysis'.

5. Z. Harcombe and T.D. Noakes, 'The universities of Stellenbosch/Cape Town low-carbohydrate diet review: Mistake or mischief?', *SAMJ* 106(12), 2016: 1179–82.

6. R. Smith, 'Peer review: a flawed process at the heart of science and journals', *Journal of the Royal Society of Medicine* 99(4), 2006: 178–82.

7. L. Isaacs, 'LCHF diet "actually works"', *Cape Times*, 20 December 2016.

8. C.E. Naudé, A. Schoonees, M. Senekal *et al.*, 'Reliable systematic review of low-carbohydrate diets shows similar weight-loss effects compared with balanced diets and no cardiovascular risk benefits: Response to methodological criticisms', *SAMJ* 107(3), 2017: 170.

9. Z. Harcombe and T.D. Noakes, 'Naudé *et al.* avoid answering the essential question: Mistake or mischief?', *SAMJ* 107(5), 2017: 360–1.

10. I. Leslie, 'The sugar conspiracy', *The Guardian*, 7 April 2016, available at https://www.theguardian.com/society/2016/apr/07/the-sugar-conspiracy-robert-lustig-john-yudkin (last accessed 4 August 2017).

11. R. Greene, 'Big Food vs. Tim Noakes: The final crusade', *The Russells*, 5 January 2017, available at https://therussells.crossfit.com/2017/01/05/big-food-vs-tim-noakes-the-final-crusade/ (last accessed 3 August 2017).

Chapter 14: Closing Arguments

1. R. Greene, 'Expert witness against Noakes to undergo investigation for ILSI ties', *The Russells*, 6 February 2017, available at https://therussells.crossfit.com/2017/02/06/expert-witness-against-noakes-to-undergo-investigation-for-ilsi-ties/ (last accessed 3 August 2017).

Chapter 15: The Verdict

1. D. Hume, *Philosophical Essays Concerning Human Understanding: An Enquiry Concerning Human Understanding* (London: A. Millar, 1748), E 10.3 SBN 110.

PART III: THE SCIENCE
Chapter 16: Once We Were Healthy

1. W. Yellowlees, *A Doctor in the Wilderness* (Perthshire: Dr W.W. Yellowlees, 2001), 166.
2. R. Bowen, 'Digestive physiology of herbivores: Basic fermentation chemistry', VIVO Pathophysiology, Colorado State University, available at http://vivo.colostate.edu/hbooks/pathphys/digestion/herbivores/ferment.html; R. Bowen, 'Digestive physiology of herbivores: Nutrient absorption and utilization in ruminants', VIVO Pathophysiology, Colorado State University, available at http://www.vivo.colostate.edu/hbooks/pathphys/digestion/herbivores/rum_absorb.html (both last accessed 4 August 2017).
3. K. Mu, 'What are chimpanzee digestive systems like compared to humans?', *Quora.com*, 3 May 2015, available at https://www.quora.com/What-are-chimpanzee-digestive-systems-like-compared-to-humans%E2%80%99 (last accessed 4 August 2017).
4. Ibid.
5. D.R. Braun, J.W. Harris, N.E. Levin *et al.*, 'Early hominin diet included diverse terrestrial and aquatic animals 1.95 Ma in East Turkana, Kenya', *Proceedings of the National Academy of Sciences* 107(22), 2010: 10002–7.
6. M.K. Georgieff, 'Nutrition and the developing brain: Nutrient priorities and measurement', *American Journal of Clinical Nutrition* 85(2), 2007: 614s–20s; S.C. Cunnane, *Survival of the Fattest: The Key to Human Brain Evolution* (Singapore: World Scientific Publishing Co., 2005).
7. P.T. Schoenemann, 'Chapter 2: Human Neuroanatomical Evolution', Indiana University Bloomington, 1997, available at http://www.indiana.edu/~brainevo/publications/dissertation/Dissertationch2.htm (last accessed 4 August 2017).
8. Cunnane, *Survival of the Fattest: The Key to Human Brain Evolution*; C.W. Marean, 'When the sea saved humanity', *Scientific American*, August 2010: 55–61; C.W. Marean, 'The origins and significance of coastal resource use in Africa and Western Eurasia', *Journal of Human Evolution* 77, 2014: 17–40.
9. Schoenemann, 'Chapter 2: Human Neuroanatomical Evolution'.
10. M. Ben-Dor, A. Gopher, I. Hershkovitz *et al.*, 'Man the fat hunter: The demise of *Homo erectus* and the emergence of a new hominin lineage in the Middle Pleistocene (ca. 400 kyr) Levant', *PLoS One* 6(12), 2011: e28689.
11. J.D. Speth, 'Protein selection and avoidance strategies of contemporary and ancestral foragers: Unresolved issues', *Philosophical Transactions of the Royal Society of London Series B, Biological Sciences* 334(1270), 1991: 265–9; discussion 69–70.
12. J. Brink, *Imagining Head-smashed-in: Aboriginal Buffalo Hunting on the Northern Plains* (Toronto: UBC Press, 2008), 34.

13. R.L. Kelly, *The Lifeways Of Hunter-Gatherers: The Foraging Spectrum* (Cambridge: Cambridge University Press, 2013), 74.
14. J.D. Speth, *Big-Game Hunting: Protein, Fat, or Politics? The Paleoanthropology and Archaeology of Big-Game Hunting* (New York: Springer, 2012), 149–61, xiii.
15. M. Ben-Dor, 'The key role of dietary fat in paleolithic human subsistence and behavior', unpublished.
16. M.K. Georgieff, 'Nutrition and the developing brain: Nutrient priorities and measurement'; Cunnane, *Survival of the Fattest: The Key to Human Brain Evolution.*
17. D.M. Bramble and D.E. Lieberman, 'Endurance running and the evolution of Homo', *Nature* 432(7015), 2004: 345–52; M.P. Mattson, 'Evolutionary aspects of human exercise – born to run purposefully', *Ageing Research Reviews* 11(3), 2012: 347–52.
18. L.A. O'Hearn, 'Optimal weaning from an evolutionary perspective', YouTube video, 12 August 2016, available at https://www.youtube.com/watch?v=hbksU68KkzI (last accessed 4 August 2017).
19. Ibid.
20. Z. Xue, W. Zhang, L. Wang *et al.*, 'The bamboo-eating giant panda harbors a carnivore-like gut microbiota, with excessive seasonal variations', *mBio* 6(3), 2015: e00022–15.
21. H. Devlin, 'Hard to bear: Pandas poorly adapted for digesting bamboo, scientists find', *The Guardian*, 19 May 2015, available at https://www.theguardian.com/science/2015/may/19/hard-to-bear-pandas-poorly-adapted-for-digesting-bamboo-scientists-find (last accessed 4 August 2017).
22. Ibid.
23. Ibid.
24. T.D. Noakes, *Waterlogged: The Serious Problem of Overhydration in Endurance Sports* (Champaign, IL: Human Kinetics, 2012).
25. J. Diamond, 'The worst mistake in the history of the human race', *Discover*, May 1987, http://discovermagazine.com/1987/may/02-the-worst-mistake-in-the-history-of-the-human-race (last accessed 4 August 2017).
26. The Neolithic Revolution, 'Agriculture slowly spreads: What do you notice about the core areas?', posted by Shannon Beyer on *SlideShare.net*, 10 September 2011, available at https://www.slideshare.net/darkyla/neolithic-revolution (last accessed 4 August 2017).
27. Y.N. Harari, *Sapiens: A Brief History of Humankind* (London: Harvill Secker, 2014), 83.
28. Ben-Dor, Gopher, Hershkovitz *et al.*, 'Man the fat hunter: The demise of *Homo erectus* and the emergence of a new hominin lineage in the Middle Pleistocene (ca. 400 kyr) Levant'.
29. A. Watts, '90% of the last million years, the normal state of the Earth's climate has been an ice age', *Watts Up With That?*, 13 May 2009, available at https://wattsupwiththat.com/2009/05/13/90-of-the-last-million-years-the-normal-state-of-the-earths-climate-has-been-an-ice-age/ (last accessed 4 August 2017).
30. 'Where woolly mammoths used to roam – Range at their peak, *Brilliant Maps*, 21 July 2015, available at http://brilliantmaps.com/woolly-mammoths/ (last accessed 4 August 2017).

31. M.R. Eades and M.D. Eades, *Protein Power* (New York: Bantam Books, 1996).
32. M. Henneberg, 'Decrease of human skull size in the Holocene', *Human Biology* 60(3), 1988: 395–405.
33. M.R. Eades and M.D. Eades, *Protein Power*, 15.
34. M.A. Ruffer, 'On arterial lesions found in Egyptian mummies (1580BC–525AD)', *The Journal of Pathology* 15(4), 1911: 453–62.
35. J. McCann, 'Maize and grace: History, corn, and Africa's new landscapes, 1500–1999', *Comparative Studies in Society and History* 43(2), 2001: 246–72.
36. Ibid.
37. A. Greaves, *Isandlwana* (Johannesburg: Jonathan Ball, 2001), 43.
38. M.K. Mutowo, 'Animal diseases and human populations in colonial Zimbabwe: The rinderpest epidemic of 1896–1898', *Zambezia* 28(1), 2001: 6.
39. M. Poland, D. Hammond-Tooke and L. Voight, *The Abundant Herds: A Celebration of the Nguni Cattle of the Zulu People* (Cape Town: Fernwood Press, 2006), 106.
40. R. Mack, 'The great African cattle plague epidemic of the 1890s', *Tropical Animal Health and Production* 2, 1970: 210–9.
41. C. van Onselen, 'Reactions to rinderpest in Southern Africa 1896–97', *Journal of African History* 13(3), 1972: 488.
42. R.H. Steckel and J.M. Prince, 'Tallest in the world: Native Americans of the Great Plains in the nineteenth century', *American Economic Review* 91(1), 2001: 287–94.
43. A. Debo, *A History of the Indians of the United States* (London: The Folio Society, 2003), 297.
44. Ibid., 295.
45. E. Lipski, 'Traditional non-Western diets', *Nutrition in Clinical Practice* 25(6), 2010: 587–8.
46. K.M. Venkat Narayan, 'Diabetes mellitus in Native American: The problem and its implications' in G.D. Sandefur, R.R. Rindfuss and B. Cohen (eds), *Changing Numbers, Changing Needs: American Indian Demography and Public Health* (Washington, DC: National Academy Press, 1996), 262–88.
47. P. Clayton and J. Rowbotham, 'How the mid-Victorians worked, ate and died', *International Journal of Environmental Research and Public Health* 6(3), 2009: 1235–53; P. Clayton and J. Rowbotham, 'An unsuitable and degraded diet? Part one: Public health lessons from the mid-Victorian working class diet', *Journal of the Royal Society of Medicine* 101(6), 2008: 282–9; P. Clayton and J. Rowbotham, 'An unsuitable and degraded diet? Part two: Realities of the mid-Victorian diet', *Journal of the Royal Society of Medicine* 101(7), 2008: 350–7; J. Rowbotham and P. Clayton, 'An unsuitable and degraded diet? Part three: Victorian consumption patterns and their health benefits', *Journal of the Royal Society of Medicine* 101(9), 2008: 454–62.
48. Clayton and Rowbotham, 'How the mid-Victorians worked, ate and died'.
49. Ibid., 1240.
50. R. McCarrison, *Nutrition and Health* (London: The McCarrison Society, 1982); R. McCarrison, *Studies in Deficiency Disease* (London: Henry Frowde and Hodder & Stoughton, 1945).
51. McCarrison, *Nutrition and Health*.
52. H.M. Sinclair, *The Work of Sir Robert McCarrison* (London: Faber and Faber Ltd, 1953), 302.

53. Ibid., 268.
54. Ibid., 267.
55. Ibid., 270.
56. Ibid., 271.
57. Ibid.
58. Ibid., 305–6.
59. S.L. Malhotra, 'Geographical aspects of acute myocardial infarction in India with special reference to patterns of diet and eating', *British Heart Journal* 29(3), 1967: 337–44.
60. S.L. Malhotra, 'Epidemiology of ischaemic heart disease in India with special reference to causation', *British Heart Journal* 29(6), 1967: 903.
61. S.L. Malhotra, 'Epidemiological study of cholelithiasis among railroad workers in India with special reference to causation', *Gut* 9(3), 1968: 290–5.
62. S.L. Malhotra, 'Peptic ulcer in India and its aetiology', *Gut* 5, 1964: 412–6; S.L. Malhotra, C.T. Majumdar and P.C. Bardoloi, 'Peptic ulcer in Assam', *Gut* 5, 1964: 355–8.
63. S.L. Malhotra, 'A comparison of unrefined wheat and rice diets in the management of duodenal ulcer', *Postgraduate Medical Journal* 54(627), 1978: 6–9.
64. S.L. Malhotra, 'Geographical distribution of gastrointestinal cancers in India with special reference to causation', *Gut* 8(4), 1967: 361–72.
65. S.L. Malhotra, 'An epidemiological study of varicose veins in Indian railroad workers from the South and North of India, with special reference to the causation and prevention of varicose veins', *International Journal of Epidemiology* 1(2), 1972: 177–83.
66. Lipski, 'Traditional non-Western diets'.
67. Ibid.
68. J.B. Orr and J.L. Gilks, *Studies of Nutrition: The Physique and Health of Two African Tribes* (London: H.M. Stationery Office, 1931).
69. A.G. Shaper, M. Jones and J. Kyobe, 'Plasma-lipids in an African tribe living on a diet of milk and meat', *The Lancet* 2(7216), 1961: 1324–7; G.V. Mann, R.D. Shaffer, R.S. Anderson *et al.*, 'Cardiovascular disease in the Masai', *Journal of Atherosclerosis Research* 4, 1964: 289–312; A.G. Shaper, K.W. Jones, M. Jones *et al.*, 'Serum lipids in three nomadic tribes in Northern Kenya', *American Journal of Clinical Nutrition* 13, 1963: 135–46; K. Biss, K.J. Ho, B. Mikkelson *et al.*, 'Some unique biologic characteristics of the Masai of East Africa', *The New England Journal of Medicine* 284(13), 1971: 694–9; A.G. Shaper, 'Cardiovascular studies in the Samburu tribe of Northern Kenya', *American Heart Journal* 63, 1962: 437–42; G.V. Mann, R.D. Shaffer and A. Rich, 'Physical fitness and immunity to heart-disease in Masai', *The Lancet* 2(7426), 1965: 1308–10; G.V. Mann, A. Spoerry, M. Gray *et al.*, 'Atherosclerosis in the Masai', *American Journal of Epidemiology* 95(1), 1972: 26–37.
70. M.J. Murray, A.B. Murray, N.J. Murray *et al.*, 'Serum cholesterol, triglycerides and heart disease of nomadic and sedentary tribesmen consuming isoenergetic diets of high and low fat content', *British Journal of Nutrition* 39(1), 1978: 159–63.
71. W. Price, *Nutrition and Physical Degeneration* (Oxford: Benediction Classics, 2010).
72. J.D. Boyd and C.L. Drain, 'The arrest of dental caries in childhood', *JAMA* 90(23), 1928: 1867–9.

73. W.A. Price, 'New light on the etiology and control of dental caries', *Journal of Dental Research* 12, 1932: 540–4.
74. T.F. Dreyer, 'Dental caries in prehistoric South Africans', *Nature* 136(3434), 1935: 302–3.
75. Price, *Nutrition and Physical Degeneration*, 268.
76. Ibid., 272.
77. Ibid., 295.
78. R. Schmid, *Primal Nutrition: Paleolithic and Ancestral Diets for Optimal Health* (Rochester: Healing Arts Press, 1987).
79. Price, *Nutrition and Physical Degeneration*, 259.
80. M. Mellanby and C.L. Pattison, 'Remarks on the influence of a cereal-free diet rich in vitamin D and calcium on dental caries in children', *British Medical Journal* 1(3715), 1932: 507–10.
81. Price, *Nutrition and Physical Degeneration*, 55.
82. V. Stefansson, *Not By Bread Alone* (New York: The Macmillan Company, 1946); V. Stefansson, *The Fat of the Land* (New York: The MacMillan Company, 1956); V. Stefansson, *The Friendly Arctic* (New York: The Macmillan Company, 1921).
83. W.S. McClellan and E.F du Bois, 'Prolonged meat diets with a study of kidney function and ketosis', *Journal of Biological Chemistry* XLV, 1930: 651–67.
84. V. Stefansson, *Cancer: Disease of Civilization? An Anthropological and Historical Study* (New York: Hill and Wang Inc., 1960).
85. Schmid, *Primal Nutrition: Paleolithic and Ancestral Diets for Optimal Health*.
86. A.R. David and M.R. Zimmerman, 'Cancer: An old disease, a new disease or something in between?', *Nature Reviews Cancer* 10(10), 2010: 728–33.
87. 'Scientists suggest that cancer is man-made', University of Manchester, 14 October 2010, available at http://www.manchester.ac.uk/discover/news/scientists-suggest-that-cancer-is-man-made/ (last accessed 4 August 2017).
88. J.J. DiNicolantonio, 'Increase in the intake of refined carbohydrates and sugar may have led to the health decline of the Greenland Eskimos', *Open Heart* 3(2), 2016: e000444.
89. Lipski, 'Traditional non-Western diets'.
90. Price, *Nutrition and Physical Degeneration*, 55.
91. N.K. McGrath-Hanna, D.M. Greene, R.J. Tavernier *et al.*, 'Diet and mental health in the Arctic: Is diet an important risk factor for mental health in circumpolar peoples? – a review', *International Journal of Circumpolar Health* 62(3), 2003: 228–41.
92. Price, *Nutrition and Physical Degeneration*, 152.
93. K. O'Dea, *The Hunter-Gatherer Lifestyle of Australian Aborigines: Implications for Health. Current Problems in Nutrition, Pharmacology and Toxicology* (London: Libbey, 1988), 26–36.
94. K. O'Dea, K. Traianedes, J.L. Hopper *et al.*, 'Impaired glucose tolerance, hyperinsulinemia, and hypertriglyceridemia in Australian Aborigines from the desert', *Diabetes Care* 11(1), 1988: 23–9; K. O'Dea, 'Westernisation, insulin resistance and diabetes in Australian aborigines', *Medical Journal of Australia* 155(4), 1991: 258–64; K. O'Dea, 'Marked improvement in carbohydrate and lipid metabolism in diabetic Australian aborigines after temporary reversion to traditional lifestyle', *Diabetes* 33(6), 1984: 596–603.

95. K. O'Dea, *The Hunter-Gatherer Lifestyle of Australian Aborigines: Implications for Health*, 28.

96. O'Dea, 'Marked improvement in carbohydrate and lipid metabolism in diabetic Australian aborigines after temporary reversion to traditional lifestyle'.

97. T.L. Cleave, *The Saccharine Disease: Conditions caused by the taking of refined carbohydrates, such as sugar and white flour* (Bristol: John Wright & Sons Ltd, 1974).

98. T.L. Cleave and G.D. Campbell, *Diabetes, Coronary Thrombosis and the Saccharine Disease* (Bristol: John Wright & Sons Ltd, 1966), 9.

99. Ibid., 46–9.

100. Ibid., 53.

101. Ibid., 59.

102. J. Yudkin, *Pure, White and Deadly* (London: Penguin Books, 1972), viii.

103. Ibid., 4.

104. J. Yudkin, 'Patterns and trends in carbohydrate consumption and their relation to disease', *Proceedings of the Nutrition Society* 23, 1964: 149–62.

105. Yudkin, *Pure, White and Deadly*, 188.

106. R. Lustig, 'Sugar: The Bitter Truth', YouTube Video, 30 July 2009, available at https://www.youtube.com/watch?v=dBnniua6-oM (last accessed 4 August 2017).

107. R.H. Lustig, *Fat Chance: Beating the Odds Against Sugar, Processed Food, Obesity and Disease* (New York: Hudson Street Press, 2013).

108. G. Taubes, *The Case Against Sugar* (New York: Alfred A. Knopf, 2016).

109. R.J. Johnson, 'The Fat Switch' (Mercola.com, 2012); R.J. Johnson, *The Sugar Fix: The High-Fructose Fallout That is Making You Fat and Sick* (New York: Rodale Press, 2008). S.E. Perez-Pozo, J. Schold, T. Nakagawa et al., 'Excessive fructose intake induces the features of metabolic syndrome in healthy adult men: Role of uric acid in the hypertensive response', *International Journal of Obesity* 34, 2010: 454–61; R. Nakagawa, H. Hu, S. Zharikov et al., 'A causal role for uric acid in fructose-induced metabolic syndrome', *American Journal of Physiology Renal Physiology* 290, 2006: F625–F631.

110. W.R. Leonard, J.J. Snodgrass and M.L. Robertson, 'Evolutionary perspectives on fat ingestion and metabolism in humans' in J.P. Montmayeur and J. le Coutre (eds), *Fat Detection: Taste, Texture, and Post Ingestive Effects* (Boca Raton: CRC Press/ Taylor & Francis, 2010), 3–18.

111. U. Toepel, J.F. Knebel, J. Hudry et al., 'The brain tracks the energetic value in food images', *NeuroImage* 44(3), 2009: 967–74.

112. Price, *Nutrition and Physical Degeneration*; Schmid, *Primal Nutrition: Paleolithic and Ancestral Diets for Optimal Health*; R. Schmid, *The Untold Story of Milk: The History, Politics and Science of Nature's Perfect Food: Raw Milk from Pasture-fed Cows* (Washington, DC: NewTrends Publishing, 2005).

Chapter 17: The Worst Mistake in the History of Medicine

1. J. le Fanu, *The Rise and Fall of Modern Medicine* (New York: Basic Books, 2012), 403.

2. G. Taubes, *Good Calories, Bad Calories* (New York: Anchor Books, 2007), 5.

3. M.G. Enig, *Know Your Fats: A Complete Primer for Understanding the Nutrition of Fats, Oils, and Cholesterol* (Bethesda: Bethesda Press, 2010); M.G. Enig, S. Atal, M. Keeney and J. Sampugna, 'Isomeric trans fatty acids in the U.S. diet', *Journal of the American*

College of Nutrition 9(5), 1990: 471–86; M.G. Enig, R.J. Munn and M. Keeney, 'Dietary fat and cancer trends – a critique', *Federation Proceedings* 37, 1978: 2215–20.

4. F.A. Kummerow and J.M. Kummerow, *Cholesterol Won't Kill You But Trans Fats Could: Separating Scientific Fact from Nutritional Fiction in What You Eat* (Victoria: Trafford Publishing, 2008); P.V. Johnston, O.C. Johnson and F.A. Kummerow, 'Occurrence of trans fatty acids in human tissue', *Science* 126, 1957: 648–9; P.V. Johnston, F.A. Kummerow and C.H. Walton, 'Origin of the trans fatty acids in human tissue', *Proceedings of the Society for Experimental Biology and Medicine* 99, 1958: 735–6.

5. R.J. Johnson, M.S. Segal, Y. Sautin *et al.*, 'Potential role of sugar (fructose) in the epidemic of hypertension, obesity and the metabolic syndrome, diabetes, kidney disease, and cardiovascular disease', *American Journal of Clinical Nutrition* 86(4), 2007: 899–906.

6. USDA, *Agriculture Fact Book 2001–2002*, March 2003: 16. Available at www.4uth.gov. ua/usa/english/trade/files/2002factbook.pdf (last accessed 4 August 2017).

7. See Figure 2 in Enig, Munn and Keeney, 'Dietary fat and cancer trends – a critique'; R.L. Rizek, B. Friend and L. Page, 'Fat in todays food supply – level of use and sources', *Journal of the American Oil Chemists' Society* 51(6), 1974: 244–50.

8. Enig, Munn and Keeney, 'Dietary fat and cancer trends – a critique'.

9. Kummerow and Kummerow, *Cholesterol Won't Kill You But Trans Fats Could: Separating scientific Fact from Nutritional Fiction in What You Eat.*

10. F.A. Kummerow, 'Viewpoint on the report of the National Cholesterol Education Program Expert Panel on the Detection, Evaluation and Treatment of High Cholesterol in Adults', *Journal of the American College of Nutrition* 12, 1993: 2–13.

11. C.R. Daniel, A.J. Cross, C. Koebnick *et al.*, 'Trends in meat consumption in the USA', *Public Health Nutrition* 14(4), 2011: 575–83.

12. USDA, *Agriculture Fact Book 2001–2002.*

13. A. Keys, 'Sucrose in the diet and coronary heart disease', *Atherosclerosis* 14(2), 1971: 193–202.

14. J. Yudkin, *Pure, White and Deadly* (London: Penguin Books, 1972).

15. J. Yudkin, 'Dietary fat and dietary sugar in relation to ischaemic heart-disease and diabetes', *The Lancet* 2(7349), 1964: 4–5.

16. T.L. Blasbalg, J.R. Hibbeln, C.E. Ramsden *et al.*, 'Changes in consumption of omega-3 and omega-6 fatty acids in the United States during the 20th century', *American Journal of Clinical Nutrition* 93(5), 2011: 950–62.

17. A. Keys, 'Atherosclerosis: A problem in newer public health', *Journal of the Mount Sinai Hospital, New York* 20(2), 1953: 118–39.

18. A. Keys, A. Menotti, M.J. Karvonen *et al.*, 'The diet and 15-year death rate in the seven countries study', *American Journal of Epidemiology* 124(6), 1986: 903–15.

19. J. Yerushalmy and H.E. Hilleboe, 'Fat in the diet and mortality from heart disease: A methodologic note', *New York State Journal of Medicine* 57(14), 1957: 2343–54.

20. P.D.P. Wood, 'A possible selection effect in medical science', *The Statistician* 30(2), 1981: 131–5.

21. Ibid.

22. T.D. Noakes, 'The 2012 University of Cape Town Faculty of Health Sciences Centenary Debate', *SAJCN* 28(1), 2016: 19–33.

23. P. Grasgruber, M. Sebera, E. Hrazdira *et al.*, 'Food consumption and the actual statistics of cardiovascular diseases: An epidemiological comparison of 42 European countries', *Food & Nutrition Research* 60, 2016.

24. P.D.P. Wood, ' A possible selection effect in medical science', 131-5.

25. P. Grasgruber *et al.*

26. Ibid., 23.

27. Ibid., 1.

28. Credit Suisse Research Institute, 'Fat: The New Health Paradigm', September 2015, available at http://publications.credit-suisse.com/tasks/render/file/index.cfm?fileid= 9163B920-CAEF-91FB-EE5769786A03D76E (last accessed 2 August 2017).

29. Ibid.

30. A. Keys, J.T. Anderson and F. Grande, 'Serum cholesterol response to changes in the diet: II. The effect of cholesterol in the diet', *Metabolism* 14(7), 1965: 759–65.

31. Z. Harcombe, 'An examination of the randomised controlled trial and epidemiological evidence for the introduction of dietary fat recommendations in 1977 and 1983: A systematic review and meta-analysis', PhD thesis, University of the West of Scotland, March 2016.

32. E. di Angelantonio, P. Gao, L. Pennells *et al.*, 'Lipid-related markers and cardiovascular disease prediction', *JAMA* 307(23), 2012: 2499–506.

33. 'Risk of fatal coronary heart disease in familial hypercholesterolaemia', Scientific Steering Committee on behalf of the Simon Broome Register Group, *BMJ* 303(6807), 1991: 893–6.

34. L. Pérez de Isla, R. Alonso, N. Mata *et al.*, 'Predicting cardiovascular events in familial hypercholesterolemia: The SAFEHEART Registry', *Circulation* 135(22), 2017: 2133–44.

35. R. Lomonaco, F. Bril, P. Portillo-Sanchez *et al.*, 'Metabolic impact of nonalcoholic steatohepatitis in obese patients with type 2 diabetes', *Diabetes Care* 39(4), 2016: 632–8; F. Bril, J.J. Sninsky, A.M. Baca *et al.*, 'Hepatic steatosis and insulin resistance, but not steatohepatitis, promote atherogenic dyslipidemia in NAFLD', *Journal of Clinical Endocrinology & Metabolism* 101(2), 2016: 644–52; F. Bril and K. Cusi, 'Nonalcoholic fatty liver disease: The new complication of type 2 diabetes mellitus', *Endocrinology and Metabolism Clinics of North America* 45(4), 2016: 765–81; F. Bril, D. Barb, P. Portillo-Sanchez *et al.*, 'Metabolic and histological implications of intrahepatic triglyceride content in nonalcoholic fatty liver disease', *Hepatology* 65(4), 2017: 1132–44.

36. M. Maersk, A. Belza, H. Stodkilde-Jorgensen *et al.*, 'Sucrose-sweetened beverages increase fat storage in the liver, muscle, and visceral fat depot: A 6-mo randomized intervention study', *American Journal of Clinical Nutrition* 95, 2012: 283–9. R.H. Lustig, K. Mulligan, S.M. Noworolski *et al.*, 'Isocaloric fructose restriction and metabolic improvement in children with obesity and metabolic syndrome', *Obesity* 24, 2016: 453–60. J-M. Schwartz, M. Clearfield and K. Mulligan, 'Conversion of sugar to fat: Is hepatic de novo lipogenesis leading to metabolic syndrome and associated chronic diseases?', *Journal of the American Osteopathic Association* 117(8), 2017: 520–7. J-M. Schwartz, S.M. Noworolski, A. Erkin-Cakmam *et al.*, 'Effects of dietary fructose restriction on liver fat, de novo lipogenesis, and insulin kinetics in children with obesity', *Gastroenterology*, 1 June 2017: pii: S0016-5085(17)35685-8. doi: 10.1053/j.gastro.2017.05.043 [epub ahead of print].

37. C.C. Duwaerts, A.M. Amin, K. Siao *et al.*, 'Specific macronutrients exert unique influences on the adipose-liver axis to promote hepatic steatosis in mice, *Cellular and Molecular Gastroenterology and Hepatology* 4(2), 2017: 223–36.

38. S. Haufe, S. Engeli, P. Kast *et al.*, 'Randomized comparison of reduced fat and reduced carbohydrate hypocaloric diets on intrahepatic fat in overweight and obese human subjects', *Hepatology* 53(5), 2011: 1504–14.

39. D.J. Unwin, D.J. Cuthbertson, R. Feinman *et al.*, 'A pilot study to explore the role of a low-carbohydrate intervention to improve GGT levels and HbA1c', *Diabesity in Practice* 4(3), 2015: 102–8.

40. E.C. Jang, D.W. Jun, S.M. Lee *et al.*, 'Comparison of efficacy of low-carbohydrate and low-fat diet education program in non-alcoholic fatty liver disease: Randomized controlled study', *Hepatology Research: The Official Journal of the Japan Society of Hepatology*, 2017, doi: 10.1111/hepr.12918; J.D. Browning, J.A. Baker, T. Rogers *et al.*, 'Short-term weight loss and hepatic triglyceride reduction: Evidence of a metabolic advantage with dietary carbohydrate restriction', *American Journal of Clinical Nutrition* 93(5), 2011: 1048–52.

41. K. Sevastianova, A. Santos, A. Kotronen *et al.*, 'Effect of short-term carbohydrate overfeeding and long-term weight loss on liver fat in overweight humans', *American Journal of Clinical Nutrition* 96(4), 2012: 727–34.

42. J.S. Volek and R.D. Feinman, 'Carbohydrate restriction improves the features of metabolic syndrome. Metabolic syndrome may be defined by the response to carbohydrate restriction', *Nutrition & Metabolism (Lond.)* 2, 2005: 31; J.S. Volek, S.D. Phinney, C.E. Forsythe *et al.*, 'Carbohydrate restriction has a more favorable impact on the metabolic syndrome than a low fat diet', *Lipids* 44(4), 2009: 297–309; J.S. Volek, M.L. Fernandez, R.D. Feinman *et al.*, 'Dietary carbohydrate restriction induces a unique metabolic state positively affecting atherogenic dyslipidemia, fatty acid partitioning, and metabolic syndrome', *Progress in Lipid Research* 47(5), 2008: 307–18.

43. S. Mark, S. du Toit, T.D. Noakes *et al.*, 'A successful lifestyle intervention model replicated in diverse clinical settings', *SAMJ* 106(8), 2016: 763–6.

44. M. Sebestjen, B. Zegura, B. Guzic-Salobir *et al.*, 'Fibrinolytic parameters and insulin resistance in young survivors of myocardial infarction with heterozygous familial hypercholesterolemia', *Wiener klinische Wochenschrift* 113(3–4), 2001: 113–8; G. DiMinno, M.J. Silver, A.M. Cerbone *et al.*, 'Increased fibrinogen binding to platelets from patients with familial hypercholesterolemia', *Arteriosclerosis (Dallas, Tex)* 6(2), 1986: 203–11.

45. S.M. Haffner, S. Lehto, T. Ronnemaa *et al.*, 'Mortality from coronary heart disease in subjects with type 2 diabetes and in nondiabetic subjects with and without prior myocardial infarction', *The New England Journal of Medicine* 339(4), 1998: 229–34.

46. W.R. Ware, 'The mainstream hypothesis that LDL cholesterol drives atherosclerosis may have been falsified by non-invasive imaging of coronary artery plaque burden and progression', *Medical Hypotheses* 73(4), 2009: 596.

47. I.M. Stratton, A.I. Adler, H.A. Neil *et al.*, 'Association of glycaemia with macrovascular and microvascular complications of type 2 diabetes (UKPDS 35): Prospective observational study', *BMJ* 321(7258), 2000: 405–12.

48. Ibid.

49. M. Moss, *Salt Sugar Fat: How the Food Giants Hooked Us* (New York: Random House, 2013).

50. S-A. Creed, D. Grier, J. Proudfoot and T.D. Noakes, *The Real Meal Revolution* (Cape Town: Quivertree, 2013), xxvi.

51. E. Cohen, M. Cragg, J. de Fonseka *et al.*, 'Statistical review of US macronutrient consumption data, 1965–2011: Americans have been following dietary guidelines, coincident with the rise in obesity', *Nutrition* 31(5), 2015: 727–32; L.S. Gross, L. Li, E.S. Ford *et al.*, 'Increased consumption of refined carbohydrates and the epidemic of type 2 diabetes in the United States: An ecologic assessment', *American Journal of Clinical Nutrition* 79(5), 2004: 774–9.

52. Ibid.

53. R. Bowen, 'Digestive physiology of herbivores: Basic fermentation chemistry', VIVO Pathophysiology, Colorado State University, available at http://vivo. colostate.edu/hbooks/pathphys/digestion/herbivores/ferment.html (last accessed 4 August 2017).

54. R. Bowen, 'Digestive physiology of herbivores: Nutrient absorption and utilization in ruminants', VIVO Pathophysiology, Colorado State University, available at http://www.vivo.colostate.edu/hbooks/pathphys/digestion/herbivores/rum_absorb. html (last accessed 4 August 2017).

55. M. Ben-Dor, A. Gopher, I. Hershkovitz *et al.*, 'Man the fat hunter: The demise of *Homo erectus* and the emergence of a new hominin lineage in the Middle Pleistocene (ca. 400 kyr) Levant', *PLoS One* 6(12), 2011: e28689.

56. M. Ben-Dor, A. Gopher and R. Barkai, 'Neandertals' large lower thorax may represent adaptation to high protein diet', *American Journal of Physical Anthropology* 160, 2016: 367–78.

57. L. Cordain, J.B. Miller, S.B. Eaton and N. Mann, 'Macronutrient estimations in hunter-gatherer diets', *American Journal of Clinical Nutrition* 72(6), 2000: 1589–92.

58. R.R. Briefel and C.L. Johnson, 'Secular trends in dietary intake in the United States', *Annual Review of Nutrition* 24, 2004: 401–31.

59. S. Lindeberg, M. Eliasson, B. Lindahl *et al.*, 'Low serum insulin in traditional Pacific Islanders: The Kitava Study', *Metabolism* 48(10), 1999: 1216–9.

60. S.L. Aronoff, P.H. Bennett, P. Gorden *et al.*, 'Unexplained hyperinsulinemia in normal and "prediabetic" Pima Indians compared with normal Caucasians: An example of racial differences in insulin secretion', *Diabetes* 26(9), 1977: 827–40; P. Zimmet, S. Whitehouse and J. Kiss, 'Ethnic variability in the plasma insulin response to oral glucose in Polynesian and Micronesian subjects', *Diabetes* 28(7), 1979: 624–8.

61. H. Kaplan, R.C. Thompson, B.C. Trumble *et al.*, 'Coronary atherosclerosis in indigenous South American Tsimane: A cross-sectional cohort study', *The Lancet* 389(10080), 2017: 1730–9.

62. G. Dowse and P. Zimmet, 'The thrifty genotype in non-insulin dependent diabetes', *BMJ* 306(6877), 1993: 532–3.

63. K.S. Rigano, J.L. Gehring, B.D. Evans Hutzenbiler *et al.*, 'Life in the fat lane: Seasonal regulation of insulin sensitivity, food intake, and adipose biology in brown bears', *Journal of Comparative Physiology B, Biochemical, Systemic, and Environmental Physiology* 187(4), 2017: 649–76.

64. A. Bentley, *Inventing Baby Food* (Oakland: University of California Press, 2014).

65. A. Fasano, 'Zonulin, regulation of tight junctions, and autoimmune diseases', *Annals of the New York Academy of Sciences* 1258, 2012: 25–33.

66. G. Reaven, 'Insulin resistance and coronary heart disease in nondiabetic individuals', *Arteriosclerosis, Thrombosis and Vascular Biology* 32(8), 2012: 1754–9.

67. Ibid.

68. A.M. Coulston, C.B. Hollenbeck, A.L. Swislocki *et al.*, 'Deleterious metabolic effects of high-carbohydrate, sucrose-containing diets in patients with non-insulin-dependent diabetes mellitus', *American Journal of Medicine* 82(2), 1987: 213–20.

69. A.M. Coulston, C.B. Hollenbeck, A.L. Swislocki *et al.*, 'Persistence of hypertriglyceridemic effect of low-fat high-carbohydrate diets in NIDDM patients', *Diabetes Care* 12(2), 1989: 94–101.

70. A. Garg, J.P. Bantle, R.R. Henry *et al.*, 'Effects of varying carbohydrate content of diet in patients with non-insulin-dependent diabetes mellitus', *JAMA* 271(18), 1994: 1421–8.

71. Volek and Feinman, 'Carbohydrate restriction improves the features of metabolic syndrome. Metabolic syndrome may be defined by the response to carbohydrate restriction'; J.W. Gofman, 'Diet in the prevention and treatment of myocardial infarction', *American Journal of Cardiology* 1(2), 1958: 271–83; L.C. Hudgins, M. Hellerstein, C. Seidman *et al.*, 'Human fatty acid synthesis is stimulated by a eucaloric low fat, high carbohydrate diet', *Journal of Clinical Investigation* 97(9), 1996: 2081–91; B.M Volk, L.J. Kunces, D.J. Freidenreich *et al.*, 'Effects of step-wise increases in dietary carbohydrate on circulating saturated fatty acids and palmitoleic acid in adults with metabolic syndrome', *PLoS One* 9(11), 2014: e113605.

72. T.E. Matsha, M. Macharia, Y.Y. Yako *et al.*, 'Gamma-glutamyltransferase, insulin resistance and cardiometabolic risk profile in a middle-aged African population', *European Journal of Preventive Cardiology* 21(12), 2014: 1541–8.

73. M. Nannipieri, C. Gonzales, S. Baldi *et al.*, 'Liver enzymes, the metabolic syndrome, and incident diabetes: The Mexico City diabetes study', *Diabetes Care* 28(7), 2005: 1757–62.

74. Matsha, Macharia, Yako *et al.*, 'Gamma-glutamyltransferase, insulin resistance and cardiometabolic risk profile in a middle-aged African population'.

75. Mark, Du Toit, Noakes *et al.*, 'A successful lifestyle intervention model replicated in diverse clinical settings'.

76. C.M. Apovian, L.J. Aronne, D.H. Bessesen *et al.*, 'Pharmacological management of obesity: an endocrine Society clinical practice guideline', *Journal of Clinical Endocrinology & Metabolism* 100(2), 2015: 342–62.

77. A.J. Scheen and P.J. Lefebvre, 'Pharmacological treatment of obesity: Present status', *International Journal of Obesity and Related Metabolic Disorders: Journal of the International Association for the Study of Obesity* 23 Suppl 1, 1999: 47–53.

78. Ibid.

79. C.L. Roumie, R.A. Greevy, C.G. Grijalva *et al.*, 'Association between intensification of metformin treatment with insulin vs sulfonylureas and cardiovascular events and all-cause mortality among patients with diabetes', *JAMA* 311(22), 2014: 2288–96; S.E. Holden, S. Jenkins-Jones, C.L. Morgan *et al.*, 'Glucose-lowering with exogenous insulin monotherapy in type 2 diabetes: Dose association with all-cause mortality, cardiovascular events and cancer', *Diabetes, Obesity & Metabolism* 17(4), 2015: 350–62.

80. M.P. Czech, 'Insulin action and resistance in obesity and type 2 diabetes', *Nature Medicine* 23, 2017: 804–14. S.M. de la Monte and J.R. Wands, 'Alzheimer's disease is type 3 diabetes: Evidence reviewed', *Journal of Diabetes Science and Technology* 2(6), 2008: 1101–13. M. Demasi, R.H. Lustig and A. Malhotra, 'The cholesterol and calorie hypotheses are both dead – it is time to focus on the real culprit: insulin resistance', *Clinical Pharmacist*, 14 July 2017, available at pharmaceutical-journal. com /opinion/insight/the-cholesterol-and-calorie-hypotheses-are-both-dead-it-is-time-to- focus-on-the-real-culprit-insulin-resistance/20203046.article (last accessed 10 August 2017). K.A. Erion and B.E. Corkey, 'Hyperinsulinemia: A cause of obesity?', *Current Obesity Reports* 6(2), 2017: 178–86. B.C. Melnik, S.M. John and G. Schmitz, 'Over-stimulation of insulin/IGF-1 signaling by western diet may promote diseases of civilization: Lessons learnt from laron syndrome', *Nutrition and Metabolism* 8, 2011: 41–4. G.M. Reaven, 'Insulin resistance/compensatory hyperinsulinemia, essential hypertension, and cardiovascular disease', *Journal of Clinical Endocrinology and Metabolism* 88(6), 2003: 2399–403. E. Tikkanen, M. Pirinen and A.P. Sarin, 'Genetic support for the causal role of insulin in coronary heart disease', *Diabetologia* 59 (11), 2016: 2369–77. T. Tsujimoto, H. Kajio and T. Sugiyama, 'Association between hyperinsulinemia and increased risk of cancer death in nonobese and obese people: A population-based observational study', *International Journal of Cancer* 141, 2017: 102–11.

81. M.R. Law, J.K. Morris and N.J. Wald, 'Use of blood pressure lowering drugs in the prevention of cardiovascular disease: Meta-analysis of 147 randomised trials in the context of expectations from prospective epidemiological studies', *BMJ* 338, 2009: b1665.

82. Mark, Du Toit, Noakes *et al.*, 'A successful lifestyle intervention model replicated in diverse clinical settings'.

83. N.J. Schork, 'Personalized medicine: Time for one-person trials', *Nature* 520(7549), 2015: 609–11.

84. B.H. Roberts, *The Truth About Statins* (New York: Pocket Books, 2012); P.J. Rosch, Z. Harcombe, M. Kendrick *et al.*, *Fat and Cholesterol Don't Cause Heart Attacks and Statins are Not the Solution* (Cwmbran: Columbus Publishing Ltd, 2016).

85. S.M. de la Monte and J.R. Wands, 'Alzheimer's disease is type 3 diabetes-evidence reviewed', *Journal of Diabetes Science and Technology* 2(6), 2008: 1101–13.

86. 'Remote care promotes low carbohydrate diet adherence and glycemic control allowing medication reduction in type 2 diabetes – abstract', *Virta Health*, 14 June 2017; A.L. McKenzie, S.J. Hallberg, B.C. Creighton *et al.*, 'A novel intervention including individualized nutritional recommendations reduces hemoglobin A1c level, medication use, and weight in type 2 diabetes', *JMIR Diabetes* 2(1), 2017: e5.

87. CDC, 'United States Cancer Statistics: 2013 Technical Notes', *OnLine Journal of Biological Sciences*, 2013, available at https://www.cdc.gov/cancer/npcr/uscs/pdf/uscs-2013-technical-notes.pdf (last accessed 6 August 2017).

Closure

1. T. Christofferson, *Tripping Over the Truth* (South Carolina: CreateSpace Independent Publishing Platform, 2014), xxii.

2. N.F. Krebs, M. Mazariegos, A. Tshefu *et al.*, 'Meat consumption is associated with

less stunting among toddlers in four diverse low-income settings', *Food and Nutrition Bulletin* 32(3), 2011: 185–91.

3. M. Tang and N.F. Krebs, 'High protein intake from meat as complementary food increases growth but not adiposity in breastfed infants: A randomized trial', *American Journal of Clinical Nutrition* 100(5), 2014: 1322–8.

4. N.F. Krebs, J.E. Westcott, N. Butler *et al.*, 'Meat as a first complementary food for breastfed infants: Feasibility and impact on zinc intake and status', *Journal of Pediatric Gastroenterology and Nutrition* 42(2), 2006: 207–14.

5. N.F. Krebs, L.G. Sherlock, J. Westcott *et al.*, 'Effects of different complementary feeding regimens on iron status and enteric microbiota in breastfed infants', *Journal of Pediatrics* 163(2), 2013: 416–23.

6. Ibid.

7. B.E. Young and N.F. Krebs, 'Complementary feeding: Critical considerations to optimize growth, nutrition, and feeding behavior', *Current Pediatrics Reports* 1(4), 2013: 247–56.

8. Krebs, Mazariegos, Tshefu *et al.*, 'Meat consumption is associated with less stunting among toddlers in four diverse low-income settings'.

9. L.L. Iannotti, C.K. Lutter, C.P. Stewart *et al.*, 'Eggs in early complementary feeding and child growth: A randomized controlled trial', *Pediatrics*, June 2017: e20163459.

10. H.H. Vorster, '"Make starchy foods part of most meals": A food-based dietary guideline for South Africa', *SAJCN* 26(3), 2013: S28–S35.

11. H.H. Vorster, 'The new South African food-based dietary guidelines in perspective', *Nutrition Society of South Africa*, available at http://www.nutritionsociety.co.za/index.php/11-useful-information/26-the-new-south-african-food-based-dietary-guidelines-in-perspective (last accessed 3 August 2017).

12. B. Kubheka, 'Ethical and legal perspectives on the medical practitioners use of social media', *SAMJ* 107(5), 2017: 387.

13. D. Ilbury, *Tim Noakes: The Quiet Maverick* (Cape Town: Penguin Books, 2017).

14. G. Watson, 'On Tim Noakes and bullsh*t, *Health24*, 13 January 2014, available at http://www.news24.com/MyNews24/On-Tim-Noakes-and-Bullsht-20140113 (last accessed 8 September 2017).

15. J. Burne, 'Cuddly dietitians in cosy embrace of industry fat cats', *Health Insight UK*, 16 March 2015, available at http://healthinsightuk.org/2015/03/16/cuddly-dietitians-in-cosy-embrace-of-industry-fat-cats/ (last accessed 3 August 2017).

The Noakes Foundation

The Noakes Foundation is a public benefit organisation founded by the Noakes family. The foundation aims to advance medical science's understanding of the benefits of a healthy low-carbohydrate, high-fat diet by providing evidence-based information on optimum nutrition. Through their research, the foundation aims to change the way humans think about food and nutrition, and consequently tackle the epidemics of obesity and type-2 diabetes – diseases which are set to cripple national healthcare within the next 10 years. The Noakes Foundation relies on funding to carry out this mandate; all royalties for the book received by Professor Noakes will be donated to The Noakes Foundation, helping the organisation continue with the important work it is doing. For more information about the foundation, visit www.thenoakesfoundation.org.

The Noakes Foundation actively promotes the Eat Better South Africa! campaign, which aims to show South Africans – especially those in poorer communities – that it is possible to eat a healthy LCHF/Banting diet on as little as thirty rand per day, with major health gains for individuals and communities.

Index

Page numbers in *italics* indicate figures and tables. Stars (*) indicate footnotes.